Cardiac CT

Guest Editor

JILL E. JACOBS, MD

RADIOLOGIC CLINICS OF NORTH AMERICA

www.radiologic.theclinics.com

Consulting Editor
FRANK H. MILLER, MD

July 2010 • Volume 48 • Number 4

SAUNDERS an imprint of ELSEVIER, Inc.

W.B. SAUNDERS COMPANY
A Division of Elsevier Inc.

1600 John F. Kennedy Boulevard • Suite 1800 • Philadelphia, Pennsylvania 19103-2899

http://www.theclinics.com

RADIOLOGIC CLINICS OF NORTH AMERICA Volume 48, Number 4
July 2010 ISSN 0033-8389, ISBN 13: 978-1-4377-2594-0

Editor: Barton Dudlick
Developmental Editor: Donald Mumford

Radiologic Clinics of North America (ISSN 0033-8389) is published bimonthly by Elsevier Inc., 360 Park Avenue South, New York, NY 10010-1710. Months of issue are January, March, May, July, September, and November. Periodicals postage paid at New York, NY and additional mailing offices. Subscription prices are USD 361 per year for US individuals, USD 545 per year for US institutions, USD 176 per year for US students and residents, USD 421 per year for Canadian individuals, USD 684 per year for Canadian institutions, USD 520 per year for international individuals, USD 684 per year for international institutions, and USD 253 per year for Canadian and foreign students/residents. To receive student and resident rate, orders must be accompanied by name of affiliated institution, date of term and the signature of program/residency coordinatior on institution letterhead. Orders will be billed at individual rate until proof of status is received. Foreign air speed delivery is included in all Clinics subscription prices. All prices are subject to change without notice. **POSTMASTER:** Send address changes to Radiologic Clinics of North America, Elsevier Health Sciences Division, Subscription Customer Service, 3251 Riverport Lane, Maryland Heights, MO63043. **Customer Service: Telephone: 1-800-654-2452** (U.S. and Canada); **1-314-447-8871** (outside U.S. and Canada). **Fax: 1-314-447-8029. E-mail: journalscustomerservice-usa@ elsevier.com** (for print support); **journalsonlinesupport-usa@elsevier.com** (for online support).

Reprints. For copies of 100 or more of articles in this publication, please contact the Commercial Reprints Department, Elsevier Inc., 360 Park Avenue South, New York, New York 10010-1710. Tel.: (+1) 212-633-3812; Fax: (+1) 212-462-1935; E-mail: reprints@elsevier.com.

Radiologic Clinics of North America also published in Greek Paschalidis Medical Publications, Athens, Greece.

Radiologic Clinics of North America is covered in *MEDLINE/PubMed (Index Medicus), EMBASE/Excerpta Medica, Current Contents/Life Sciences, Current Contents/Clinical Medicine, RSNA Index to Imaging Literature, BIOSIS, Science Citation Index,* and *ISI/BIOMED*.

Printed in the United States of America.

Contributors

CONSULTING EDITOR

FRANK H. MILLER, MD
Professor of Radiology; Chief, Body Imaging
Section and Fellowship Program and GI
Radiology; and Medical Director MRI,
Department of Radiology, Northwestern
University Feinberg School of Medicine,
Chicago, Illinois

GUEST EDITOR

JILL E. JACOBS, MD
Associate Professor of Radiology, Chief,
Department of Radiology, Cardiac Imaging,
New York University Langone Medical Center,
New York, New York

AUTHORS

SUHNY ABBARA, MD
Associate Professor, Director, Cardiovascular
Imaging Section, Harvard Medical School,
Massachusetts General Hospital, Boston,
Massachusetts

NANDAN S. ANAVEKAR, MD
Division of Cardiovascular Diseases,
Mayo Clinic College of Medicine,
Rochester, Minnesota

PHILIP A. ARAOZ, MD
Division of Cardiovascular Diseases,
Mayo Clinic College of Medicine,
Rochester, Minnesota

ELISABETH ARNOLDI, MD
Department of Radiology and Radiological
Science, Medical University of South Carolina,
Charleston, South Carolina; Department
of Clinical Radiology, University Hospitals
Munich—Grosshadern Campus,
Ludwig-Maximilians University,
Munich, Germany

OMER AWAN, MD
Department of Diagnostic Radiology,
University of Maryland, Baltimore, Maryland

GORKA BASTARRIKA, MD, PhD
Department of Radiology and Radiological
Science, Medical University of South Carolina,
Charleston, South Carolina; Department
of Radiology, University of Navarra,
Pamplona, Spain

ANDREW BLUM, MD
Cardiovascular Imaging Fellow, Harvard
Medical School, Massachusetts General
Hospital, Boston, Massachusetts

CRYSTAL R. BONNICHSEN, MD
Division of Cardiovascular Diseases,
Mayo Clinic College of Medicine,
Rochester, Minnesota

JEROME F. BREEN, MD
Division of Cardiovascular Diseases,
Mayo Clinic College of Medicine,
Rochester, Minnesota

HERSH CHANDARANA, MD
Assistant Professor of Radiology, Department of Radiology, New York University School of Medicine, New York, New York

JOSEPH JEN-SHO CHEN, MD
Department of Diagnostic Radiology, University of Maryland, Baltimore, Maryland

CLAUS D. CLAUSSEN, MD
Department of Diagnostic and Interventional Radiology, University Hospital Tuebingen, Eberhard-Karls-University Tuebingen, Tuebingen, Germany

JAMES P. EARLS, MD
Fairfax Radiology Consultants PC, Fairfax, Virginia

ELLIOT K. FISHMAN, MD
Professor of Radiology, Surgery and Oncology, Director of Diagnostic Imaging and Body CT, The Russell H. Morgan Department of Radiology and Radiological Science, Johns Hopkins Hospital, Baltimore, Maryland

THOMAS A. FOLEY, MD
Division of Cardiovascular Diseases, Mayo Clinic College of Medicine, Rochester, Minnesota

JAMES F. GLOCKNER, MD
Division of Cardiovascular Diseases, Mayo Clinic College of Medicine, Rochester, Minnesota

ARI GOLDBERG, MD, PhD
Assistant Professor of Radiology and Fellow, Cardiovascular Imaging Section, Department of Radiology, Hospital of the University of Pennsylvania, Philadelphia, Pennsylvania

THOMAS HENZLER, MD
Department of Radiology and Radiological Science, Medical University of South Carolina, Charleston, South Carolina; Department of Clinical Radiology and Nuclear Medicine, University Medical Center Mannheim, Medical Faculty Mannheim-Heidelberg University, Mannheim, Germany

DOUGLAS HUGHES JR, MD
Mallinckrodt Institute of Radiology, Washington University School of Medicine, Saint Louis, Missouri

JILL E. JACOBS, MD
Associate Professor of Radiology, Chief, Department of Radiology, Cardiac Imaging, New York University Langone Medical Center, New York, New York

PAMELA T. JOHNSON, MD
Assistant Professor of Radiology, The Russell H. Morgan Department of Radiology and Radiological Science, Johns Hopkins Hospital, Baltimore, Maryland

DOMINIK KETELSEN, MD
Department of Diagnostic and Interventional Radiology, University Hospital Tuebingen, Eberhard-Karls-University Tuebingen, Tuebingen, Germany

RENEE KREML, MD
Lecturer, Division of Cardiothoracic Radiology, Department of Radiology, Cardiovascular Center, University of Michigan Medical School, University of Michigan Health System, Ann Arbor, Michigan

JONATHON LEIPSIC, MD
Department of Radiology, University of British Columbia, Vancouver, British Columbia, Canada

HAROLD I. LITT, MD, PhD
Chief, Cardiovascular Imaging Section, Department of Radiology, Hospital of the University of Pennsylvania, Philadelphia, Pennsylvania

MINH LU, MD
Department of Diagnostic Radiology, University of Maryland, Baltimore, Maryland

MATTHEW W. MARTINEZ, MD
Division of Cardiovascular Diseases, Mayo Clinic College of Medicine, Rochester, Minnesota

DYLAN V. MILLER, MD
Division of Cardiovascular Diseases, Mayo Clinic College of Medicine, Rochester, Minnesota

MICHAEL F. MORRIS, MD
Division of Cardiovascular Diseases, Mayo Clinic College of Medicine, Rochester, Minnesota

KONSTANTIN NIKOLAOU, MD
Department of Clinical Radiology, University Hospitals Munich—Grosshadern Campus, Ludwig-Maximilians University, Munich, Germany

SMITA PATEL, MD
Associate Professor, Division of Cardiothoracic Radiology, Department of Radiology, Cardiovascular Center, University of Michigan Medical School, University of Michigan Health System, Ann Arbor, Michigan

U. JOSEPH SCHOEPF, MD
Department of Radiology and Radiological Science, Medical University of South Carolina; Division of Cardiology, Department of Medicine, Medical University of South Carolina, Charleston, South Carolina

MARILYN J. SIEGEL, MD
Mallinckrodt Institute of Radiology, Washington University School of Medicine, Saint Louis, Missouri

MONVADI B. SRICHAI, MD
Assistant Professor of Radiology and Medicine, Departments of Radiology and Medicine (Cardiology Division), New York University School of Medicine, New York, New York

BASKARAN SUNDARAM, MD
Assistant Professor, Division of Cardiothoracic Radiology, Department of Radiology, Cardiovascular Center, University of Michigan Medical School, University of Michigan Health System, Ann Arbor, Michigan

CAROLYN M. TAYLOR, MD, MPH
Clinical Assistant Professor of Medicine, Division of Cardiology, University of British Columbia, St Paul's Hospital, Vancouver, British Columbia, Canada

CHRISTIAN THILO, MD
Department of Radiology and Radiological Science, Medical University of South Carolina; Division of Cardiology, Department of Medicine, Medical University of South Carolina, Charleston, South Carolina

JENS VOGEL-CLAUSSEN, MD
Department of Diagnostic and Interventional Radiology, University Hospital Tuebingen, Eberhard-Karls-University Tuebingen, Tuebingen, Germany; Russel H. Morgan Department of Radiology and Radiological Science, The Johns Hopkins Hospital, Baltimore, Maryland

CHARLES S. WHITE, MD
Professor of Radiology and Medicine and Chief of Thoracic Radiology, Department of Diagnostic Radiology, University of Maryland, Baltimore, Maryland

ERIC E. WILLIAMSON, MD
Division of Cardiovascular Diseases, Mayo Clinic College of Medicine, Rochester, Minnesota

Contents

Coronary computed tomography angiography (CCTA) has become an important tool in the assessment of coronary artery disease. It is considered an appropriate test for several indications, including the evaluation of symptomatic patients with low to intermediate probability of obstructive coronary disease. Since its first applications in 1999 using 4-slice CT there have been numerous technological advancements, enabling excellent submillimeter spatial resolution and significant improvements in temporal resolution. This article reviews these advancements in CT technology and the current status and recent developments in cardiac CT with regards to spatial, temporal and contrast resolution and z-axis (volume) coverage. The article also describes the many techniques and new technologies available for dose reduction in cardiac CT.

Cardiac computed tomographic angiography (CCTA) is a unique diagnostic modality that can provide a comprehensive assessment of cardiac anatomy. Rapid advances in scanner and software technology have resulted in the ability to noninvasively image the coronary arteries. However, careful patient preparation and scanning technique is required to ensure optimal image quality while minimizing radiation dose delivered. Important components of patient preparation include knowledge of the indications and contraindications for CCTA, patient screening, patient premedication, patient positioning, prescan instruction, and electrocardiograph lead placement. Scanning technique should be determined on a patient by patient basis and tailored according to age and radiation risk, body mass index and chest circumference, heart rate and variability, presence of stents, and coronary calcification.

Careful protocol design is essential to successfully perform coronary computed tomographic (CT) angiography, from patient preparation, to gating, to contrast infusion, to data acquisition, to data reconstruction parameters. The emergence of newer generation scanners with even larger numbers of detector arrays and dual tubes has further improved dataset quality. However, it is only with tailored interpretation of these datasets that the true value of the newest scanners will be implemented. Unless the user becomes skilled at analyzing CT data, the full potential of new technology will be minimized. This article presents experience based guidance on postprocessing techniques, from axial review to two-dimensional renderings to three dimensional reconstructions, to optimize analysis of cardiac CT data.

Accurate interpretation of cardiac computed tomography requires fundamental knowledge of the normal cardiac anatomy and its common variations. This article reviews the normal anatomy of the coronary arteries, cardiac chambers, and cardiac valves.

Coronary artery anomalies (CAA) are uncommon congenital variations in coronary anatomy, occurring in 0.2% to 1.2% of the general population, the majority of which are detected incidentally and have little clinical significance. A minority of CAA, primarily due to an interarterial course, is clinically significant, and may present with symptoms of myocardial ischemia, malignant ventricular arrhythmias, and even sudden cardiac death. Until recently, CAA were primarily detected at catheter coronary angiography. With recent advances in multidetector computed tomography (CT) technology and the use of electrocardiographic gating, coronary CT angiography provides an exquisite omnidimensional display of the anomalous coronary arteries and their relation to the adjacent structures noninvasively, and is the diagnostic test of choice. Understanding CAA morphology and clinical significance of CAA is important for establishing a diagnosis, and is essential for appropriate patient management and treatment planning.

Cardiac CT scan has emerged from a research tool to a widely used clinical modality in the diagnostic management of coronary artery disease. Based on evidence of numerous clinical studies coronary CT angiography (cCTA) has emerged as a fast, accurate, and noninvasive alternative to conventional angiography in selected patient populations. A major strength of cCTA is its ability to combine information on the coronary artery anatomy, the vessel lumen, and atherosclerotic lesions. Recent investigations on the application of cCTA in myocardial perfusion imaging suggest that cCTA may allow analysis of the hemodynamic relevance of detected stenosis. Data is accumulating that supports its relevance for patient management and outcome. This article examines the role of cCTA for the evaluation of plaques and stenosis.

The past decade has brought rapid advances in CT technology, which allows increasingly precise application to the study of coronary arteries and acute chest pain. The literature has expanded to lend quantifiable justification to the intuitive appeal of a rapid, reproducible, 3D study of the heart and vasculature. More complete analysis of efficacy and costs on broader populations will further refine our understanding of how best to implement what may become the new gold standard. Meanwhile, evolving technology promises to further challenge radiologists and clinicians to optimize approach and diagnosis to acute chest pain.

Although conventional coronary angiography is used to evaluate the patency of coronary artery bypass grafts, it is invasive and has associated risks. The evolution of the multidetector CT (MDCT) has enabled accurate, noninvasive visualization of graft patency. This article identifies and describes typical MDCT findings in bypass grafts and native coronary arteries.

GOAL STATEMENT
The goal of the *Radiologic Clinics of North America* is to keep practicing radiologists and radiology residents up to date with current clinical practice in radiology by providing timely articles reviewing the state of the art in patient care.

ACCREDITATION
The *Radiologic Clinics of North America* is planned and implemented in accordance with the Essential Areas and Policies of the Accreditation Council for Continuing Medical Education (ACCME) through the joint sponsorship of the University of Virginia School of Medicine and Elsevier. The University of Virginia School of Medicine is accredited by the ACCME to provide continuing medical education for physicians.

The University of Virginia School of Medicine designates this educational activity for a maximum of 15 *AMA PRA Category 1 Credits*™ for each issue, 90 credits per year. Physicians should only claim credit commensurate with the extent of their participation in the activity.

The American Medical Association has determined that physicians not licensed in the US who participate in this CME activity are eligible for a maximum of *15 AMA PRA Category 1 Credits*™ for each issue, 90 credits per year.

Credit can be earned by reading the text material, taking the CME examination online at http://www.theclinics.com/home/cme, and completing the evaluation. After taking the test, you will be required to review any and all incorrect answers. Following completion of the test and evaluation, your credit will be awarded and you may print your certificate.

FACULTY DISCLOSURE/CONFLICT OF INTEREST
The University of Virginia School of Medicine, as an ACCME accredited provider, endorses and strives to comply with the Accreditation Council for Continuing Medical Education (ACCME) Standards of Commercial Support, Commonwealth of Virginia statutes, University of Virginia policies and procedures, and associated federal and private regulations and guidelines on the need for disclosure and monitoring of proprietary and financial interests that may affect the scientific integrity and balance of content delivered in continuing medical education activities under our auspices.

The University of Virginia School of Medicine requires that all CME activities accredited through this institution be developed independently and be scientifically rigorous, balanced and objective in the presentation/discussion of its content, theories and practices.

All authors/editors participating in an accredited CME activity are expected to disclose to the readers relevant financial relationships with commercial entities occurring within the past 12 months (such as grants or research support, employee, consultant, stock holder, member of speakers bureau, etc.). The University of Virginia School of Medicine will employ appropriate mechanisms to resolve potential conflicts of interest to maintain the standards of fair and balanced education to the reader. Questions about specific strategies can be directed to the Office of Continuing Medical Education, University of Virginia School of Medicine, Charlottesville, Virginia.

The faculty and staff of the University of Virginia Office of Continuing Medical Education have no financial affiliations to disclose.

The authors/editors listed below have identified no financial or professional relationships for themselves or their spouse/partner:
Nandan S. Anavekar, MD; Elisabeth Arnoldi, MD; Omer Awan, MD; Andrew Blum, MD; Crystal R. Bonnichsen, MD; Jerome F. Breen, MD; Hersh Chandarana, MD; Joseph Jen-Sho Chen, MD; Claus D. Claussen, MD; Barton Dudlick (Acquisitions Editor); Tom A. Foley, MD; James F. Glockner, MD; Ari Goldberg, MD, PhD; Thomas Henzler, MD; Douglas Hughes, Jr., MD; Jill E. Jacobs, MD (Guest Editor); Pamela T. Johnson, MD; Theodore E. Keats, MD (Test Author); Dominik Ketelsen, MD; Renee Kreml, MD; Minh Lu, MD; Matthew W. Martinez, MD; Dylan V. Miller, MD; Frank H. Miller, MD (Consulting Editor); Michael F. Morris, MD; Konstantin Nikolaou, MD; Smita Patel, MD; Monvadi B. Srichai, MD; Baskaran Sundaram, MD; Carolyn M. Taylor, MD, MPH; Christian Thilo, MD; Jens Vogel-Claussen, MD; and Charles S. White, MD.

The authors/editors listed below have identified the following financial or professional relationships for themselves or their spouse/partner:
Suhny Abbara, MD is a consultant for Siemens, Perceptive Informatics, and Magellan Health, owns stock in Merck, Partners Imaging, and Amirsys, receives royalty income from Amirsys and Elsevier, and is an industry funded research/investigator for Bracco.
Philip A. Araoz, MD is a consultant for Medtronic.
Gorka Bastarrika, MD, PhD is on the Speakers' Bureau for Bayer-Schering, General Electric, Medrad, and Siemens.
James P. Earls, MD is an industry funded research/investigator and serves on the Speakers Bureau for GE Healthcare.
Elliot K. Fishman, MD, FACR is an industry funded research/investigator and a consultant, and is on the Advisory Committee/Board, for GE Healthcare and Siemens Medical Solutions; and owns stock in Hipgraphics, Inc.
Jonathon Leipsic, MD is a consultant and is on the Advisory Committee/Board for GE Healthcare.
Harold I. Litt, MD, PhD is an industry funded research/investigator for Siemens Medical Solutions, Acorn Cardiovascular, and Rcadia, and serves on the Advisory Committee for Siemens Medical Solutions.
U. Joseph Schoepf, MD is an industry funded research/investigator, consultant, and serves on the Speakers Bureau for Bayer-Schering/Medrad, Bracco, General Electric, and Siemens.
Marilyn J. Siegel, MD is on the Speakers' Bureau for Siemens.
Eric E. Williamson, MD is a consultant for Siemens Medical.

Disclosure of Discussion of Non-FDA Approved Uses for Pharmaceutical Products and/or Medical Devices.
The University of Virginia School of Medicine, as an ACCME provider, requires that all faculty presenters identify and disclose any off-label uses for pharmaceutical and medical device products. The University of Virginia School of Medicine recommends that each physician fully review all the available data on new products or procedures prior to clinical use.

TO ENROLL
To enroll in the Radiologic Clinics of North America Continuing Medical Education program, call customer service at 1-800-654-2452 or sign up online at http://www.theclinics.com/home/cme. The CME program is available to subscribers for an additional annual fee USD 245.

Radiologic Clinics of North America

THE CLINICS ARE NOW AVAILABLE ONLINE!

Access your subscription at:
www.theclinics.com

Preface
Cardiac CT

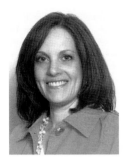

Jill E. Jacobs, MD
Guest Editor

With recent advances in computed tomographic (CT) technology, noninvasive CT imaging of the heart has become a reality. In this issue of *Radiologic Clinics of North America*, a renowned group of cardiac CT imagers addresses the important components of performing and interpreting cardiac CT examinations. One's diagnostic capabilities are dependent on acquisition of a motion-free, optimally enhanced CT data set using suitable CT equipment and on accurate interpretation of the appropriately postprocessed images. Because of this, a thorough understanding of proper patient selection and preparation, optimization of CT scanning protocols, and knowledge of postprocessing techniques is mandatory when performing an optimized cardiac CT examination. These important topics are therefore initially addressed in this issue.

It is also vitally important to monitor radiation dose when performing cardiac CT studies. As for all radiologic examinations that use ionizing radiation, attention to the ALARA principle (using a dose that is as low as reasonably achievable) is mandatory. Therefore, the first article of this issue discusses the critically important topic of how to achieve diagnostic image quality while minimizing radiation dose. Many radiation reduction strategies including tube-current modulation, tube voltage optimization, the use of prospective ECG triggering versus retrospective ECG gating, and the use of statistical iterative image reconstruction are discussed, and the relationship between heart rate and radiation dose is explored.

Of course, accurate interpretation of the cardiac CT examination first requires knowledge of both the normal cardiac anatomy and its many variants. Once this is achieved, knowledge of common coronary artery anomalies and their clinical implications is necessary. These topics are addressed as a prelude to exploring articles about arterial pathology including diagnosis of coronary artery disease, evaluation of the acute chest pain patient, and evaluation of coronary artery bypass grafts and stents. Assessment of extra-arterial cardiac structures is also obligatory when interpreting a cardiac CT study. Therefore, this issue also addresses evaluation of myocardial abnormalities and ischemia, evaluation of the cardiac valves, and evaluation of cardiac masses and pseudotumors. Last, but certainly not least, is an article on the anatomic variations and common complications that are seen when evaluating congenital heart disease in adults.

I hope you agree that the contributors to this issue have done an excellent job discussing the major components of performing and interpreting a cardiac CT examination. For those readers already performing cardiac CT studies, this issue will hopefully provide some additional pointers to optimize image acquisition and study interpretation. For those readers not yet performing cardiac CT studies, it is my hope that this issue will spur you on to begin performing these examinations in your practice.

Jill E. Jacobs, MD
Department of Radiology Cardiac Imaging
NYU Langone Medical Center
560 First Avenue
TCH HW205, New York
NY 10016-6497, USA

E-mail address:
jill.jacobs@nyumc.org

Radiol Clin N Am 48 (2010) xiii
doi:10.1016/j.rcl.2010.06.013

Cardiac Computed Tomography Technology and Dose-reduction Strategies

James P. Earls, MD[a],*, Jonathon Leipsic, MD[b]

KEYWORDS
- Cardiac computed tomography • Dose reduction
- Angiography

Coronary computed tomography angiography (CCTA) has become an important tool in the assessment of coronary artery disease. It is considered an appropriate test for several indications, including the evaluation of symptomatic patients with low to intermediate probability of obstructive coronary disease.[1–3] The development of CCTA has been rapid, from a research application to a commonly used clinical tool in one decade. Since its first applications in 1999 using 4-slice CT there have been numerous technological advancements, enabling excellent submillimeter spatial resolution and significant improvements in temporal resolution. This article reviews these important advancements in CT technology. The article reviews current status and recent developments in cardiac CT with regards to the 3 major keys to image quality: spatial, temporal and contrast resolution, as well as z-axis (volume) coverage.

Alongside the technological advancements came increases in the mean effective dose of the examinations. Because of the high doses associated with some cardiac CT scans there has been much concern about increasing radiation risks.[4–6] The second portion of this article describes the many techniques and new technologies available for dose reduction in cardiac CT.

HISTORICAL PERSPECTIVE

Before multislice CCTA, electron-beam CT[7,8] was used widely for coronary artery calcium scoring. The development of cardiac CT was driven by the introduction of multidetector row CT in 1998.[9,10] Since 1999, 4-slice CT systems with 4 × 1 mm or 4 × 1.25 mm collimation and 0.5-second gantry rotation time have been clinically used for electrocardiographic (ECG)-triggered or ECG-gated multidetector row CT (MDCT) examinations at low to moderate heart rates. Although 4-slice CT offered many advances, there were limitations because of motion artifacts, limited spatial resolution, and the long breath hold times of up to 40 seconds.[10]

In 2001, 16-slice CT systems with submillimeter collimation (16 × 0.5 mm, 16 × 0.625 mm) and gantry rotation times of 375 milliseconds were introduced and significantly improved temporal resolution and a reduction in examination times and breath holds.[11] These advancements resulted in improvements in the quality and diagnostic accuracy of CCTA.[12–15] Advances in temporal resolution increased the percentage of evaluable vessel segments, shortened overall scan times, and enabled higher-contrast vessel attenuation with lower-contrast volumes.[16,17]

Disclosures: James Earls is on the Speakers Bureau. Jonathon Leipsic is on the Speakers Bureau for GE Healthcare.
[a] Fairfax Radiology Consultants PC, 2272 Merrilee, Fairfax, VA 22031, USA
[b] Department of Radiology, University of British Columbia, Vancouver, BC, Canada
* Corresponding author. 5553 Rockpointe Drive, Clifton, VA 20124.
E-mail address: jpearls@yahoo.com

Radiol Clin N Am 48 (2010) 657–674
doi:10.1016/j.rcl.2010.04.003

Sixty-four–row multislice CT scanners were introduced in 2004, marking a coming of age for CCTA. These systems enabled simultaneous acquisition of 64 slices with 0.5-mm, 0.6-mm, or 0.625-mm collimated slice width at gantry rotation times down to 0.33 seconds. The wider coverage with thinner slices shortened the scan time to 6 to 12 seconds,[18] a feasible breath hold time even for patients with limited ability to cooperate. This step forward allowed a significant increase in the diagnostic accuracy of CCTA. However, image quality at higher heart rates, in calcified and stented segments, and in large patients remained limited.[19–22]

Vendor development of CT platforms remained in lockstep through the development of the 64-row scanners but has gone in varied directions to attempt to solve lingering limitations in clinical CCTA (Fig. 1).

SPATIAL RESOLUTION

In-plane spatial resolution is determined by the number of detector channels in a detector row and the width of each detector aperture. Routinely 700 to 900 detector channels cover a scan field of view (FOV) of approximately 500 mm, the in-plane distance between 2 detector channels or the in-plane sampling distance is 0.56 to 0.71 mm in the isocenter of the scanner.[23] This strategy results in excellent spatial resolution typically in the range of 0.5 to 0.625 mm in the z-axis and approximately 0.5 mm in the x- and y-axes. Spatial resolution is the same in all directions and allows for isotropic resolution. Isotropic voxels enable

excellent multiplanar capabilities required for cardiac CT. Although spatial resolution of CT is excellent and superior to other noninvasive modalities like magnetic resonance (MR) imaging, it still limits coronary evaluation, particularly in grading of stenosis beyond a binary scale of less or greater than 50%.[24]

Additional improvements in scanner technology, like quarter detector offset or in-plane flying focal spots, are used to double the number of samples acquired and decrease the sampling distance to 0.28 to 0.36 mm. In practice, it cannot be used to its fullest extent in CCTA because of increased image noise and streak artifacts from high-contrast structures.[23] For routine imaging with standard body convolution kernels, CCTA in-plane resolution of 0.5 mm is not exceeded. Whereas in-plane resolution is limited and has not changed drastically over the last few years, through-plane (z-axis) resolution has improved considerably as thinner collimation has become available for clinical use.

Modern 64-slice systems are a significant advance from 16-slice systems (Fig. 2). They provide 0.5- to 0.625-mm collimated slice width for cardiac examinations, resulting in through-plane resolution of approximately 0.4 mm. This exceptional isotropic spatial resolution is typically used when attempting to achieve detailed visualization of calcified coronary arteries and stented segments. The inherent limitation of increased noise with harder convolution kernels and higher isotropic resolution has remained an Achilles heel of CCTA. Noise limits the evaluation of smaller stents,[25] heavily calcified segments,[26] accurate

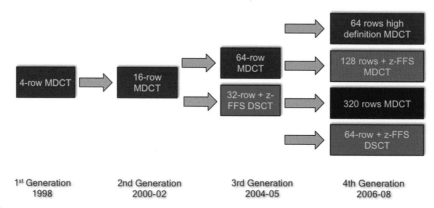

Fig. 1. Cardiac CT systems initially followed a similar developmental pathway for the first and second generation. The DSCT uses a z-flying focal spot (zFFS) that alternates between 2 z-positions of the radiograph focal spot, acquiring 2 slices per detector row, which results in double sampling in the z direction. With the fourth generation, each of the 4 CT vendors has taken distinct pathways to improve cardiac imaging to include a 64-MDCT with higher resolution and new detectors, a 128-row MDCT with zFFS (256 MDCT), a 320-row MDCT, and a 64-row DSCT with zFFS (128-DSCT).

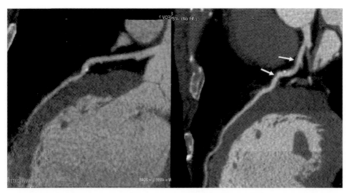

Fig. 2. Improvements in image quality can be seen in images of the left anterior descending (LAD) coronary artery in a 48-year-old man imaged initially on a 16-MDCT (*left*) then 6 months later on a 64-MDCT (*right*). Non-obstructing soft plaque (*arrows*) is depicted on the 64-NDCT and is not seen on the 16-MDCT.

grading of coronary stenoses, and the accurate characterization of plaque. Blooming from calcification and partial volume averaging artifacts seen in stent imaging are caused largely by insufficient spatial resolution.

Historically, increasing spatial resolution has led to increased image noise. Noise increases linearly with through-plane (z-axis) resolution and with the third power of the in-plane resolution.[23] As a result, to maintain the desired contrast-to-noise ratio (CNR) and double the resolution, the tube current (and therefore the radiation dose) has to be increased by a factor of 2^4 (16-fold increase). This increase would be unacceptable given growing concerns regarding effective radiation dose in cardiac CT; however, not increasing radiation dose and improving spatial resolution would result in excessive noise and degradation of image quality, limiting the evaluation of small coronary arteries and plaques.[27]

Developments in image reconstruction have shown promise in improving high-contrast resolution without increasing image noise in the low-contrast areas. CT images have historically been reconstructed using filtered back projection (FBP). FBP is computationally fast, enabling robust image reconstruction for clinical use. Further improvements in spatial resolution are limited by increased noise from FBP reconstruction. Iterative reconstruction (IR) techniques help to overcome these issues and attempts to decouple spatial resolution and image noise.[28]

IR reconstructs CT data sets by fully modeling the system statistics and system optics. The reconstruction process is iterative to overcome the mathematical complexity introduced by the added modeling.[29] IR techniques do not assume the measured signal is free of noise, but uses more accurate statistical modeling during the reconstruction process. IR enables improved

image noise properties, while maintaining spatial resolution and other image quality parameters (**Fig. 3**).

IR has the potential to enhance spatial resolution, particularly of high-contrast objects and to reduce noise in low-contrast ones. Initial experiences with IR have shown improvement in segmental interpretability compared with FBP when performing CCTA at lower tube current and improved diagnostic accuracy in calcified and stented coronary segments.[30]

IR is more computationally intensive and demanding than FBP and requires more time for image reconstruction. There is also a different noise texture in the reconstructed images, yielding a different appearance compared with FBP. Despite these limitations, IR techniques represent the most promising approach to improving spatial resolution and dealing with heavily calcified segments, which have been among the major limitations of CCTA.

TEMPORAL RESOLUTION

Cardiac CT requires synchronization of the data acquisition with the patient's ECG with optimal image quality occurring when data are acquired in a motion-free fashion. Whether the study is performed with prospective ECG triggering or retrospectively ECG-gated spiral CT, partial scans data segments are used for image reconstruction to decrease exposure time and optimize temporal resolution. Partial scanning consists of 180° of fan-beam data plus the total fan angle of the detector for a typical minimum total of approximately 230 to 250°. Within the center of the scan rotation, where the heart is typically located, 180° of scan data is adequate for image reconstruction. As a result, temporal resolution equals half the gantry rotation time. The first-generation 4-slice systems had

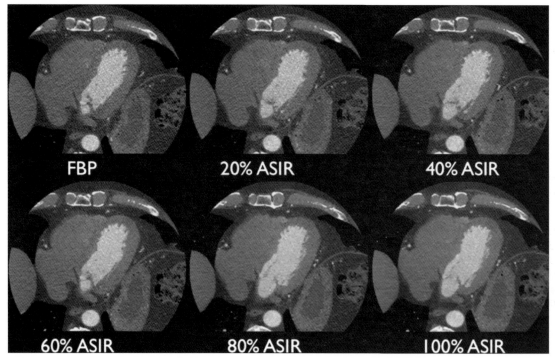

Fig. 3. In its current release, use of ASIR generates images that contain a weighted blend of FBP with ASIR. A single image of the ventricles was processed in 6 different ways: 100% FBP and in increasing amounts of ASIR (and decreasing FBP) up to 100% ASIR. There is a visible reduction in image noise going from 100% FBP to 100% ASIR.

temporal resolution of 250 milliseconds, which has improved to 165 milliseconds on standard 64-slice technology, resulting in improved image quality even at higher heart rates.[26,31] However, this does not approach the temporal resolution of angiography (1–10 ms) and is inferior to MR imaging (20–50 ms).[32,33]

Multiple techniques and technological advancements have been developed to further improve temporal resolution. Multisegment reconstruction improves the temporal resolution by dividing the half-scan data into 2 to 4 subsegments over multiple cardiac cycles. Clinical use of technique is usually limited to patients with high resting heart rates and irregular rhythms caused by interpolation error. Multisegment reconstruction relies on a regular rhythm to synchronize and seamlessly fuse data acquired from different heartbeats. Multisegment reconstruction is also limited by higher effective radiation dose, which correlates directly with the number of cardiac cycles used for reconstruction.

Development of the dual-source system was the most significant improvement in temporal resolution. Dual-source CT (DSCT) arrived in 2006 with a design that reflects an early prototype design concept called the dynamic spatial reconstructor.[34] DSCT enables enhanced temporal

resolution without a faster gantry rotation by using 2 radiograph tubes and 2 detectors.[35] Tubes and detectors are mounted perpendicularly within the same gantry. The configuration allows adequate projection data for full image reconstruction during a quarter rotation, unlike the typical half-rotation required in single-source systems. With this approach, temporal resolution is improved to one quarter of the gantry rotation time or 83 milliseconds.[35] This technology has been validated in several clinical studies, showing the potential to accurately rule out significant coronary artery disease and stenoses at higher heart rates.[36–38] The second-generation DSCT scanner released in 2009 further improved temporal resolution. This scanner has a gantry rotation time of 280 milliseconds, which results in a temporal resolution of 75 milliseconds.[39]

VOLUME COVERAGE

Technological advances in cardiac CT enabling z-axis coverage have also been occurring at a rapid rate (**Fig. 4**). Recently, 256- and 320-row single-source systems and 128-row DSCT scanners have been developed.[40,41] These larger detectors have helped to eliminate detector misregistration artifacts and banding, which are often seen with the

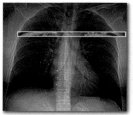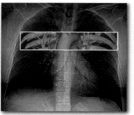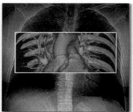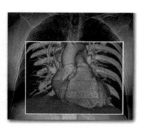

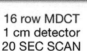

16 row MDCT	64 row MDCT	128 row MDCT	320 row MDCT
1 cm detector	4 cm detector	8 cm detector	16 cm detector
20 SEC SCAN	4-8 SEC SCAN	2-4 SEC SCAN	1-3 SEC SCAN

Fig. 4. Increasing detector width of new cardiac CT systems has led to a significant decrease in scan acquisition time.

traditional 4-cm 64-slice detector. With increasing detector z-coverage the number of heartbeats contributing to the image data decreases, thereby decreasing the likelihood of banding artifact. This system has been shown in several recent publications to be a robust tool in CCTA.[40,42]

Limitations with increasing detector width include data distortion related to arrhythmia or ectopic beats during scan acquisition, and increased radiograph scatter,[41] which may cause hypodense or streak artifacts. Scattered radiation may also reduce CNR, further limiting their application. The scatter resulting from large detector scanners increases in magnitude in a linear fashion with increasing z-width of the detector. With DSCT using 2 128-row detectors there is an additional issue of cross-scattered radiation, resulting from scatter from 1 radiograph tube being detected by the other detector offset by 90°. Compared with a scatter-free case, this method results in CNR degradation on the order of 5% to 10% for a single-source system and likely an even greater negative effect on CNR using DSCT.[43] This scatter-induced CNR reduction translates to a requirement of 5% to 25% more radiation to restore the CNR.[43]

A new DSCT scan technique increases z-axis coverage and scans the entire heart in less than one cardiac cycle. A high-pitch helical algorithm uses a pitch of up to 3.4 and can cover the heart in approximately 260 milliseconds of scan time.[39,44–47] Radiation dose-reduction benefits of this new technique are discussed further in the following section.

RADIATION DOSE ISSUES IN CARDIAC CT

The use of CT for general diagnostic purposes and for dedicated cardiac indications has come under significant scrutiny in recent years.[4–6] Mounting concern has arisen from the increased use of CT, with more than 70 million scans performed in the

United States in 2007, as well as increasing radiation dose.

The international Prospective Multicenter Study On RadiaTion Dose Estimates Of Cardiac CT AngIOgraphy I (PROTECTION I) Trial is the largest multicenter study of radiation dose and techniques used in CCTA.[27] The investigators collected data on approximately 2000 CCTA scans from 50 centers worldwide and reported a median estimated effective dose of 12 mSv. Most reported scans were performed with retrospective gating. Use of prospective gating was limited to 6% of studies because the data were collected before widespread clinical release of this technique.

Radiation risk is a controversial topic in CT. A direct link between radiation from medical imaging and development of solid-organ cancers has never been established in the less than 20 mSv effective dose range encountered in cardiac CT. However, most physicians take a conservative approach and adhere to the as low as reasonably achievable (ALARA) principle. It is the physician's responsibility to keep radiation exposure at a minimum for each examination and to maintain diagnostic efficacy.

Benefits of the information obtained from CCTA must be carefully balanced with the potential risk of the radiation used to generate the images. If there is no proven benefit to performing an examination, regardless of the radiation dose, then the risk is too high and it should not be performed. Lowering radiation dose of an appropriately ordered CT to a point at which the scan loses diagnostic capability also does not ultimately benefit the patient. Likewise, use of greater amounts of radiation than needed likely does not add significantly to the diagnostic ability of the study.

Techniques used for dose reduction in cardiac CT can be grouped into optimized selection of scanning parameters and use of newer dose-reduction technology. Optimal user selectable options include methods such as tube current dependent on weight or body mass index (BMI, calculated as weight in kilograms divided by the square of height in meters), use of lower tube voltage,[48,49] minimization of the scan length (z-axis), and reduction in the number of phases or series performed. Newer scanning technology include use of ECG-dependent tube current modulation,[50] prospective ECG gating[51–55] high-pitched spiral acquisition,[39,44–47] and use of noise-reduction algorithms such as IR.[28,56,57]

Depending on the CT scanner and software version available, many different tools may be available to lower radiation dose, maintaining diagnostic image quality. Many of the following techniques are often used in conjunction for additional dose reduction. Raff and colleagues[58] recently showed that a combination of dose-reduction factors could be used concurrently to great effect in clinical practice. These investigators evaluated 4995 sequential patients and used a straightforward best-practice CCTA scan model, which included minimized scan range, heart-rate reduction, ECG-gated tube current modulation, and reduced tube voltage in suitable patients. Compared with the control period, patients' estimated median radiation dose was reduced by 53.3% (effective dose from 21 mSv to 10 mSv) and overall image quality was maintained.

Measuring Radiation Dose

Radiation dose is proportional to tube current, exposure time, and the square of tube voltage and is inversely proportional to the pitch for helical acquisition. Estimated radiation doses for CCTA examinations can be expressed in numerous terms. Conventional units of radiation dose (rads and rems) have been replaced with SI units of Grays (Gy) and Sieverts (Sv). Special measures for radiation done on CT have been developed, the volume computed tomography dose index (CTDI$_{vol}$ [in Gy]), dose length product (DLP [in mGy × cm]), and effective dose (ED [in mSv]).

The CTDI$_{vol}$ averages radiation dose over the x, y, and z directions. This figure is used to express the average dose delivered to the scan volume (three-dimensional CT slice) for a specific examination. The DLP is defined as the CTDI$_{vol}$ times scan length and is an indicator of the integrated radiation dose of an entire CT examination. The CTDI$_{vol}$ and DLP are now reported by most CT systems in current use. ED reflects the nonuniform radiation absorption within the body and is determined from dose to individual organs and the associated relative radiation risk assigned to each organ. A reasonable approximation of the ED for a patient is obtained by multiplying DLP

by a conversion factor, k (in mSv/mGy'cm), which varies dependent on the body region that is imaged. The current recommended conversion coefficient for CCTA is 0.014 mSv/mGy'cm.[59]

SPECIFIC TECHNIQUES FOR DOSE REDUCTION
Tube Current Optimization

Current cardiac capable CT scanners have significantly greater tube power than earlier machines. Cardiac protocols require greater tube current delivered in a significantly shorter period of time than is routinely used for other CT protocols. Maximum power of the radiograph tube reaches 100 kW, and radiation dose may exceed 100 mGy. This power is useful for rapid cardiac scanning of individuals with high BMI. However, if protocols are not individually adjusted, it may result in needlessly high radiation doses.

Radiation dose can be reduced by use of anatomy-adapted tube-current modulation. This effective technique is not fully compatible with the ECG-dependent dose-modulation technique currently used in CCTA. Manual selection of tube current for each individual case is essential in cardiac CT scanning. The current is tailored according to the patient's BMI, chest circumference, and estimated muscle and breast mass (**Fig. 5**). Reliance on a standard CT protocol without altering mA leads to excessive radiation doses for thin patients and potentially poor image quality in patients with a high BMI. A 5-cm difference in thoracic diameter corresponds to a factor of 2 or more in the dose required to maintain similar image quality.[60] Jung and colleagues[61] found use of weight-adapted mA reduced dose by 17.9% for men and 26.3% for women and that constant image noise is achieved and image quality preserved. In patients with a high BMI, increasing contrast volume can be used to offset the expected decrease in coronary artery attenuation.[62]

In the PROTOCOL study, LaBounty and colleagues[63] prospectively evaluated 449 patients undergoing 64-detector CCTA at 3 centers and compared patients before (n = 247) and after initiation (n = 202) of a standardized BMI and heart rate-based protocol that incorporated multiple dose-reduction strategies including gating technique, tube voltage, current, padding duration, and scan length. In multivariate analysis, a 20% reduction in radiation dose was associated with every 100-mA reduction in tube current.

Tube Voltage Optimization

Radiation dose varies with the square of the kilovoltage, which means mall reductions in tube

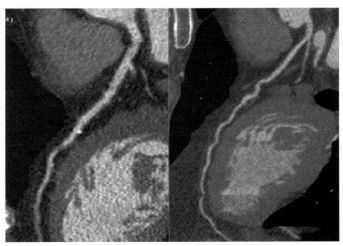

Fig. 5. Tube current (mA) should ideally be adjusted based on the patient's weight, size, and/or BMI. These 2 prospective studies with similar image quality were performed using 64-MDCT. The study on the left was obtained in a thin 53-year-old woman with a BMI of 18 kg/m^2; 275 mA was used and the examination had an ED of 0.6 mSv. The study on the right was obtained in a obese 51-year-old man with a BMI of 50 kg/m^2; 800 mA was used and the examination had an ED of 6.9 mSv.

voltage allow for a substantial reduction in ED **(Fig. 6)**.[48,64–66] Abada and colleagues[48] reduced the kilovoltage in CCTA from the traditional 120 to 80 kV in patients with a low BMI undergoing CCTA and found up to an 88% dose reduction. Use of 100 kV in the PROTECTION I study resulted in a 53% reduction in dose, and image quality was maintained.[67] However, one must be careful lowering the kV in CCTA examinations; although the signal improves, image noise also increases. High image noise and blurring at the edge of the

coronary artery wall have been reported, making assessment of coronary plaque more difficult in some cases.[48]

Decreasing voltage to 100 or 80 kV has the added benefit of increasing opacification of vessels because of an increase in the photoelectric effect and a decrease in Compton scattering. Intraluminal CT attenuation (HU) of the coronary arteries is significantly higher at 100 kV compared with 120 kV (Feuchtner). Because of this increase in opacification, the iodine dose can be reduced safely.[65,68]

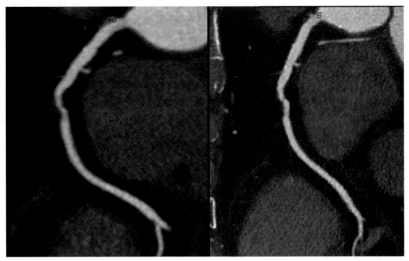

Fig. 6. There is no visible image quality degradation from lowering the kV from 120 to 100 in this 54-year-old woman with midright coronary artery plaque. In these prospectively gated examinations, decreasing the kV resulted in a reduction of the ED by 48% from 4.2 mSv to 2.2 mSv.

Scan Coverage Optimization

Radiation dose is directly proportional to z-axis coverage. Accurate fine-tuning of coverage is important to minimize dose. If the scan length is too long, unnecessary radiation is delivered to the upper chest and abdominal organs. If the length is too short, part of the coronary tree may be excluded. When minimum z-axis coverage is prescribed there is risk of excluding anatomy if the patient does not perform an identical breath hold to the one performed for planning purposes. Coaching the patient in appropriate breathing techniques to ensure standardization of breath holding is imperative to prevent truncation of anatomy because of irregular breath holding.

Minimization of z-axis is important. In the PROTOCOL study, multivariate analysis showed a 5% reduction in ED for every 1 cm of reduced z-axis scan length.[63] To minimize z-axis coverage but ensure adequate anatomy is imaged, we prescribe the z-axis from review of the calcium-scoring scan, if performed, or we perform a low dose axial scout. CCTA scanning starts 20 mm above the left main origin and concludes 10 mm below the cardiac apex. Other investigators prefer to plan coverage from the scout topogram to prescribe a volume beginning at the bifurcation of the trachea. However, use of the scout film has been shown to be inaccurate for determining the precise origin of the coronary arteries.[69]

FOV

Limitation of the FOV (x-y plane) helps minimize radiation and potentially improves quality. The size of the imaging voxel is reduced as the FOV is decreased, improving spatial resolution. Use of a bowtie filter allows for reduced radiation exposure by limiting the scatter toward the detectors. These filters are optimized for patient size. Most cardiac studies can be imaged with a small bowtie filter that is most efficient at reducing dose. Budoff and colleagues[70] reported a 40% dose reduction by using a small bowtie filter rather than larger filters. Routine use of small bowtie filters and small FOV is prudent to minimize dose of cardiac CT studies.

Bismuth Shielding

Bismuth shields are of small sheets of bismuth-impregnated latex that are placed over radiosensitive organs during CT scanning.[71] Bismuth shielding reduces exposure to these superficial radiosensitive organs such as the breast, thyroid gland, and orbits. Significant radiation dose reduction to these organs has been reported, ranging from 29% to 57%.[72,73] They reduce radiation exposure by attenuating photons only when the shields are positioned between the organ and radiograph tube; photons originating from other directions may have undergone some filtration and attenuation as they passed through the CT table, the posterior chest wall, and the mediastinum.

Limited data exist on the use of these shields during cardiac CT and concerns exist about the effect of bismuth shields on image quality. During coronary calcium scoring bismuth breast shielding provided a 37% decrease in radiation dose to the breast.[74] In our experience the effect of using breast bismuth shields on image noise, signal-to-noise ratio (SNR) and CNR seems to be minimal and we use these routinely at our centers; however, more formal analysis has yet to be performed.

ECG-controlled Tube Current Modulation

Scan data used for diagnosis are most commonly from the diastolic phase, which implies that a high tube current is required only during the diastolic phase and that a low tube current is acceptable during the remaining cardiac phase. Reduction of the tube current during the less critical portions of the cardiac cycle (usually systole) is achieved using ECG-gated tube current modulation. ECG-gated tube current modulation reduces radiation exposure without decreasing diagnostic image quality. Using this technique, full tube current is on during the most optimal phases of the cardiac cycle (usually portions of diastole) and is then reduced during the remaining phases.

ECG-gated tube current modulation algorithms vary the length of the full tube current plateau depending on heart rate. Some newer versions can detect arrhythmias and automatically maintain full tube current for the arrhythmic cardiac cycles. Depending on heart rate, ECG-gated tube current modulation can reduce overall effective radiation dose by 20% to 48%.[48,50,64] The effects of dose reduction are more pronounced for lower heart rates. In the PROTECTION I study, a 25% dose reduction was noted when ECG-gated tube current modulation was used, and it was used in 73% of studies.[27]

Benefits of ECG dose modulation are dependent on patient heart rate. At higher heart rates, there is less time to rapidly change the tube current and a less substantial reduction in ED is obtained (Fig. 7). In addition, because reconstruction of the coronary arteries in late systole is often of use at higher heart rates, a longer peak current plateau may be advantageous, although it increases dose. At higher rates some centers choose to either extend the time of full tube current

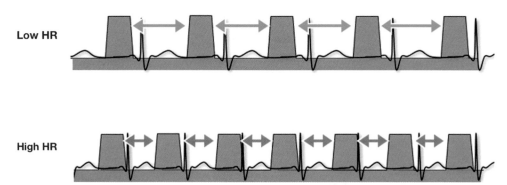

Fig. 7. Benefit of ECG dose modulation is dependent on patient heart rate. At higher heart rates, there is less time (*red arrows*) compared with lower heart rates (*green arrows*) to rapidly change the tube current and a less substantial reduction in ED is obtained.

or forgo its use altogether, increasing the relative dose. In patients with irregular heart rate, ECG-gated tube current modulation may inadvertently reduce tube current during the optimal imaging phase, yielding reduced image quality and diagnostic usefulness.[64]

Prospective Triggering

The use of prospectively ECG-triggered CCTA has shown the largest ED reduction compared with other methods discussed in this article.[51–53,55,75–78] Prospective ECG triggering is also referred to as step-and-shoot or sequential scanning technique. Using this technique, the table is stationary during image acquisition and moves to the next location for another scan that is initiated by the subsequent cardiac cycle. There is little overlap between the scans, resulting in a considerable reduction in radiation dose. The method takes advantage of the larger volume coverage available with newer 64 and higher detector row CT scanners. Complete coverage of the heart can be performed in as little as a single heartbeat for wide detector scanners,[40,42,79,80] 2 to 3 heartbeats with 128-detector DSCT,[81,82] or in 5 to 8 heart beats on a 64-row system.[51]

Prospective ECG triggering enables acquisition of CCTA at doses generally in the 1- to 4-mSv range.[51–53,55,75–78] We reported the first clinical use of this technique for MDCT CCTA.[51] The mean ED for prospectively triggered examinations was 2.8 mSv, 83% less than the retrospective helical technique (mean 18.4 mSv). Despite the reduced dose, the image quality score was significantly greater for images obtained with the prospectively triggered technique. Many other studies have since evaluated the use of prospective gating for CCTA (**Table 1**). In the PROTECTION I study, prospective ECG triggering was used in only 6% of studies, but when used it led

to a 71% reduction in effective radiation dose compared with the standard spiral scan technique.[27] The 6% figure reflects the PROTECTION I data accumulated before widespread release of prospective triggering protocols. Current use of prospective triggering is likely higher, but no formal survey has been performed.

Prospective gating is currently performed on all currently available MDCT and DSCT cardiac capable scanners including those with 64, 128, 256, and 320 detector rows (see **Table 1**). Prospective gating also reduces dose of other types of cardiac studies, including postcoronary artery bypass graft (post-CABG) scans (79.5% reduction from 31.2 mSv retrospective gating to 6.4 mSv).[77] In the emergency department, Shuman and colleagues[52] reported that the use of prospective triggering for triple rule-out studies reduced the mean ED from 31.8 ± 5.1 mSv (retrospective gating) to 9.2 ± 2.2 mSv (prospective triggering). In that study 99.5% of coronary segments imaged with prospective triggering were evaluable and prospectively triggered images were 2.2 (95% confidence interval [CI], 1.1–4.5) times as likely as retrospectively gated images to receive a high image quality score (P<.05).

Several studies have evaluated the diagnostic accuracy of prospectively triggered CCTA compared with conventional angiography (CA). Scheffel and colleagues[78] studied 120 patients and reported overall patient-based sensitivity, specificity, positive predictive value (PPV) and negative predictive value (NPV) for the diagnosis of significant stenoses were 100%, 93%, 94%, and 100%. Stolzmann and colleagues[83] reported overall sensitivity, specificity, PPV, and NPV were 98%, 99%, 95%, and 100%, respectively. Dewey and colleagues[79] evaluated 320-MDCT before same-day CA and reported per-patient sensitivity and specificity for CT compared with CA were 100% and 94%, respectively.

Table 1
Summary of CT studies performed using prospective triggering; published studies as of January 2010

Author	Journal	Year	PG (n)	RG (n)	PG Dose (mSv)	Change (%)	Segments Diagnostic (%)	Major Findings
MDCT-64								
Earls et al[51]	Radiology	2008	121	82	2.8	−83	98.6	IQ PG > RG; segment assessability PG = RG
Shuman et al[52]	Radiology	2008	50	50	4.2	−77	98.9	IQ PG > RG but = when adjusted for chest diameter
Husmann et al[76]	Eur Heart J	2008	41		2.1		95.0	98.9% segment assessable <HR 63, 85% >HR 63
Hirai et al[55]	Radiology	2008	75	75	4.1	−79	98.9	IQ, stenosis detection, and grade PG = RG
Gopal[89]	Int J Cardiovasc Imaging	2008	149	45	3.5	−83		Use of 100 kVp reduced dose 41.5%
Maruyama[90]	J Am Coll Cardiol	2008	76	97	4.3	−80	96.6	PG similar accuracy and % assessability as RG
Earls and Schrack[77]	Int J Cardiovasc Imag	2009	1822	156	3.1	−82		PG used in 92.1% CCTA; CABG PG 6.4 mSv versus RG 30.8 mSv
DeFrance[91]	Int J Cardiovasc Imag	2009	57	25	6.9	−59	99.3	IQ excellent 90%, good 8%, acceptable 1% noninterpretable 1%
Einstein[92]	Am J Cardiol	2009	225	138	3.4	−78		IQ greater for PG in sequential-if-appropriate strategy
Herzog et al[85]	Acad Radiol	2009	129		2.2			HR <62 less nondiagnostic segments on ROC (2% vs 14%)
Herzog[93]	Heart	2009	42		2.1		97	Estimated dose 8.5 mSv CA 2.1 mSv CTCA
Husmann[94]	Eur Heart J	2009	100	100	2.2	−89		Combined imaging with stress-only SPECT
Husmann et al[54]	AJR	2009	140		2.2			Used BMI adapted contrast volumes successfully
Husmann[95]	Acad Radiol	2009	61		2.1			Specificity and PPV improved by combining it with CS
Klass[96]	Eur Radiol	2009	20	20	3.7	−80		IQ no difference
Ko et al[86]	Int J Cardiovasc Imag	2009	85	93	3.8	−64	97.4	IQ inversely related to HR and HR variability

Study	Journal	Year						Comments
Tatsugami et al[62]	AJR	2009	101		2.1		94.5	BMI based kV & mA: noise unchanged; vessel HU lower high BMI
MDCT-256-320								
Weigold[97]	Int J Cardiovasc Imag	2009	77	12	4	−65		First experience 256 cardiac
Efstathopoulos[98]	Phys Med Biol	2009	15	10	3.2	−76		2 axial acquisitions performed with 256 MDCT
MDCT-320								
Rybicki et al[40]	Int J Cardiovasc Imaging	2008	34	6	6.7	−50	99.8	Initial PG with 320 scanner; used wide phase window
Steigner et al[42]	Int J Cardiovasc Imaging	2009	41		6.7			Phase window 10% yields diagnostic IQ >90% of patients
Dewey et al[79]	Circulation	2009	30		4.2		100	Dose CT 4.2 versus 8.5 CCA
Hoe & Toh[80]	J Cardiovasc Comput Tomogr	2009	200		7.9			1-beat acquisition HR < 65, >65 higher dose and 2–3 HB acquisition
DSCT-64								
Gutstein et al[75]	J Cardiovasc Comput Tomogr	2008	42	162	3.1	−85		Initial DSCT use
Scheffel et al[78]	Heart	2008	120		2.8		98.0	First accuracy study
Stolzmann et al[53]	Radiology	2008	90		2.6		97.9	HR and HR variability increase artifacts
Stolzmann et al[83]	AJR	2008	89		2.6		96.0	Accuracy compared with low- and high-calcium groups no different
Blankstein[99]	Am J Cardiol	2009	42	188	3.2			IQ no different
Hein[100]	Int J Cardiovasc Imag	2009	119	394	3.4	−55	97.6	IQ no different
Xu et al[87]	Eur J Radiol	2009	50	50	5.1	−57	99.7	All HR 70–110 bpm: adaptive PG same IQ and assessability as RG
Zhao[101]	Eur J Radiol	2009	30	30	2.2	−85		Stent assessability, accuracy, image quality no change compared with RG
DSCT-128								
Anders et al[81]	Rofo	2009	20		3.6			Initial PG on 128-MDCT 75 ms temporal resolution
Arnoldi et al[82]	Eur Radiol	2009	20	60	3.0	−67		IQ no different

Abbreviations: HR, heart rate; IQ, image quality; PG, prospective gating; RG, retrospective gating; SPECT, single photon emission-computed tomography.

Some versions of this technique allow for a user-defined broadening of acquisition window, known as padding. This technique acquires additional phase information on either side of the targeted phase, which can at times be useful if image quality of the target phase is suboptimal. The broadened acquisition window comes with a substantial increased radiation dose because of prolonged tube on time.[77] In theory use of padding increases the diagnostic usefulness of the examination. However, Leipsic and colleagues[84] prospectively evaluated 886 patients at 3 centers and concluded that use of reduced or no padding was associated with a substantial reduction in radiation dose, with preserved study interpretability.

There are limitations to the use of prospective ECG triggering. Because data are acquired only during a limited portion of the cardiac cycle there is no capability to evaluate cardiac function. Image quality degrades at higher heart rates. Most studies performed with prospective triggering have used upper heart rate criteria of between 65 and 70 beats per minute (bpm). Husmann and colleagues[76] reported that 98.9% of the coronary segments were clinically assessable for heart rates less than 63 bpm; however, this dropped to 85% at higher heart rates. Other studies have reported similar inverse correlation between image quality or segment assessability and heart rate.[53,85,86] Heart rate variability has also been independently correlated with overall image quality for prospectively triggered CCTA.[53,85,86] Newer techniques and faster CT systems may be helpful in increasing the upper heart rate limitation. Using DSCT, Xu and colleagues[87] evaluated patients with heart rate of 70 to 110 bpm using a new adaptive prospectively gated technique and compared results with retrospective gating. These investigators found coronary assessability of the prospectively triggered scan was 99.7%, similar to 98.7% with retrospective gating.

Most centers currently rely on use of β-blockers to lower the heart rate, enabling use of prospective triggering and yielding examinations with excellent image quality and low ED. Despite the heart rate limitation and lack of functional data associated with prospective triggering, it can still be a commonly used technique for CCTA. In our clinical practice we preferentially use prospective triggering for all clinical cases as long as 3 criteria are met: (1) heart rate is less than 70 bpm, (2) heart rate variability is less than 10 bpm, and (3) functional data are not required. We evaluated data on 2124 consecutive clinical examinations.[77] Without any β-blockade, approximately 50% of patients failed one or more of the listed criteria. However, with careful heart rate control, 95.0% of patients had a heart rate of less than 70 bpm, 93.7% had less than 10 bpm of observed heart rate variability, and 90.5% met both criteria. As a result prospective triggering was used for 1822 of 1978 (92.1%) CCTAs and 121 of 146 (83.2%) of CCTAs following CABG.

High-pitch Spiral Prospectively Gated DSCT

If the pitch is of a retrospectively gated CCTA is increased, there is less overlap and reduction in radiation exposure; however, if the pitch is increased to greater than 1.5 data gaps occur, resulting in critical artifacts. As stated earlier high-pitch data acquisitions can now be performed on DSCT platforms with 2 radiograph tubes and 2 detectors.[39,44–47] Using this high-pitch spiral dual-source technique, a pitch of 3.2 or 3.4, and the new broader 128 × 0.6 mm DSCT detector, enough data are acquired to cover the heart during a single heartbeat.[44,46,47] Because of the short subsecond radiation exposure and little overlap between spiral acquisitions, considerable reduction in radiation dose has been found.

Achenbach and colleagues[44] evaluated high-pitch spiral technique in 50 consecutive patients weighing 100 kg or less and with heart rate of 60 bpm or less (**Fig. 8**). Data acquisition lasted a mean of 258 milliseconds, was prospectively triggered at 60% of the R-R interval, 99.5% of coronary artery segments were interpretable, and the mean ED was 0.87 mSv. Lell and colleagues[46] reported that 99.4% of coronary segments were evaluable and found a mean dose of 1.0 mSv. Sommer and colleagues[47] evaluated its use in a triple rule-out

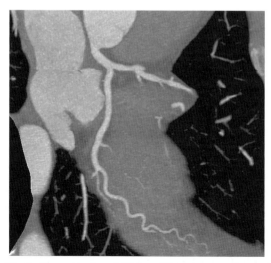

Fig. 8. Example of an LAD in a 79-kg man performed with 100 kV, 320 mAs using a high-pitch spiral acquisition technique on a 128-DSCT system. ED was 0.85 mSv. (*Courtesy of* Stephen Achenbach MD.)

protocol in 31 patients with acute chest pain; dose was 4.08 mSv with 84.7% of segments interpretable, compared with 20.4 mSv and 92.9% with retrospective technique, respectively.

There are limitations, no functional data are available, and it is susceptible to artifacts because of ectopy. Use of high-pitch spiral technique has been limited to heart rates of less than 60 bpm and it has been primarily used with nonobese (<100 kg) patients. Proof of concept trials were initially performed on the 64-DSCT system; however, the recently published larger series have been using the more modern 128-detector row DSCT platform. Nevertheless, early clinical results show good potential and the technique represents yet another method for performing low-dose CCTA.

IR

Statistical iterative image reconstruction is a new technique that may be used to lower radiation exposure of all CT studies, including cardiac.[28,56,57,88] FBP has limitations that can negatively affect image quality and require higher tube current to achieve adequate SNRs. IR provides greater flexibility for accurate noise modeling and geometric system description.[57] Initial experience suggests that these new methods allow for improvements in image quality and lower image noise and thus seem to be particularly promising for low-radiation dose cardiac CT.[57]

Recently, adaptive statistical IR (ASIR) was introduced as a novel reconstruction algorithm for CT.[28,56,88] ASIR uses iterative comparisons of each acquired image to a synthesized projection incorporating modeling of system optics and system statistics. Compared with FBP, images reconstructed with ASIR have lower image noise. ASIR is used to help deal with one of the primary issues of dose and tube current reduction for CCTA with FBP: increased image noise with decreased tube current. By using ASIR to reduce image noise, tube current can be reduced and relative image noise maintained, achieving lower radiation doses.

Hara and colleagues[28] reported use of ASIR was associated with 32% to 65% ED reductions compared with FBP without degradation of image quality for abdominal imaging. In CCTA Leipsic and colleagues[30] evaluated 62 patients using an ASIR-capable 64-detector scanner and a low-dose CCTA technique. Compared with FBP (0% ASIR), increasing ASIR reduced image noise up to 43% but there was no effect on signal. Reconstruction using 40% or 60% ASIR significantly improved image quality and the proportion of interpretable segments when using a low mA technique.

Use of ASIR was recently reported in a multicenter analysis in 1202 consecutive patients in 3 arms: routine 64-detector CCTA with FBP (n = 753), 64-detector CCTA with ASIR (n = 247), and the latter following initiation of a protocol using 100 kV (in patients with a BMI <30 kg/m^2) and a BMI-based mA protocol (n = 202).[63] The mean effective radiation of the 3 groups was 3.8, 2.6, and 1.3 mSv, respectively. Despite the reduced radiation dose, image interpretability and SNR of post-protocol ASIR and FBP were similar. Independent of patient parameters, ASIR was associated with reduced current use (↓ 169 mA, P < .001). The implementation of a common ASIR protocol permitted CCTA examinations with a median of 1.3 mSv of radiation.

SUMMARY

Cardiac CT technology continues to evolve. Although there has been substantial improvement in spatial and temporal resolution, significant challenges remain. Increasing concern about the effects of radiation has promoted accelerated development of new CT systems and techniques capable of imaging the heart at a lower radiation dose than previously possible. Use of optimized user-defined scan parameters as well as newly available technologies can be used concurrently to substantially lower radiation dose without negatively affecting image quality.

REFERENCES

1. Budoff MJ, Achenbach S, Blumenthal RS, et al. Assessment of coronary artery disease by cardiac computed tomography: a scientific statement from the American Heart Association Committee on Cardiovascular Imaging and Intervention, Council on Cardiovascular Radiology and Intervention, and Committee on Cardiac Imaging, Council on Clinical Cardiology. Circulation 2006;114(16):1761–91.
2. Fox K, García MA, Ardissino D, et al. [Guidelines on the management of stable angina pectoris. Executive summary]. Rev Esp Cardiol 2006;59(9):919–70 [in Spanish].
3. Hendel RC, Patel MR, Kramer CM, et al. ACCF/ACR/SCCT/SCMR/ASNC/NASCI/SCAI/SIR 2006 appropriateness criteria for cardiac computed tomography and cardiac magnetic resonance imaging: a report of the American College of Cardiology Foundation Quality Strategic Directions Committee Appropriateness Criteria Working Group, American College of Radiology, Society of

Cardiovascular Computed Tomography, Society for Cardiovascular Magnetic Resonance, American Society of Nuclear Cardiology, North American Society for Cardiac Imaging, Society for Cardiovascular Angiography and Interventions, and Society of Interventional Radiology. J Am Coll Cardiol 2006;48(7):1475–97.

4. Brenner DJ, Hall EJ. Computed tomography–an increasing source of radiation exposure. N Engl J Med 2007;357(22):2277–84.

5. Einstein AJ, Henzlova MJ, Rajagopalan S. Estimating risk of cancer associated with radiation exposure from 64-slice computed tomography coronary angiography. JAMA 2007;298(3):317–23.

6. Smith-Bindman R, Lipson J, Marcus R, et al. Radiation dose associated with common computed tomography examinations and the associated lifetime attributable risk of cancer. Arch Intern Med 2009;169(22):2078–86.

7. Boyd D, Lipton M. Cardiac computed tomography. Proc IEEE 1983;71(3):298–307.

8. Lipton MJ, Higgins CB, Farmer D, et al. Cardiac imaging with a high-speed Cine-CT Scanner: preliminary results. Radiology 1984; 152(3):579–82.

9. Achenbach S, Ulzheimer S, Baum U, et al. Noninvasive coronary angiography by retrospectively ECG-gated multislice spiral CT. Circulation 2000; 102(23):2823–8.

10. Becker CR, Knez A, Ohnesorge B, et al. Imaging of noncalcified coronary plaques using helical CT with retrospective ECG gating. AJR Am J Roentgenol 2000;175(2):423–4.

11. Flohr T, Ohnesorge B, Bruder H, et al. Image reconstruction and performance evaluation for ECG-gated spiral scanning with a 16-slice CT system. Med Phys 2003;30(10):2650–62.

12. Nieman K, Cademartiri F, Lemos PA, et al. Reliable noninvasive coronary angiography with fast submillimeter multislice spiral computed tomography. Circulation 2002;106(16):2051–4.

13. Ropers D, Baum U, Pohle K, et al. Detection of coronary artery stenoses with thin-slice multidetector row spiral computed tomography and multiplanar reconstruction. Circulation 2003; 107(5):664–6.

14. Mollet NR, Cademartiri F, Nieman K, et al. Multislice spiral computed tomography coronary angiography in patients with stable angina pectoris. J Am Coll Cardiol 2004;43(12):2265–70.

15. Kuettner A, Trabold T, Schroeder S, et al. Noninvasive detection of coronary lesions using 16-detector multislice spiral computed tomography technology: initial clinical results. J Am Coll Cardiol 2004;44(6): 1230–7.

16. Dewey M, Hoffmann H, Hamm B. CT coronary angiography using 16 and 64 simultaneous detector rows: intraindividual comparison. Rofo 2007; 179(6):581–6.

17. Burgstahler C, Reimann A, Brodoefel H, et al. Quantitative parameters to compare image quality of non-invasive coronary angiography with 16-slice, 64-slice and dual-source computed tomography. Eur Radiol 2009;19(3):584–90.

18. Hamon M, Morello R, Riddell JW, et al. Coronary arteries: diagnostic performance of 16- versus 64-section spiral CT compared with invasive coronary angiography–meta-analysis. Radiology 2007; 245(3):720–31.

19. Flohr T, Stierstorfer K, Raupach R, et al. Performance evaluation of a 64-slice CT system with z-flying focal spot. Rofo 2004;176(12):1803–10.

20. Herzog C, Nguyen SA, Savino G, et al. Does two-segment image reconstruction at 64-section CT coronary angiography improve image quality and diagnostic accuracy? Radiology 2007; 244(1):121–9.

21. Halliburton SS, Stillman AE, Flohr T, et al. Do segmented reconstruction algorithms for cardiac multi-slice computed tomography improve image quality? Herz 2003;28(1):20–31.

22. Budoff MJ, Dowe D, Jollis JG, et al. Diagnostic performance of 64-multidetector row coronary computed tomographic angiography for evaluation of coronary artery stenosis in individuals without known coronary artery disease: results from the prospective multicenter ACCURACY (Assessment by Coronary Computed Tomographic Angiography of Individuals Undergoing Invasive Coronary Angiography) trial. J Am Coll Cardiol 2008;52(21): 1724–32.

23. Flohr TG, Raupach R, Bruder H, et al. Cardiac CT: how much can temporal resolution, spatial resolution, and volume coverage be improved? J Cardiovasc Comput Tomogr 2009;3(3):143–52.

24. Cheng V, Gutstein A, Wolak A, et al. Moving beyond binary grading of coronary arterial stenoses on coronary computed tomographic angiography: insights for the imager and referring clinician. JACC Cardiovasc Imaging 2008;1(4): 460–71.

25. Schuijf JD, Pundziute G, Jukema JW, et al. Evaluation of patients with previous coronary stent implantation with 64-section CT. Radiology 2007;245(2): 416–23.

26. Raff GL, Gallagher MJ, O'Neill WW, et al. Diagnostic accuracy of noninvasive coronary angiography using 64-slice spiral computed tomography. J Am Coll Cardiol 2005;46(3):552–7.

27. Hausleiter J, Meyer T, Hermann F, et al. Estimated radiation dose associated with cardiac CT angiography. JAMA 2009;301(5):500–7.

28. Hara AK, Paden RG, Silva AC, et al. Iterative reconstruction technique for reducing body radiation

dose at CT: feasibility study. AJR Am J Roentgenol 2009;193(3):764–71.

29. Nuyts J, De Man B, Dupont P, et al. Iterative reconstruction for helical CT: a simulation study. Phys Med Biol 1998;43(4):729–37.

30. Leipsic J, LaBounty J, Heilborn B, et al. Multicenter validation of noise reduction and image quality using ASIR in cardiac CT. Presented at the North American Society of Cardiovascular Imaging Annual Meeting. Orlando (FL), October 30, 2009.

31. Flohr T, Ohnesorge B. Heart rate adaptive optimization of spatial and temporal resolution for electrocardiogram-gated multislice spiral CT of the heart. J Comput Assist Tomogr 2001;25(6):907–23.

32. Mahesh M, Cody DD. Physics of cardiac imaging with multiple-row detector CT. Radiographics 2007;27(5):1495–509.

33. Lee V. Cine gradient echo imaging. In: Lee VS, editor. Cardiovascular MRI: physical principles to practical protocols. Philadelphia: Lippincott, Williams & Wilkins; 2006. p. 283–306.

34. Wood EH. Noninvasive three-dimensional viewing of the motion and anatomical structure of the heart, lungs, and circulatory system by high speed computerized X-ray tomography. CRC Crit Rev Biochem 1979;7(2):161–86.

35. Flohr TG, McCollough CH, Bruder H, et al. First performance evaluation of a dual-source CT (DSCT) system. Eur Radiol 2006;16(2):256–68.

36. Johnson TRC, Nikolaou K, Busch S, et al. Diagnostic accuracy of dual-source computed tomography in the diagnosis of coronary artery disease. Invest Radiol 2007;42(10):684–91.

37. Matt D, Scheffel H, Leschka S, et al. Dual-source CT coronary angiography: image quality, mean heart rate, and heart rate variability. AJR Am J Roentgenol 2007;189(3):567–73.

38. Leber AW, Johnson T, Becker A, et al. Diagnostic accuracy of dual-source multi-slice CT-coronary angiography in patients with an intermediate pretest likelihood for coronary artery disease. Eur Heart J 2007;28(19):2354–60.

39. Achenbach S, Marwan M, Schepis T, et al. High-pitch spiral acquisition: a new scan mode for coronary CT angiography. J Cardiovasc Comput Tomogr 2009;3(2):117–21.

40. Rybicki FJ, Otero HJ, Steigner ML, et al. Initial evaluation of coronary images from 320-detector row computed tomography. Int J Cardiovasc Imaging 2008;24(5):535–46.

41. Dewey M, Zimmermann E, Laule M, et al. Three-vessel coronary artery disease examined with 320-slice computed tomography coronary angiography. Eur Heart J 2008;29(13):1669.

42. Steigner ML, Otero HJ, Cai T, et al. Narrowing the phase window width in prospectively ECG-gated single heart beat 320-detector row coronary CT angiography. Int J Cardiovasc Imaging 2009; 25(1):85–90.

43. Engel KJ, Herrmann C, Zeitler G. X-ray scattering in single- and dual-source CT. Med Phys 2008; 35(1):318–32.

44. Achenbach S, Marwan M, Ropers D, et al. Coronary computed tomography angiography with a consistent dose below 1 mSv using prospectively electrocardiogram-triggered high-pitch spiral acquisition [Internet]. Eur Heart J 2009; Available at: http://www.ncbi.nlm.nih.gov/pubmed/19897497. Accessed January 4, 2010.

45. Hausleiter J, Bischoff B, Hein F, et al. Feasibility of dual-source cardiac CT angiography with high-pitch scan protocols. J Cardiovasc Comput Tomogr 2009;3(4):236–42.

46. Lell M, Marwan M, Schepis T, et al. Prospectively ECG-triggered high-pitch spiral acquisition for coronary CT angiography using dual source CT: technique and initial experience. Eur Radiol 2009; 19(11):2576–83.

47. Sommer WH, Schenzle JC, Becker CR, et al. Saving dose in triple-rule-out computed tomography examination using a high-pitch dual spiral technique [Internet]. Invest Radiol 2009; Available at: http://www.ncbi.nlm.nih.gov/pubmed/20027121. Accessed January 13, 2010.

48. Abada HT, Larchez C, Daoud B, et al. MDCT of the coronary arteries: feasibility of low-dose CT with ECG-pulsed tube current modulation to reduce radiation dose. AJR Am J Roentgenol 2006;186(6 Suppl 2): S387–90.

49. Leschka S, Stolzmann P, Schmid FT, et al. Low kilovoltage cardiac dual-source CT: attenuation, noise, and radiation dose. Eur Radiol 2008; 18(9):1809–17.

50. Jakobs TF, Becker CR, Ohnesorge B, et al. Multislice helical CT of the heart with retrospective ECG gating: reduction of radiation exposure by ECG-controlled tube current modulation. Eur Radiol 2002;12(5):1081–6.

51. Earls JP, Berman EL, Urban BA, et al. Prospectively gated transverse coronary CT angiography versus retrospectively gated helical technique: improved image quality and reduced radiation dose. Radiology 2008;246(3):742–53.

52. Shuman WP, Branch KR, May JM, et al. Prospective versus retrospective ECG gating for 64-detector CT of the coronary arteries: comparison of image quality and patient radiation dose. Radiology 2008;248(2):431–7.

53. Stolzmann P, Leschka S, Scheffel H, et al. Dual-source CT in step-and-shoot mode: noninvasive coronary angiography with low radiation dose. Radiology 2008;249(1):71–80.

54. Husmann L, Herzog BA, Burkhard N, et al. Low-dose coronary CT angiography with prospective

ECG triggering: validation of a contrast material protocol adapted to body mass index. AJR Am J Roentgenol 2009;193(3):802–6.

55. Hirai N, Horiguchi J, Fujioka C, et al. Prospective versus retrospective ECG-gated 64-detector coronary CT angiography: assessment of image quality, stenosis, and radiation dose. Radiology 2008; 248(2):424–30.

56. Marin D, Nelson RC, Schindera ST, et al. Low-tube-voltage, high-tube-current multidetector abdominal CT: improved image quality and decreased radiation dose with adaptive statistical iterative reconstruction algorithm–initial clinical experience. Radiology 2010;254(1):145–53.

57. Thibault J, Sauer KD, Bouman CA, et al. A three-dimensional statistical approach to improved image quality for multislice helical CT. Med Phys 2007;34(11):4526–44.

58. Raff GL, Chinnaiyan KM, Share DA, et al. Advanced Cardiovascular Imaging Consortium Co-Investigators. Radiation dose from cardiac computed tomography before and after implementation of radiation dose-reduction techniques. JAMA 2009;301(22):2340–8.

59. European_Guidelines_Quality_Criteria_Computed_Tomography_Eur_16252.pdf [Internet]. Available at: http://w3.tue.nl/fileadmin/sbd/Documenten/Leergang/BSM/European_Guidelines_Quality_Criteria_Computed_Tomography_Eur_16252.pdf. Accessed January 6, 2010.

60. Starck G, Lönn L, Cederblad A, et al. A method to obtain the same levels of CT image noise for patients of various sizes, to minimize radiation dose. Br J Radiol 2002;75(890):140–50.

61. Jung B, Mahnken AH, Stargardt A, et al. Individually weight-adapted examination protocol in retrospectively ECG-gated MSCT of the heart. Eur Radiol 2003;13(12):2560–6.

62. Tatsugami F, Husmann L, Herzog BA, et al. Evaluation of a body mass index-adapted protocol for low-dose 64-MDCT coronary angiography with prospective ECG triggering. AJR Am J Roentgenol 2009;192(3):635–8.

63. LaBounty TM, Earls J, Leipsic J, et al. Estimated radiation dose of coronary computed tomography angiography using adaptive statistical iterative reconstruction: a multicenter study. Circulation 2009;120:S334.

64. Hausleiter J, Meyer T, Hadamitzky M, et al. Radiation dose estimates from cardiac multislice computed tomography in daily practice: impact of different scanning protocols on effective dose estimates. Circulation 2006;113(10): 1305–10.

65. Sigal-Cinqualbre AB, Hennequin R, Abada HT, et al. Low-kilovoltage multi-detector row chest CT in adults: feasibility and effect on image quality and iodine dose. Radiology 2004;231(1): 169–74.

66. Paul J, Wartski M, Caussin C, et al. Late defect on delayed contrast-enhanced multi-detector row CT scans in the prediction of SPECT infarct size after reperfused acute myocardial infarction: initial experience. Radiology 2005;236(2): 485–9.

67. Bischoff B, Hein F, Meyer T, et al. Impact of a reduced tube voltage on CT angiography and radiation dose: results of the PROTECTION I study. JACC Cardiovasc Imaging 2009;2(8):940–6.

68. Wintersperger B, Jakobs T, Herzog P, et al. Aorto-iliac multidetector-row CT angiography with low kV settings: improved vessel enhancement and simultaneous reduction of radiation dose. Eur Radiol 2005;15(2):334–41.

69. Bakhsheshi H, Mao S, Budoff MJ, et al. Preview method for electron-beam CT scanning of the coronary arteries. Acad Radiol 2000;7(8): 620–6.

70. Budoff M. Maximizing dose reductions with cardiac CT. (formerly Cardiac Imaging). Int J Cardiovasc Imaging 2009;25(0):279–87.

71. Gunn ML, Kanal KM, Kolokythas O, et al. Radiation dose to the thyroid gland and breast from multidetector computed tomography of the cervical spine: does bismuth shielding with and without a cervical collar reduce dose? J Comput Assist Tomogr 2009; 33(6):987–90.

72. Fricke BL, Donnelly LF, Frush DP, et al. In-plane bismuth breast shields for pediatric CT: effects on radiation dose and image quality using experimental and clinical data. AJR Am J Roentgenol 2003;180(2):407–11.

73. Hopper KD, King SH, Lobell ME, et al. The breast: in-plane x-ray protection during diagnostic thoracic CT–shielding with bismuth radioprotective garments. Radiology 1997;205(3):853–8.

74. Yilmaz MH, Yaşar D, Albayram S, et al. Coronary calcium scoring with MDCT: the radiation dose to the breast and the effectiveness of bismuth breast shield. Eur J Radiol 2007;61(1):139–43.

75. Gutstein A, Wolak A, Lee C, et al. Predicting success of prospective and retrospective gating with dual-source coronary computed tomography angiography: development of selection criteria and initial experience. J Cardiovasc Comput Tomogr 2008;2(2):81–90.

76. Husmann L, Valenta I, Gaemperli O, et al. Feasibility of low-dose coronary CT angiography: first experience with prospective ECG-gating. Eur Heart J 2008;29(2):191–7.

77. Earls JP, Schrack EC. Prospectively gated low-dose CCTA: 24 months experience in more than 2,000 clinical cases. Int J Cardiovasc Imaging 2008;25(S2):177–87.

78. Scheffel H, Alkadhi H, Leschka S, et al. Low-dose CT coronary angiography in the step-and-shoot mode: diagnostic performance. Heart 2008;94(9): 1132–7.

79. Dewey M, Zimmermann E, Deissenrieder F, et al. Noninvasive coronary angiography by 320-row computed tomography with lower radiation exposure and maintained diagnostic accuracy: comparison of results with cardiac catheterization in a head-to-head pilot investigation. Circulation 2009;120(10):867–75.

80. Hoe J, Toh KH. First experience with 320-row multidetector CT coronary angiography scanning with prospective electrocardiogram gating to reduce radiation dose. J Cardiovasc Comput Tomogr 2009;3(4):257–61.

81. Anders K, Baum U, Gauss S, et al. [Initial experience with prospectively triggered, sequential CT coronary angiography on a 128-slice scanner]. Rofo 2009;181(4):332–8 [in German].

82. Arnoldi E, Johnson TR, Rist C, et al. Adequate image quality with reduced radiation dose in prospectively triggered coronary CTA compared with retrospective techniques. Eur Radiol 2009; 19(9):2147–55.

83. Stolzmann P, Scheffel H, Leschka S, et al. Influence of calcifications on diagnostic accuracy of coronary CT angiography using prospective ECG triggering. AJR Am J Roentgenol 2008;191(6):1684–9.

84. Labounty TM, Leipsic J, Min J, et al. Effect of padding duration on radiation dose and image interpretation in prospectively ECG-triggered coronary CT angiography. AJR Am J Roentgenol 2010; 194(4):933–7.

85. Herzog BA, Husmann L, Burkhard N, et al. Low-dose CT coronary angiography using prospective ECG-triggering: impact of mean heart rate and heart rate variability on image quality. Acad Radiol 2009;16(1):15–21.

86. Ko SM, Kim NR, Kim DH, et al. Assessment of image quality and radiation dose in prospective ECG-triggered coronary CT angiography compared with retrospective ECG-gated coronary CT angiography [Internet]. Int J Cardiovasc Imaging 2009; Available at: http://www.ncbi.nlm. nih.gov/pubmed/20033490. Accessed January 4, 2010.

87. Xu L, Yang L, Zhang Z, et al. Low-dose adaptive sequential scan for dual-source CT coronary angiography in patients with high heart rate: Comparison with retrospective ECG gating. Eur J Radiol 2009. [Internet] Available at: http://www.ncbi.nlm.nih.gov/pubmed/19595528. Accessed January 4, 2010.

88. Silva AC, Lawder HJ, Hara A, et al. Innovations in CT dose reduction strategy: application of the adaptive statistical iterative reconstruction algorithm. AJR Am J Roentgenol 2010;194(1):191–9.

89. Gopal A, Mao SS, Karlsberg D, et al. Radiation reduction with prospective ECG-triggering acquisition using 64-multidetector Computed Tomographic angiography. Int J Cardiovasc Imaging 2009;25(4):405–16.

90. Maruyama T, Takada M, Hasuike T, et al. Radiation dose reduction and coronary assessability of prospective electrocardiogram-gated computed tomography coronary angiography: comparison with retrospective electrocardiogram-gated helical scan. J Am Coll Cardiol 2008;52(18):1450–5.

91. DeFrance T, Dubois E, Gebow D, et al. Helical prospective ECG-gating in cardiac computed tomography: radiation dose and image quality. Int J Cardiovasc Imaging 2010;26(1):99–107.

92. Einstein AJ, Wolff SD, Manheimer ED, et al. Comparison of image quality and radiation dose of coronary computed tomographic angiography between conventional helical scanning and a strategy incorporating sequential scanning. Am J Cardiol 2009;104(10):1343–50.

93. Herzog BA, Husmann L, Burkhard N, et al. Low-dose CT coronary angiography using prospective ECG-triggering: impact of mean heart rate and heart rate variability on image quality. Acad Radiol 2009;16(1):15–21.

94. Husmann L, Herzog BA, Gaemperli O, et al. Diagnostic accuracy of computed tomography coronary angiography and evaluation of stress-only single-photon emission computed tomography/ computed tomography hybrid imaging: comparison of prospective electrocardiogram-triggering vs. retrospective gating. Eur Heart J 2009;30(5): 600–7.

95. Husmann L, Herzog BA, Burger IA, et al. Usefulness of additional coronary calcium scoring in low-dose CT coronary angiography with prospective ECG-triggering impact on total effective radiation dose and diagnostic accuracy. Acad Radiol 2010;17(2):201–6.

96. Klass O, Jeltsch M, Feuerlein S, et al. Prospectively gated axial CT coronary angiography: preliminary experiences with a novel low-dose technique. Eur Radiol 2009;19(4):829–36.

97. Weigold W, Olszewski M, Walker M, et al. Low-dose prospectively gated 256-slice coronary computed tomographic angiography. Int J Cardiovasc Imaging 2009;25:217–30.

98. Efstathopoulos EP, Kelekis NL, Pantos I, et al. Reduction of the estimated radiation dose and associated patient risk with prospective ECG-gated 256-slice CT coronary angiography. Phys Med Biol 2009;54(17):5209–22.

99. Blankstein R, Shah A, Pale R, et al. Radiation dose and image quality of prospective triggering with dual-source cardiac computed tomography. Am J Cardiol 2009;103(8):1168–73.

100. Hein F, Meyer T, Hadamitzk M, et al. Prospective ECG-triggered sequential scan protocol for coronary dual-source CT angiography: initial experience. Int J Cardiovasc Imaging 2009;25: 231–9.

101. Zhao L, Zhang Z, Fan Z, et al. Prospective versus retrospective ECG gating for dual source CT of the coronary stent: comparison of image quality, accuracy, and radiation dose. Eur J Radiol 2009. [Epub ahead of print].

Patient Preparation and Scanning Techniques

Carolyn M. Taylor, MD, MPH[a],*, Andrew Blum, MD[b],
Suhny Abbara, MD[b]

KEYWORDS
- Scanning techniques • Patient preparation • Artifacts

Cardiac computed tomography angiography (CCTA) is a unique diagnostic modality that can provide a comprehensive assessment of cardiac anatomy. Rapid advances in scanner and software technology have resulted in the ability to noninvasively image the coronary arteries. Given that coronary arteries are subject to cardiac contractile motion and generally have diameters of less than 5 mm, this represents a formidable achievement. However, despite dramatic technological advances, limitations exist. To ensure appropriate application of CCTA with diagnostic image quality and optimal use of radiation saving techniques, patient preparation and prescan planning is critical.

PATIENT PREPARATION
Patient Screening

Indications
Appropriate indications for CCTA were outlined in the 2006 ACCF/ACR/SCCT/SCMR/ASNC/NASCI/SCAI/SIR Appropriateness Criteria document.[1] There are currently 13 clinical indications for which the use of CCTA is felt to be appropriate, comprising 4 indications for the detection of coronary artery disease (CAD) and 9 non-CAD indications.

Current indications for CCTA in the detection of CAD include:

1. Symptomatic patients at intermediate pretest probability of CAD with either an uninterpretable electrocardiogram (ECG) or inability to exercise
2. Patients with a chest pain syndrome and an uninterpretable or equivocal stress test
3. Acute chest pain patients with intermediate pretest probability of CAD without ECG changes and with serial negative cardiac biomarkers
4. Evaluation of coronary arteries in patients with new-onset heart failure to assess etiology.

Additional (non-CAD detection) indications include:

1. Suspected pulmonary embolism
2. Suspected aortic dissection or thoracic aortic aneurysm
3. Evaluation of a cardiac mass when nonradiating imaging modalities (transthoracic echocardiography [TTE], transesophageal echocardiography [TEE], magnetic resonance [MR] imaging) are technically limited
4. Evaluation of pericardial conditions when nonradiating imaging modalities (TTE, TEE, MR imaging) are technically limited.
5. Evaluation of pulmonary vein anatomy prior to atrial fibrillation radiofrequency ablation
6. Evaluation of cardiac venous anatomy prior to biventricular pacing
7. Coronary arterial mapping (including internal mammary artery) prior to repeat cardiac surgical revascularization

[a] Division of Cardiology, University of British Columbia, St Paul's Hospital, 1081 Burrard Street, Room B344, Vancouver, British Columbia V6Z 1Y6, Canada
[b] Cardiovascular Imaging Section, Harvard Medical School, Massachusetts General Hospital, 55 Fruit Street, GRB-295, Boston, MA 02114, USA
* Corresponding author.
E-mail address: cmtaylor@providencehealth.bc.ca

Radiol Clin N Am 48 (2010) 675–686
doi:10.1016/j.rcl.2010.04.011
0033-8389/10/$ – see front matter © 2010 Elsevier Inc. All rights reserved.

8. Assessment of complex congenital heart disease
9. Suspected coronary anomalies in symptomatic patients.

It is important to recognize that the current expert consensus criteria require that a patient either have new-onset heart failure or be symptomatic for the evaluation of CAD with CCTA. Using CCTA to noninvasively detect CAD in *asymptomatic* patients is not generally considered to be appropriate (inappropriate in low and intermediate pretest probability patients and of uncertain appropriateness in high pretest probability patients). In symptomatic patients at low and high pre-test probability of CAD the use of CCTA is currently of uncertain appropriateness. The current guidelines emerged with (1) a focus on avoiding the use of a radiating modality in patients amenable to alternative diagnostic strategies, and (2) avoiding unnecessary/inappropriate testing in those at very low risk (who are less likely to benefit from additional testing) and very high risk (who may be better served by an invasive diagnostic modality that offers improved stenosis quantification and allows for simultaneous revascularization if required). While the 2006 Appropriateness Criteria are useful guidelines, CCTA is evolving rapidly with dramatic reductions in radiation dose,[2,3] and the accepted indications for the technology may expand significantly in the near future.

Contraindications and special considerations
Contraindications to CCTA include pregnancy, prior severe/anaphylactic contrast reaction, inability of patients to cooperate with scanning instructions and perform sufficient breath-hold, renal insufficiency, and clinically unstable patients. Although generally contraindicated in these conditions, exceptions exist for which CCTA may be considered. The risks of scanning must be weighed according to potential benefits (or risks associated with not scanning). Alternative imaging modalities available for diagnosis should be carefully reviewed. In the case of contraindications, CCTA should be reserved for cases not amenable to alternative, noncontraindicated modalities and where the potential benefits of CCTA are felt to outweigh the risks.

Special attention should be devoted to conditions associated with reduced diagnostic image quality. Conditions in which prescan nitroglycerin (such as severe aortic stenosis, hypertrophic cardiomyopathy, and recent phosphodiesterase [PDE]-5 inhibitor use) and β-blockade (such as asthma, decompensated heart failure, and significant atrioventricular [AV] block) is contraindicated

should be identified. Although CCTA can be performed in the absence of nitrates or β-blockade, diagnostic image quality may be significantly reduced. Marked heart rate variability or arrhythmia (including sinus arrhythmia, premature contractions, and atrial fibrillation) can result in significant motion artifacts and limit diagnostic image quality. Similarly, markedly elevated baseline heart rates may be difficult to appropriately rate control, resulting in reduced scan interpretability.

Although obesity is not an absolute contraindication to CCTA, weight restrictions for scanner dimensions and abilities exist. Most modern-day scanners are capable of scanning patients with a body weight of up to 450 pounds (204 kg). However, even with body weights well below scanner limits, image quality may be negatively affected, with increased noise and a reduction in interpretable segments and specificity, despite an increased tube current.[4] The maximum x-ray tube output may be reached in patients with wide anterior-posterior (AP) diameters without achieving an adequate signal to noise ratio.[5] "Obesity protocols" now exist, with increased tube voltage (140 kV) and current associated with an improvement in image quality at the expense of radiation dose.[6]

Patients unable to raise their arms above their head should be identified. Raising the arms during scanning has been shown to reduce radiation dose delivered[7] and avoids artifacts resulting from the humeri. A patient's ability to hold breath, maintain position, and avoid movement is of importance in terms of minimizing motion artifact. Alternative imaging modalities should be considered when either ability or cooperation with these mentioned factors is of concern. If CCTA is felt to be clinically required, an increase in artifacts and risk of reduced interpretability must be anticipated.

While a common and important imaging modality, it must be remembered that computed tomography (CT) is associated with ionizing radiation exposure. A stochastic relationship between radiation exposure and risk of cancer induction is presumed to exist. Monte Carlo simulation models suggest that radiation doses employed in modern-day CCTA are associated with a nonnegligible lifetime attributable risk of cancer and that the risk is increased among women and younger age groups.[8] Several radiation dose reduction techniques can be employed,[3] with radiation doses varying widely by center.[9] The anticipated radiation dose and risk-benefit ratio must be weighed in all individuals referred for CCTA. In individuals at high risk of radiation exposure (pregnant patients, young patients, multiple radiation procedures to date, and so forth), the anticipated radiation dose from CCTA must be carefully considered and non-radiating (or lower radiation dose) alternatives reviewed.

The presence of high-density material (contrast, metal, calcium, bone) can result in beam hardening, blooming, and streaking artifacts (**Fig. 1**). In addition, any effect of motion artifact on image interpretability is more pronounced in the setting of high-density materials. The presence of metallic pacemaker leads (**Fig. 2**), implantable cardioverter-defibrillator (ICD) leads, and mechanical heart valves can prove to be problematic in terms of metal artifact. While artifacts should be anticipated, the presence of pacemakers, ICDs, and mechanical valves do not constitute contraindications to CCTA.

Although CCTA can play a role in ruling out significant in-stent restenosis (**Fig. 3**), visualization of the stent lumen may be limited due to beam hardening, and is highly dependent on stent diameter.[10–12] The Society of Cardiovascular Computed Tomography (SCCT) does not currently recommend the routine application of CCTA to assess coronary stents.[13] However, the most recent expert consensus document[14] suggests that CCTA may be a reasonable alternative to invasive angiography to rule out significant in-stent restenosis (ISR) in patients at low to intermediate pre-test probability for ISR who are known to have larger stents, providing high image quality is anticipated. CCTA can be a useful tool in the assessment of coronary artery bypass grafting (CABG)[15]; however, the ability to assess the native coronary arteries in patients post CABG is limited due to the generally severe underlying coronary

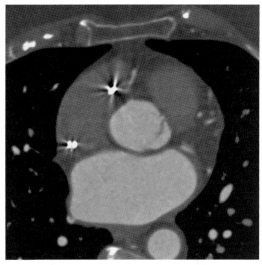

Fig. 2. Dual-chamber (right atrial and right ventricular) pacemaker leads resulting in beam hardening/metal streak artifact. Although artifacts should be anticipated, the presence of a pacemaker is not a contraindication to CCTA.

calcification. One must be aware of the limitations likely to arise when imaging patients with stents and prior bypass surgery.

Patients with cardiac arrhythmias (including atrial fibrillation, sinus arrhythmia, premature ventricular contractions [PVCs], intermittent cardiac pacing, and sinus tachycardia) are problematic in terms of motion artifact. Using

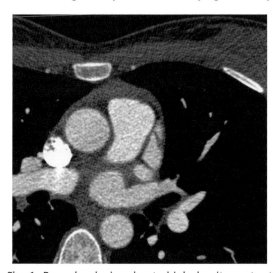

Fig. 1. Beam hardening due to high-density contrast bolus. High-density material (contrast, metal, calcium, bone) can result in beam hardening, blooming, and streak artifacts.

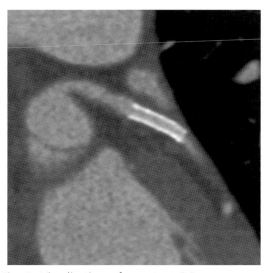

Fig. 3. Visualization of a patent 3.5-mm coronary stent in a ramus intermedius branch. Although CCTA can play a role in ruling out significant in-stent restenosis, visualization of the stent lumen may be limited due to beam hardening, partial volume averaging and motion, and is highly dependent on stent diameter.

retrospective gating, most vendors offer processing tools to aid in the management of arrhythmia. However, in coronary assessment the presence of significant arrhythmia (ventricular bigeminy, atrial fibrillation, and so forth) commonly results in severe motion artifact and uninterpretable segments. Although generally excluded from CCTA for coronary assessment purposes, much work is currently ongoing in the CCTA assessment of patients with atrial fibrillation.[16]

Prescan patient instructions

Patients should be advised of the standard instructions appropriate for all contrast enhanced studies including (1) avoidance of solids for a minimum of 4 hours before the scan, (2) maintaining oral hydration with clear fluids up to 1 hour before the scan, and (3) the need to hold metformin for a minimum of 48 hours following the scan. In addition, all patients should be screened for prior contrast reactions. Severe anaphylactic contrast reactions in the past are a contraindication for repeat scanning, unless for emergency indications where alternative noncontrast imaging modalities are not appropriate. Patients with non-severe reactions in the past for whom CCTA is felt to be clinically required should receive pretreatment to minimize the risk of recurrent contrast reaction. A premedication strategy of prednisone, 50 mg by mouth 13 hours, 7 hours, and 1 hour prior to scan, and oral diphenhydramine (Benadryl), 50 mg 1 hour prior to scan, is employed in many radiology departments.[17]

Given that optimal heart rate control is desirable for diagnostic image quality and radiation dose reduction, caffeine products should not be consumed within 12 hours of CCTA. In contrast to other contrast enhanced scans, CCTA generally includes the administration of nitrates before scanning. A dangerous interaction between phosphodiesterase (PDE)-5 Inhibitors and nitrates can occur, resulting in severe hypotension. Patients should be advised to abstain from PDE-5 inhibitors for a minimum of 24 to 48 hours before scan; a minimum of 24 hours' abstinence with sildenafil (Viagra) and vardenafil (Levitra); and 48 hours' abstinence with tadalafil (Cialis).[18,19] Patients should be advised to continue taking all of their usual cardiovascular medications. **Box 1** outlines suggested prescanning instructions for patients and referring physicians.

Intravenous Access

Intravenous (IV) access should be established once patient screening has been completed and contraindications excluded. It should be anticipated that a study with high diagnostic image

---

Box 1
CCTA standard prescan instructions

Patient instructions:

No solids for 4 hours before the scan

Maintain hydration with clear fluids up to 1 hour before the scan (no caffeine)

Hold metformin for 48 hours following the scan

Inform the radiology department and referring physician ahead of time if history of contrast allergy or known renal dysfunction

No caffeine products for 12 hours before scan (including coffee, tea, soda pop, energy drinks, caffeine pills, Tylenol 3, energy pills, and diet pills)

Abstinence from PDE-5 inhibitors for a minimum of 24 to 48 hours before scan (minimum of 24 hours abstinence with sildenafil and vardenafil; 48 hours with tadalafil)

Continue taking all cardiac medications as per usual

Suggested instructions for referring physician:

Consider outpatient prescription for prescan β-blockade where appropriate and safe (resting heart rate >60 beats/min and no evidence of AV block, hypotension, asthma, severe heart failure; consider metoprolol 50 mg by mouth the morning of scan)

In at-risk* patients, assess renal function. If estimated glomerular filtration rate <60 mL/min/m^2, consider alternative noncontrast imaging modality. (*Patients at risk of reduced renal function should be determined based on age and history. Individuals with preexisting renal dysfunction, diabetes, congestive heart failure, volume depletion, hypotension, low body mass index, concurrent nephrotoxin use, and advanced age are at increased risk of contrast-induced nephropathy).

Screen patient for prior contrast allergy. If present, review alternative noncontrast-enhanced imaging options. If contrast scan felt to be clinically required and allergy not severe/anaphylactic, consider pretreatment (prednisone 50 mg by moth 13 hours, 7 hours, and 1 hour before scan and oral diphenhydramine 50 mg 1 hour before scan).

Patient should be in sinus rhythm. The presence of arrhythmias (atrial fibrillation, frequent ventricular ectopy, ventricular bigeminy, and so forth) should alert the referring physician to consider alternate imaging modalities, as significant reductions in diagnostic image quality and/or significantly higher radiation doses are anticipated.

quality is likely to be achievable; this often requires heart rate control, and some centers await heart rate control before inserting an IV. The IV cannula size and position must allow for the high flow rates of a power injector, and an 18-gauge IV catheter is recommended (although a 20-gauge may be sufficient in smaller patients).[20] Because of a more direct course to the heart, the right antecubital vein is preferable, followed by the left antecubital vein. Venous access in the hand generally does not allow for adequate flow rates for CCTA and should be avoided. Central IV access lines, unless specifically tested and labeled for power injections, should not be used.

Patient Premedication

All patients without contraindications should have nitroglycerin (recommended dose: 0.6–0.8 mg sublingual) administered immediately before CCTA. Nitroglycerin results in coronary vasodilation via vascular smooth muscle relaxation. Nitroglycerin administration typically results in a 20% increase in coronary artery diameter,[21] which may be of critical importance especially in the assessment of distal coronary vessels. Potential side effects of nitrates include hypotension, headache, and dizziness. Severe aortic stenosis, hypertrophic cardiomyopathy, acute right ventricular infarction, raised intracranial pressure, cardiac tamponade, constrictive pericarditis, volume depletion, and recent use of PDE-5 inhibitors (sildenafil, vardenafil, tadalafil) represent contraindications to nitrate use.

Limitations in temporal resolution exist with modern-day CCTA scanners, and heart rate control is typically required for coronary evaluation. Target heart rate varies by scanner type (dual vs single source), gantry speed, and information required (coronary vs noncoronary anatomy). In addition to slowing the heart rate, minimizing heart rate variability is of critical importance[22] in terms of diagnostic quality. β-Blockers (BB) have been routinely recommended to achieve a target heart rate below 60 to 65 beats per minute,[23] and the use of BB has been associated with a reduction in mean heart rate and variability.[22] Various protocols for BB administration exist, with the majority of American centers employing oral BB followed by supplemental IV BB if required based on heart rate.[24] Major side effects of BB use include worsening heart failure, heart block, hypotension, bradycardia, and bronchospasm. Based on their negative chronotropic effects, BB are contraindicated in individuals with decompensated heart failure, second-degree AV block, hypotension, and asthma. In patients with contraindications to

BB, calcium channel blockade (CCB) with verapamil, 240 mg orally has been employed,[25] with varying success.[26] Studies using the I_f current blocking agent, ivabradine, with heart rate reduction through sinoatrial node depression, are underway. Although dual-source scanners provide improved diagnostic accuracy over single-source scanners in the setting of high heart rates, potential advantages exist in segment evaluability with heart rate control even with dual-source scanning.[6,27,28]

Patient Positioning

Patients should be asked to lie supine on the CT scan table with their heart located in the center of the gantry (slightly lateral to midline). Table height should be adjusted until the horizontal laser (marking the gantry center in y-axis) is located one-third of the way down on the anterior portion of the chest. Taking care to center the heart in the gantry (in both x- and y-axes) optimizes both spatial and temporal resolution.[29,30] Whenever able, patients should be asked to lift their arms above their head (out of the field of view surrounding the heart). Artifact from the humeri may result if the patient's arms are not appropriately raised (**Fig. 4**). Caution should be taken to avoid kinking of the IV access; ideally the IV arm should be kept as straight as possible. The IV line and contrast pump should be positioned cranially in such a way that the line does not cross through the gantry thus resulting in streak artifact. A trial run of passing the patient through the gantry for a distance of the planned scanned range ensures that the patient and lines pass unobstructed, and allows the patient to prepare for the anticipated table motion. **Fig. 5** demonstrates ideal positioning of a patient for CCTA.

Electrocardiogram Lead Placement

ECG leads should be positioned outside of the field of view to avoid artifact from the ECG electrodes and cables. Lead placement should include left arm (positioned under the left clavicle), right arm (positioned under right clavicle), and lower left pelvic/left hip lead. **Fig. 6** illustrates optimal lead placement. An example of artifact resulting from improper lead placement is shown in **Fig. 7**. A reliable trace must be acquired for both retrospective gated and prospective triggered scans. Optimal electrode contact requires alcohol preparation (followed by a period of aeration to facilitate drying) and abrasion of the underlying skin. In some men, shaving at the site of anticipated electrode placement may be required.

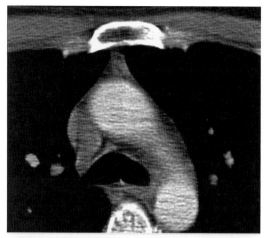

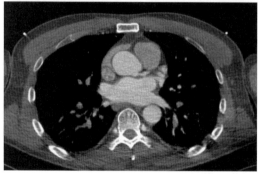

Fig. 4. High noise level despite thin patient and sufficient tube output, due to inability to raise the arms. Patients should be asked to raise their arms above their head (out of the field of view surrounding the heart) to avoid unnecessary excessive image noise caused by artifact from the humeri.

Patient Instruction

Respiratory and musculoskeletal motion can impose significant artifacts and result in noninterpretable image quality. In most cases these artifacts are avoidable with careful patient coaching and preparation. Breath-hold instructions should be practiced with the patient ahead of time. Caution must be undertaken to ensure that patients are not in fact slowly exhaling (due to failing to close their glottis) while breath-holding. In addition to preparing the patient for the length of breath-hold required and ensuring breath-holding ability, the imaging physician and technician can gain useful information with respect to heart rate response to breath-holding. In patients with a marked heart rate response and good breath-hold ability, consideration for commencing the scan once the heart rate has stabilized (after 4–5 cardiac cycles) can be undertaken.[31] The importance of lying motionless throughout scanning should be emphasized to patients. Patients

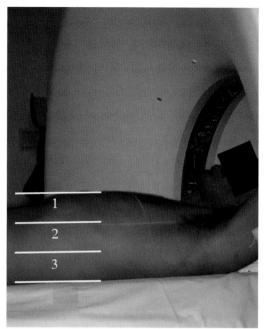

Fig. 5. Ideal patient positioning. Patients should be asked to lie supine on the CT scan table with their heart located in the center of the gantry (slightly lateral to midline). Table height should be adjusted until the horizontal laser (marking the gantry center in y-axis) is located one-third of the way down on the anterior portion of the chest. Patients should be asked to raise their arms above their head to avoid artifact arising from the humeri. The IV arm should be kept as straight as possible. The IV line and contrast pump should be positioned cranially in such a way that the line does not cross through the gantry, resulting in streak artifact. (*From* Halliburton SS, Abbara S. Practical tips and tricks in cardiovascular computed tomography: patient preparation for optimization of cardiovascular CT data acquisition. J Cardiovasc Comput Tomogr 2007;1:64; with permission.)

should be warned in advance of table motion, gantry noise, and contrast warmth. Intravenous access should be tested to ensure painless injection.

SCANNING TECHNIQUES
Goals

Achieving images of diagnostic quality while adhering to ALARA (As Low As Reasonably Achievable) requires thoughtful patient preparation and scanning technique. Patient-specific factors such as age, chest circumference, body mass index (BMI; weight in kilograms divided by height in meters squared), radiation risk, presence of stents, coronary calcification, and heart rate/variability should be considered in the determination of scanning technique.

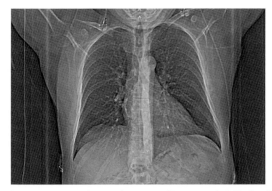

Fig. 6. Appropriate electrocardiogram (ECG) lead placement. ECG leads should be positioned outside of the field of view to avoid artifact from the ECG electrodes and cables. Lead placement should include left arm (positioned under the left clavicle), right arm (positioned under right clavicle) and lower left (and sometimes right) hip lead.

Scan Range/Anterior-Posterior Projection Image

The scan range should be determined from an initial AP projection image, also known as a "scout" or "topogram." CCTA scans are generally oriented with the tracheal bifurcation or main pulmonary arteries acting as the beginning, and just below the diaphragm acting as the ending of the scan range (approximately 12–15 cm in z-axis). However, certain indications (ie, assessment of internal mammary bypass grafts or aortic assessments) require longer scan ranges. Regardless of scan indication, z-axis range should be limited tightly to the structures of interest to minimize radiation dose.

Coronary Artery Calcium Scan

A coronary artery calcium scan may be performed following determination of the scan range. Noncontrast images with prospective ECG triggering (typically between 65% and 80% of the R-R interval)[20] are obtained. Performing a coronary artery calcium scan can aid in further optimizing the scan range and may also be useful in planning CCTA. In patients with a high degree of calcium burden there is an increased chance of nonevaluable segments.[32,33] In response to dense calcium burden on noncontrast images, some laboratories will increase the amount of padding employed with

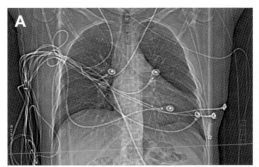

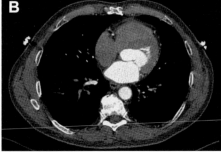

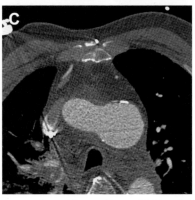

Fig. 7. Inappropriate ECG lead placement and resulting artifacts. ECG leads should be positioned beyond the field of view to avoid artifact from the ECG electrodes and cables. (A) Scout image with external ECG leads in place. These leads should be temporarily removed whenever possible. (B) Inappropriately positioned lead clips were placed within the field of view, resulting in greater artifact than just a lead wire. Due to the far lateral position, these artifacts do not cause significant image degradation of the heart, although the overall image noise is minimally increased. (C) Inappropriately placed lead clip close to the heart causes streak artifact that involves the heart, especially when in line with a pacing lead.

prospective triggering or widen the pulsing window with retrospective gating. Certain vendors provide "high definition/high resolution" scanning modes reported to improve spatial resolution in the setting of calcification and stents; however, evidence supporting this novel technology is awaited. Note that all of these techniques, while potentially offering additional phases or improved spatial resolution for image interpretation, are associated with an increased radiation dose. Certain centers avoid performing CCTA in patients with calcium scores above 600 to 1000[20] because of concerns regarding image interpretability. Other centers have abandoned performing calcium scores prior to CCTA given the additional radiation exposure, which ranges significantly (effective dose range 0.8–10.5 mSv) depending on protocol.[34,35]

Contrast Transit Time

Coronary CT angiography requires accurate timing of the arrival of the IV contrast agent to the coronary arteries, with coronary enhancement maintained throughout data acquisition. Even short timing errors (5–10 seconds) can result in significantly reduced enhancement of the coronary arteries. Two acceptable methods exist for determining the contrast transit time: automatic scan triggering ("bolus tracking" or "smart prep") and test bolus.

Automatic scan triggering (also referred to as bolus tracking or smart prep of the aorta) involves sampling a region of interest (ROI) within the ascending or descending aorta (usually every 2 seconds after the initiation of the contrast agent) and "triggering" the breathing instructions/scan once the contrast density in the ROI reaches a predetermined threshold (eg, 100 HU). Advantages of automatic scan triggering include the potential for a reduced contrast dose delivered (as contrast is not "wasted" for a test bolus). However, disadvantages exist with the risk of delivering the entire contrast dose without ever reaching optimal opacification.

An alternative method for assessing the contrast transit time employs a test bolus. A small amount of contrast (typically 10–20 mL) is injected followed by a saline bolus (approximately 50 mL) at whatever flow rate is planned for CCTA. An ROI in the ascending aorta is sampled (usually every 1–2 seconds) to identify the timing of maximum contrast density. Two to three seconds should be added to allow for maximal filling of the coronary arteries. This delay time is then used for the ensuing CCTA. Advantages of a test bolus include the ability to assess a patient's heart rate response to contrast administration, assess IV access issues, and identify patients likely to have contrast dilution problems without employing a large amount of contrast. In addition, suboptimal opacification with a low flow rate seen on test bolus can be addressed by increasing the flow rate. Radiation dose can be minimized by performing a test bolus with reduced tube voltage and current. Disadvantages of a test bolus include the fact that an additional 10 to 20 mL of contrast is used in performing a test bolus.

Data Acquisition

Scan protocol

Scan protocol will depend on scanner type and ability. In determining scan acquisition mode, the question to be addressed, pretest probability of CAD, and patient-specific factors (radiation exposure risk and heart rate variability) should be reviewed.

Two modes of ECG-gated acquisition may be employed: retrospective gating and prospective triggering. Retrospective ECG gating is achieved with helical acquisition and the x-ray tube turned on throughout the cardiac cycle. Data from the most motion-free phase is then reconstructed. Advantages of retrospective ECG gating include the ability to reconstruct alternate phases in case of cardiac motion artifact. In addition, functional analysis can generally be performed. A significant radiation dose, due to the spiral mode of acquisition, has been the main limitation.

By contrast, prospective ECG triggering involves axial acquisition whereby the x-ray tube is only on for a predetermined period of the cardiac cycle. Prospective scanning is associated with a significant savings in radiation dose (77%–87% reduction)[36–42]; however, options for additional image reconstruction in case of motion artifact are limited. Functional analysis is not possible, as only a portion of the cardiac cycle is imaged. Despite the inability to reconstruct multiple distinct phases (end-systole and end-diastole), prospective triggering provides reduced radiation dose with minimal reduction in diagnostic performance.[43] Imaging the entire heart in one cardiac cycle is now possible with 320 slice scanners. Novel scanning modes, including the "Flash Spiral" (high-pitch helical acquisition with dual-source imaging that covers the entire volume of the heart in one cardiac cycle and is prospectively triggered), are constantly evolving in a race to improve temporal and spatial resolution while reducing radiation dose.[44]

Contrast flow rate

Contrast to noise ratio (CNR) is an important component of image quality. Injection rates of 4 to 7 mL/s for CCTA are generally required to achieve adequate CNR. Patients with an increased BMI (and an anticipation of greater noise) may benefit from faster flow rates (7 mL/s). Higher injection rates at lower pressures can be achieved through the warming of contrast (which aids in reducing viscosity). Contrast volumes range between 50 and 120 mL, and are dependent on flow rate and duration. The injection duration should approximate the anticipated scan duration (ie, as long as if not slightly longer than).

Contrast injection protocols

Several contrast injection protocols exist. Biphasic or triphasic protocols are recommended. Biphasic injections require a dual-head contrast pump and deliver contrast followed by saline. A biphasic injection aids in contrast differentiation between the venous and arterial anatomy. However, the opacification of the structures of the right heart may suffer. A triphasic protocol commences with contrast injection followed by a mixture of contrast and saline. In settings where right heart analysis is required, a triphasic injection protocol may be preferable.

Tube current modulation

A tool for retrospective ECG-gated studies, tube current modulation reduces the number of photos emitted from the x-ray tube during nonoptimal phases of the cardiac cycle. Tube current modulation results in approximately 25% reduction in radiation dose and is a commonly employed dose reduction tool.[9] Image reconstruction is performed in motion-free phases of the cardiac cycle (typically end-diastole and end-systole). Motion artifacts often plague additional phases of the cardiac cycle. Tube current modulation attempts to minimize radiation dose delivered during these motion-plagued phases. The operator preselects the window beyond which tube current will be reduced (ie, pulse 35%–75% of the R-R cycle where tube current will be reduced between 76% and 34% of the cardiac cycle; **Fig. 8**). More optimal heart rates with minimal variability and no arrhythmia may be amenable to more aggressive tube current modulation (ie, 60%–70%). The image quality beyond the pulsing window will likely not be of sufficient image quality for coronary evaluation; however, ventricular function can generally still be assessed. Tube current modulation is most effective as a radiation dose–saving tool among patients with optimal heart rate control for whom

relatively short periods of full tube current/high radiation can be employed.

Padding

In prospectively triggered CCTA, the operator selects the desired phase for data acquisition (typically 70% or 75% of the cardiac cycle). The x-ray tube can be programmed for an additional 0 to 200 milliseconds of time surrounding the selected phase, a feature referred to as "padding." Padding can provide additional data from which to reconstruct images, in case of cardiac motion. The use of padding is associated with an increase in radiation dose (from an effective dose of 2.15 mSv with 0 ms of padding to 7.89 mSv with 200 ms).[45] If additional cardiac phases are desirable, retrospective gating must be employed. In contrast to tube current modulation employed in retrospective gating, in prospective scanning the tube current remains off beyond periods of padding. Whether the use of padding is associated with an improvement in diagnostic accuracy remains to be determined.

Tube voltage

Patient characteristics such as BMI, amount of tissue (breast, muscle, fat) surrounding the chest wall, and age should be considered in determining tube voltage. Tube voltage should be minimized to the lowest possible setting that preserves acceptable image quality while avoiding unnecessary radiation. Radiation dose delivered is approximately proportional to the square of the change tube voltage.[46] Therefore, a small reduction in tube voltage can result in significant radiation savings (reducing tube voltage from 120 to 100 kV is associated with approximately 50% reduction in radiation dose delivered).[9,47] In nonobese patients (BMI <30 kg/m^2 or body weight <85–90 kg) the use of 100 kV should be strongly considered. Preliminary work[48] suggests that in individuals of normal weight, greater reductions in tube voltage (80 kV) may be feasible. Some centers employ an "obesity protocol" and administer 140 kV tube voltage in patients with BMI >30 kg/m^2. While noise reduction results, a significant increase in radiation dose occurs and 140 kV tube voltage should be avoided if possible.

Tube current

In contrast to tube voltage, tube current has a relatively linear relationship with effective radiation dose. Regardless, significant radiation savings can still result by minimizing tube current to the minimum possible allowing for acceptable image quality. The use of higher tube current is associated with noise reduction. In patients with obesity and abundant chest wall tissue, a higher

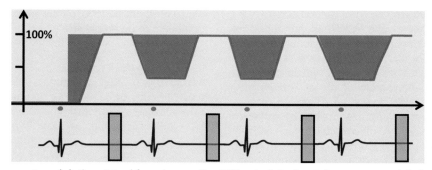

Fig. 8. Tube current modulation. A tool for retrospective ECG-gated studies, tube current modulation reduces the number of photos emitted from the x-ray tube during nonoptimal phases of the cardiac cycle. Tube current modulation results in a heart rate dependent on up to 50% reduction in radiation dose (sum of shaded areas) and is a commonly employed dose reduction tool. Tube current modulation attempts to minimize radiation dose delivered during these motion-plagued phases. The operator preselects the window beyond which tube current will be reduced. Here the tube current is modulating with pulsing at 35% to 75% of the R-R cycle (where tube current will be reduced between 76% and 34% of the next cardiac cycle).

milliamperage may be required to facilitate diagnostic image quality. Tube current may be manually selected or protocolized based on BMI and chest circumference, and generally ranges between 300 and 800 mA.[45]

SUMMARY

CCTA provides a noninvasive assessment of the coronary arteries with excellent negative predictive value in ruling out CAD. Software and scanner technology are rapidly advancing. To ensure optimal image quality, however, careful attention must be devoted to patient preparation and scanning technique. Whenever possible, radiation dose should be minimized. With thoughtful screening, preparation, and prescan planning, a high level of diagnostic image quality can be achieved without excessive radiation dose.

REFERENCES

1. Hendel RC, Patel MR, Kramer CM, et al. ACCF/ACR/SCCT/SCMR/ASNC/NASCI/SCAI/SIR 2006 appropriateness criteria for cardiac computed tomography and cardiac magnetic resonance imaging: a report of the American College of Cardiology Foundation Quality Strategic Directions Committee Appropriateness Criteria Working Group, American College of Radiology, Society of Cardiovascular Computed Tomography, Society for Cardiovascular Magnetic Resonance, American Society of Nuclear Cardiology, North American Society for Cardiac Imaging, Society for Cardiovascular Angiography and Interventions, and Society of Interventional Radiology. J Am Coll Cardiol 2006;48(7):1475–97.
2. Achenbach S, Marwan M, Ropers D, et al. Coronary computed tomography angiography with a consistent dose below 1 mSv using prospectively electrocardiogram-triggered high-pitch spiral acquisition. Eur Heart J 2009. DOI:10.1093/eurheartj/ehp470. [Epub ahead of print].
3. Raff GL, Chinnaiyan KM, Share DA, et al. Radiation dose from cardiac computed tomography before and after implementation of radiation dose–reduction techniques. JAMA 2009;301(22):2340–8.
4. Leschka S, Stinn B, Schmid F, et al. Dual source CT coronary angiography in severely obese patients: trading off temporal resolution and image noise. Invest Radiol 2009;44(11):720–7.
5. Yoshimura N, Sabir A, Kubo T, et al. Correlation between image noise and body weight in coronary CTA with 16-row MDCT. Acad Radiol 2006;13:324–8.
6. Alkadhi H, Scheffel H, Desbiolles L, et al. Dual-source computed tomography coronary angiography: influence of obesity, calcium load, and heart rate on diagnostic accuracy. Eur Heart J 2008;29(6):766–76.
7. Brink M, de Lange F, Oostveen LJ, et al. Arm raising at exposure-controlled multidetector trauma CT of thoracoabdominal region: higher image quality, lower radiation dose. Radiology 2008;249:661–70.
8. Einstein AJ, Henzlova MJ, Rajagopalan S. Estimating risk of cancer associated with radiation exposure from 64-slice computed tomography coronary angiography. JAMA 2007;298:317–23.
9. Hausleiter J, Meyer T, Hermann F, et al. Estimated radiation dose associated with cardiac CT angiography. JAMA 2009;301(5):500–7.
10. Kruger S, Mahnken AH, Sinha AM, et al. Multislice spiral computed tomography for the detection of coronary stent restenosis and patency. Int J Cardiol 2003;89:167–72.
11. Van Mieghem CA, Cademartiri F, Mollet NR, et al. Multislice spiral computed tomography for the evaluation of stent patency after left main coronary artery

stenting: a comparison with conventional coronary angiography and intravascular ultrasound. Circulation 2006;114:645–53.

12. Carbone I, Francone M, Algeri E, et al. Non-invasive evaluation of coronary artery stent patency with retrospectively ECG-gated 64-slice CT angiography. Eur Radiol 2008;18:234–43.

13. Available at: http://www.scct.org/advocacy/index.cfm. Accessed December 9, 2009.

14. Mark DB, Berman DS, Budoff MJ, et al. ACCF/ACR/AHA/NASCI/SAIP/SCAI/SCCT 2010 Expert consensus document on coronary computed tomographic angiography. J Am Coll Cardiol 2010;55(23):2663–99.

15. Ropers D, Pohle FK, Kuettner A, et al. Diagnostic accuracy of noninvasive coronary angiography in patients after bypass surgery using 64-slice spiral computed tomography with 330-ms gantry rotation. Circulation 2006;114:2334–41.

16. Wolak A, Gutstein A, Cheng VY, et al. Dual-source coronary computed tomography angiography in patients with atrial fibrillation: initial experience. J Cardiovasc Comput Tomogr 2008;2(3):172–80.

17. Marshall GD Jr, Lieberman PL. Comparison of three pretreatment protocols to prevent anaphylactoid reactions to radiocontrast media. Ann Allergy 1991;67(1):70–4.

18. Cheitlin MD, Hutter AM Jr, Brindis RG, et al. ACC/AHA expert consensus document. Use of sildenafil (Viagra) in patients with cardiovascular disease. American College of Cardiology/American Heart Association. J Am Coll Cardiol 1999;33(1):273–82.

19. Kloner RA, Hutter AM, Emmick JT, et al. Time course of the interaction between tadalafil and nitrates. J Am Coll Cardiol 2003;42(10):1855–60.

20. Abbara S, Arbab-Zadeh A, Callister TQ, et al. SCCT guidelines for performance of coronary computed tomographic angiography: a report of the Society of Cardiovascular Computed Tomography Guidelines Committee. J Cardiovasc Comput Tomogr 2009;3(3):190–204.

21. Dewey M, Hoffmann H, Hamm B. Multislice CT coronary angiography: effect of sublingual nitroglycerine on the diameter of coronary arteries. Rofo 2006;178:600–4.

22. Leschka S, Wildermuth S, Boehm T, et al. Noninvasive coronary angiography with 64-section CT: effect of average heart rate and heart rate variability on image quality. Radiology 2006;241:378–85.

23. Pannu HK, Alvarez W Jr, Fishman EK. β-Blockers for cardiac CT: a primer for the radiologist. Am J Roentgenol 2006;186:S341–5.

24. Johnson PT, Eng J, Pannu HK, et al. 64-MDCT Angiography of the coronary arteries: nationwide survey of patient preparation practice. Am J Roentgenol 2008;190:743–7.

25. Roberts WT, Wright AR, Timmis JB, et al. Safety and efficacy of a rate control protocol for cardiac CT. Br J Radiol 2009;82:267–71.

26. Earls JP, Schrack EC. Prospectively gated low-dose CCTA: 24 months experience in more than 2,000 clinical cases. Int J Cardiovasc Imaging 2009;25(2):177–87.

27. Matt D, Scheffel H, Leschka S, et al. Dual-source CT coronary angiography: image quality, mean heart rate, and heart rate variability. Am J Roentgenol 2007;189:567–73.

28. Ropers U, Ropers D, Pflederer T, et al. Influence of heart rate on the diagnostic accuracy of dual-source computed tomography coronary angiography. J Am Coll Cardiol 2007;50(25):2393–8.

29. Wang G, Vannier MW. Spatial variation of section sensitivity profile in spiral computed tomography. Med Phys 1994;21:1491–7.

30. Ohnesorge B, Flohr T, Becker C, et al. Cardiac imaging by means of electrocardiographically gated multisection spiral CT: initial experience. Radiology 2000;217:564–71.

31. Horiguchi J, Shen Y, Hirai N, et al. Timing on 16-slice scanner and implications for 64-slice cardiac CT: do you start scanning immediately after breath hold? Acad Radiol 2006;13:173–6.

32. Pundziute G, Schuijf JD, Jukema JW, et al. Impact of coronary calcium score on diagnostic accuracy of multislice computed tomography coronary angiography for detection of coronary artery disease. J Nucl Cardiol 2007;14:36–43.

33. Cordeiro MA, Miller JM, Schmidt A, et al. Non-invasive half millimetre 32 detector row computed tomography angiography accurately excludes significant stenoses in patients with advanced coronary artery disease and high calcium scores. Heart 2006;92:589–97.

34. Kim KP, Einstein AJ, de Gonzalez AB. Coronary artery calcification screening: estimated radiation dose and cancer risk. Arch Intern Med 2009;169(13):1188–94.

35. Gibbons RJ, Gerber TC. Calcium scoring with computed tomography—what is the radiation risk? Arch Intern Med 2009;169(13):1185–7.

36. Husmann L, Valenta I, Gaemperli O, et al. Feasibility of low-dose coronary CT angiography: first experience with prospective ECG-gating. Eur Heart J 2008;29:191–7.

37. Shuman WP, Branch KR, May JM, et al. Prospective versus retrospective ECG gating for 64-detector CT of the coronary arteries: comparison of image quality and patient radiation dose. Radiology 2008;248:431–7.

38. Hirai N, Horiguchi J, Fujioka C, et al. Prospective versus retrospective ECG-gated 64-detector coronary CT angiography: assessment of image quality, stenosis, and radiation dose. Radiology 2008;248:424–30.

39. Gutstein A, Wolak A, Lee C, et al. Predicting success of prospective and retrospective gating

with dual-source coronary computed tomography angiography: development of selection criteria and initial experience. J Cardiovasc Comput Tomogr 2008;2:81–90.

40. Steigner ML, Otero HJ, Cai T, et al. Narrowing the phase window width in prospectively ECG-gated single heart beat 320-detector row coronary CT angiography. Int J Cardiovasc Imaging 2009;25(1): 85–90.

41. Rybicki FJ, Otero HJ, Steigner ML, et al. Initial evaluation of coronary images from 320-detector row computed tomography. Int J Cardiovasc Imaging 2008;24:535–46.

42. Scheffel H, Alkadhi H, Leschka S, et al. Low-dose CT coronary angiography in the step-and shoot mode: diagnostic performance. Heart 2008;94:1132–7.

43. Pontone G, Andreini D, Bartorelli AL, et al. Diagnostic accuracy of coronary computed tomography angiography: a comparison between prospective and retrospective electrocardiogram triggering. J Am Coll Cardiol 2009;54(4):346–55.

44. Achenbach A, Marwan M, Schepis T, et al. High-pitch spiral acquisition: a new scan mode for coronary CT angiography. J Cardiovasc Comput Tomogr 2009;3(2):117–21.

45. Earls JP, Berman EL, Urban BA, et al. Prospectively gated transverse coronary CT angiography versus retrospectively gated helical technique: improved image quality and reduced radiation dose. Radiology 2008;246:742–53.

46. Rehani MM, Bongartz G, Kalender W, et al. Managing patient dose in computed tomography. Ann ICRP 2000;30(4):7–45.

47. Bischoff B, Hein F, Meyer T, et al. Impact of a reduced tube voltage on CT angiography and radiation dose: results of the PROTECTION I study. JACC Cardiovasc Imaging 2009;2:940–6.

48. Abada HT, Larchez C, Daoud B, et al. MDCT of the coronary arteries: feasibility of low-dose CT with ECG pulsed tube current modulation to reduce radiation dose. Am J Roentgenol 2006; 186(Suppl 2):387–90.

Postprocessing Techniques for Cardiac Computed Tomographic Angiography

Pamela T. Johnson, MD[a], Elliot K. Fishman, MD[b]

KEYWORDS

- CT angiography • Postprocessing techniques
- Two-dimensional multiplanar reformations
- Three-dimensional reconstruction • Volume rendering
- Maximum intensity projection

Implementation of 64-slice multidetector computed tomography (MDCT), with unprecedented temporal resolution, made coronary artery computed tomographic angiography (CTA) a realistic and reliable diagnostic tool. Recent investigations using a range of protocols describe per patient sensitivities of 83% to 100%, specificities of 84% to 100%, negative predictive values (NPV) of 81% to 100%, and positive predictive values of 64% to 100%.[1–5] In a recent meta-analysis,[6] the high per segment and per patient NPV of 96.5% with 64-MDCT technology was noted, which has defined a role for coronary CTA in assessing patients with low clinical suspicion. The emergence of newer generation scanners with even larger numbers of detector arrays and dual tubes promises to expand the utility of CT to a broader group of patients.

Despite the volume of literature on coronary CTA, even with 64-slice MDCT, there is a paucity of published information on postprocessing and analysis of CT datasets. This article presents experience-based guidance on postprocessing techniques, from axial review to two-dimensional (2D) renderings to three-dimensional (3D) reconstructions, for interpretation of coronary CTA data. An understanding of each technique is essential to optimally use these tools in practice; pearls and pitfalls derived from our experience are also presented.

BACKGROUND

Careful protocol design is essential to successfully perform coronary CTA, from patient preparation, to gating, to contrast infusion, to data acquisition, to data reconstruction parameters. Unlike other forms of CTA, cardiac computed tomography (CT) presents the challenge of imaging a moving target; although this is becoming less of an issue because of the speed with which newer scanners acquire data. However, the tenet holds true that the quality of the display is directly related to the quality of the dataset, regardless of the postprocessing tools used. This necessitates an understanding of how to maximize spatial, temporal, and contrast resolution for the highest-quality images. Similarly, once the data are acquired, interpretation requires hands-on training to master each technique. Workflow is maximized by implementation of reliable and streamline filming, archiving, and networking.

[a] The Russell H. Morgan Department of Radiology and Radiological Science, Johns Hopkins Hospital, 601 North Caroline Street, Room 3140D, Baltimore, MD 21287, USA
[b] The Russell H. Morgan Department of Radiology and Radiological Science, Johns Hopkins Hospital, 601 North Caroline Street, Room 3251, Baltimore, MD 21287, USA
E-mail address: pjohnso5@jhmi.edu

Radiol Clin N Am 48 (2010) 687–700
doi:10.1016/j.rcl.2010.04.004
0033-8389/10/$ – see front matter © 2010 Elsevier Inc. All rights reserved.

A workstation equipped with tools for cardiac evaluation and investing the time to learn how to use these for coronary artery analysis are mandatory. This includes the standard 2D and 3D rendering programs and software specific to vascular imaging such as automated vessel segmentation, stenosis calculation software, vessel tracking software, and four-dimensional motion analysis.

Automated Vessel Segmentation

Several automated segmentation algorithms exist. Use of segmentation is generally obligatory with maximum intensity projection (MIP) rendering to isolate the vasculature from the dense contrast in the cardiac chambers, which would otherwise obscure visualization of the arteries. Our 3D rendering platform uses a region-growing algorithm to perform automated tagging of the aorta and coronary arteries, with the capacity for manual refinement (**Fig. 1**).[7] Following automated segmentation of arteries, additional analysis can be performed with any rendering algorithm and vessel tracking.

Automatic arterial segmentation using a corkscrew algorithm was described by Khan and colleagues,[8] who used 16-MDCT to evaluate 50 subjects. Color-coded volume renderings (VRs) are generated with diameter reflected by color variation from red to blue; the technique also plots vessel diameter along an x-y axis. Compared with manually generated MIP, multiplanar reconstructions (MPR), VR, and curved planar reconstructions (CPR), diagnostic accuracy and vessel detection rates were similar, but the automatic technique required significantly less time.[8]

Stenosis Calculation Software

The means by which an arterial stenosis can be quantified include visual, manual, and automated techniques. Automated calculation of the percent stenosis is performed on the CPRs (**Fig. 2**). Cardiac-specific software packages and many vessel analysis packages typically require the user to select the area of maximum narrowing and normal vessel proximal and distal to the stenosis. Once these are selected, percent stenosis is calculated automatically. These programs are not without error.

Initial studies comparing visual and automated techniques in the literature suggested that automated quantification could improve diagnostic accuracy.[7,9]

However, more recent data suggest the contrary. Using 4 vascular phantoms with stenoses between 33% and 72%, Dikkers and colleagues[10] compared the accuracy of manual measurements with those performed by 5 cardiac software packages using a 64-slice scanner. Manual measurements correlated more accurately with true diameter than any automated program, such that the authors concluded "Manual stenosis measurements are significantly more accurate compared with automatic measurements, and therefore, manual adjustments are still essential for noninvasive assessment of coronary artery stenosis."[10]

Vessel Tracking Software

Most software programs currently used for vessel tracking require minimal user interaction. For example, with the Siemens Leonardo (Siemens Medical Solutions, Malvern, PA) workstation program called Circulation, the computer tracks the vessel by calculating a centerline after the user selects start and end points on either 2D or 3D reconstructions (**Fig. 3**). Similar programs run on the GE Advantage workstation (GE Healthcare, Milwaukee, WI) and other vendors. These generate curved planar images with the artery elongated for display in a single plane that can be rotated to view from any perspective. Viewing options include classic CT windows or as an MIP. One pearl is that in cases with a gap or high-grade stenosis in the vessel, dropping additional seed points can be useful to accurately track the artery.

POSTPROCESSING TECHNIQUES FOR DISPLAY

Knowledge of the algorithm behind each postprocessing tool, their strengths and weaknesses is mandatory. Regardless of technique, to perform the best dataset analysis, it is essential that the radiologist interactively evaluates the volume. This belief is based on our experience and the literature. Interactive review of the dataset ensures that the length and branches of each coronary artery are adequately visualized from all necessary orientations and enables the radiologist to use each available technique to greatest advantage. Review of preset 2D MPRs, 3D MIPs or VRs is prone to errors in interpretation. This relates to the skill of the radiologist or technologist who performs the postprocessing, and the potential for misinterpretation of static images that may not accurately demonstrate the anatomy or depict narrowed segments.

The most comprehensive article on postprocessing, which included all types of postprocessing tools,[11] supported interactive evaluation of the dataset; the results revealed that interactive

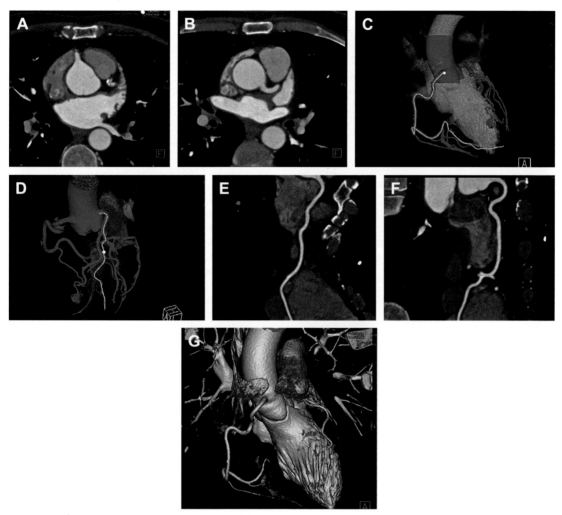

Fig. 1. A 57-year-old man with increased Agatston score but no critical coronary artery stenosis on CTA. Axial images (A, B) show calcification in the LAD and left circumflex arteries. However, segmentation of the volume (C, D) to yield CPRs (E, F) and an unsegmented color-coded VR (G) reveal that the calcification is eccentric and does not seem to cause any luminal narrowing.

interrogation of the volume had higher diagnostic accuracy. A range of interactive (1.0 × 0.5 mm transverse, oblique 1.0 mm MPR, oblique 5.0 mm MIP) and prerendered displays created by a physician (1.0 mm CPR, 3.0 mm curved MIP, segmented VRs displayed with a preset window/level that could be adjusted) were compared. Using 16 × 0.75 mm detector configuration, 40 datasets were reviewed by 6 radiologists. The greatest accuracy (91%) resulted from interactive oblique MPR, enabling the highest percentage of evaluable segments among the 2D and 3D techniques.[11] The authors concluded that "Interactive evaluation of multidetector CT coronary angiography data sets on a workstation should thus be the preferred way of interpretation."[11]

The importance of interactive rendering has been shown in 2 additional investigations.[12,13] Cademartiri and colleagues used 16 × 0.75 mm technology to compare 5 standardized views to interactive volume interrogation. Their first study[12] included 47 patients and used the following standardized views generated by an experienced radiographer: axial 1.0 × 0.5 sections, paraaxial and paracoronal 3.0 × 0.5 mm MIPs, plus parasagittal and paracoronal 1.0 × 0.5 mm MPRs. In their second study,[13] a different set of 5 standardized views was created from 44 datasets: axial 1.0 × 0.5 mm sections, plus axial, paraxial, parasagittal, and paracoronal 3.0 × 1.5 mm MIPs. These were compared with interactive interpretation at the workstation by a physician using axial, MPR,

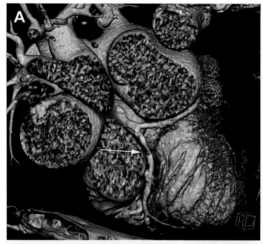

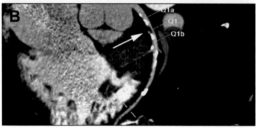

Fig. 2. A 76-year-old man with a 5-cm ascending thoracic aortic aneurysm and extensive calcified and noncalcified plaque in the LAD, shown on color-coded VR (A). A focal severe stenosis caused by lipid-laden plaque in the proximal LAD (arrows), visually estimated at 70%, is seen with VR (A) and CPR (B). Using automated stenosis calculation software on the CPR (B), the degree of diameter reduction was estimated at 80%.

CPR, MIP, and VR.[12,13] Although the standard display required significantly less time for interpretation, interactive interpretation was significantly more sensitive for lesions with 50% stenosis or more on a per-segment basis (standard with MIP and MPRs 58% vs interactive 96%[13]; standard with mostly MIPs 54% vs interactive 93%). Interobserver agreement was higher with the interactive protocol (kappa = 0.79) compared with the standard (kappa = 0.55).[13]

Cardiac MDCT interpretation can be performed interactively with various display techniques (**Fig. 4**): review of axial sections, MPRs including short- and long-axis views, CPRs, MIP, and VR. Each of these techniques is described, highlighting advantages and weaknesses. Interactive interrogation of the volume enables the interpreting radiologist to tailor postprocessing to the individual case, taking into consideration the degree of contrast enhancement, presence of artifacts, and vascular calcification to dictate the optimal techniques.

Axial Review

Although routine interpretation of coronary CTA includes MPRs and 3D renderings, review of the axial images is crucial. During axial review, the initial step is to determine the quality of the study in terms of contrast enhancement and motion artifacts, and to confirm that the optimal phase has been selected to display each of the coronary arteries with the least motion artifact. An overview of the heart should be performed, evaluating cardiac chambers, valves, pericardium, aorta, pulmonary arteries, and vena cavae. Subsequently, the anatomy of the coronary arteries is defined, identifying the origin of each vessel and its branching pattern. The axial view is often optimal for visualizing the sinoatrial nodal and atrioventricular nodal branches. Following anatomic mapping, evaluation for calcified or noncalcified plaque is performed (**Fig. 5**). The presence and extent of calcified and noncalcified plaque are important for determining the best postprocessing tools.

Pearls

1. Axial images are usually viewed as slabs in the acquisition plane; however, one helpful hint is that the best axial display of the coronary arteries can be produced by drawing a line through the plane of the aortic valve and scrolling up and down through this plane.
2. In the presence of extensive calcification, view the axial sections with a wide window.

Pitfalls

1. Full evaluation of a single artery may require review of 200 to 350 individual slices. Because of their off-axis courses, coronary arteries are best defined in orientations beyond the axial plane (**Fig. 6**). Comparison of axial review with a combination of axial, interactive MPR, MIP, and preset CPR showed that the latter combination of techniques was 98% sensitive and 94% accurate, compared with 86% sensitive and 78% accurate for axial images alone.[14]
2. Referring physicians, particularly cardiologists, prefer display similar to catheter angiography, which cannot be produced by postprocessing the axial sections.

MPRs

Although coronal and sagittal reconstructions are widely used to evaluate the arteries in other CTA applications, MPRs are best suited for evaluation of the individual cardiac chambers, aorta, and pulmonary vasculature with cardiac CT. The

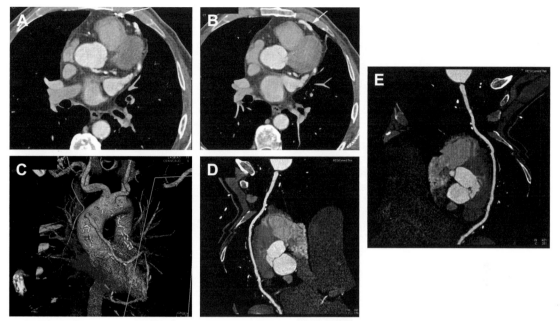

Fig. 3. A 64-year-old man status after median sternotomy and coronary artery bypass surgery with a left internal mammary artery (LIMA) graft and several venous grafts. Axial images (*A, B*) show clips in the left anterior chest from the LIMA procedure and a short segment of the saphenous vein graft (*arrows*). From a coronal color-coded VR (*C*), vessel tracking software was used to generate CPRs (*D, E*) of the graft. The saphenous graft, approximately 8 mm in diameter, arises from the anterior aspect of the aorta at the level of the arch and tracks anterior to the pulmonary artery, to communicate with the posterior coronary artery. The venous graft not only supplies what seems to be the inferior aspect of the heart via the posterior coronary artery, but also reconstitutes the occluded LAD distally, as well as the left circumflex. This widely patent saphenous vein graft is the key to this patient's patency of the coronary system.

nonlinear pathway of the coronary arteries results in only short segments being analyzed at a time with MPRs. When the left anterior descending (LAD) coronary artery is analyzed with a coronal or axial display, the angle of the reconstruction plane must be changed constantly to follow the vessel. Although this can be done interactively, it introduces potential for error and is less useful to display the length of an artery. On the other hand, MPRs are well suited for selective evaluation of a short segment (**Figs. 6** and **7**). If a narrowing is suspected on axial views, display in coronal or sagittal orientations can confirm the presence of a stenosis.

Pearls

1. Interactivity is essential because of the limitations of MPRs.
2. Oblique planes often prove valuable for interpretative difficulties on axial sections.

Pitfalls

1. Most workstations enable interactive adjustment of the thickness of the reconstruction.

However, when slabs are reduced to less than a few millimeters, images become fuzzy.

2. MPRs are best for larger vessels. Because of the small vessel caliber (typically 3–5 mm) and ectatic course of the coronary vessels, preprocessed batched coronal and sagittal images at 1- to 3-mm intervals are not as useful as with other thoracic and abdominal applications.

3. Grading of a stenosis is not advisable with coronal, sagittal, or oblique reconstructions alone, because of partial averaging.

CPRs

CPR addresses the inability to track complicated pathways of the coronary arteries using standard coronal and sagittal reconstructions. The technique of generating a CPR is described in the section on vessel tracking. Unlike axial sections and standard MPRs, the course of a vessel can be tracked using CPR regardless of the complexity or plane (see **Fig. 3**). In addition, CPR is used to identify and quantify the degree of stenosis without being hindered by partial averaging. In practice, we consider CPR an obligatory component of the coronary CTA dataset analysis.

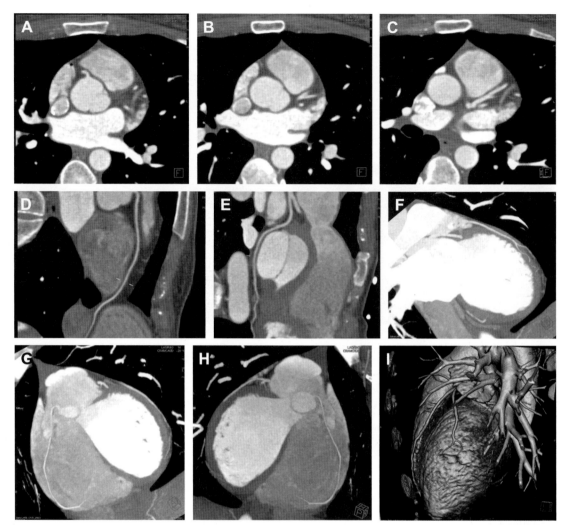

Fig. 4. Normal coronary vasculature in a 29-year-old woman to demonstrate the range of postprocessing tools available. Axial images (*A–C*), CPRs (*D, E*), MIP (*F*), coronal oblique VRs (*G, H*), and sagittal color-coded VR (*I*) depict normal coronary arteries with no calcification or stenosis.

Pearls

1. Optimal arterial enhancement (adequate contrast-to-noise and homogeneous enhancement) is essential for high-quality CPR. Poor opacification leads to errors of omission and commission. Values of 250 HU and above are ideal, and current protocols generally yield mean enhancement levels in the range of 300 to 350 HU for right and left coronary arteries.[15,16]

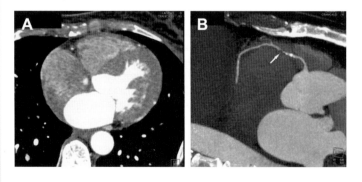

Fig. 5. A 48-year-old woman with 70% narrowing of the right coronary artery (RCA) caused by noncalcified plaque. Axial image (*A*) shows the noncalcified plaque (*arrow*). Using an MIP rendering (*B*), the region of narrowing is clearly shown; however, because the algorithm only selects the highest attenuation voxels, the noncalcified plaque within the artery is not demonstrated on the 2D image.

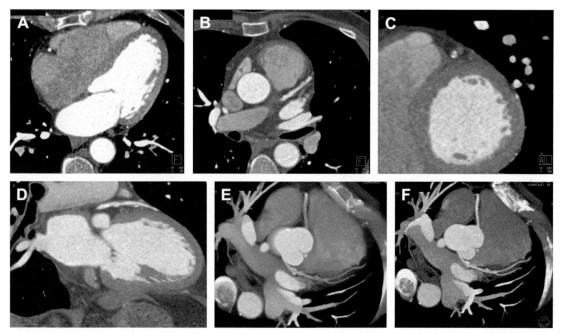

Fig. 6. A 52-year-old man with calcification in LAD and RCA, and an increased Agatston score for age (49.8). Data-set analysis was performed with a combination of axial images (*A, B*), MPRs (*C, D*), VR (*E*), and MIP (*F*). The LAD has multiple eccentric plaques present, including discrete plaques at its bifurcation, and near first septal and diagonal branches. In the mid LAD, noncalcified plaque results in less than 50% diameter reduction. The constellation of findings suggests that this patient will need to be further managed aggressively.

2. Nonetheless, CPR is especially valuable in defining the degree of stenosis in the presence of dense calcification. Interactivity is key because rotation of the vessel around 360° will reveal whether the calcification is mainly eccentric (causing positive remodeling) or creates a critical stenosis.

Pitfalls

1. Accurate assessment for stenosis requires correct centerline placement. Because of the small caliber of the coronary arteries (2–5 mm), off-axis centerline placement may result in misinterpretation of stenosis. This most commonly occurs in the presence of heavy arterial calcification.
2. Using automated vessel tracking, the resulting vascular map must be evaluated for accuracy. A few reports describe the use of automated techniques requiring significantly less time to create 2D CPR compared with manual methods. These techniques involve some user interaction to yield CPR and MPR or cross-sectional views. In 1 study, the proportion of main coronary arteries identified automatically ranged from 50% to 79% and nearly 80% of automated CPRs required user override to replace missing sections.[17] For identification

of stenoses of 50% or more with 16-MDCT, diagnostic accuracy of manual and automated techniques was not significantly different, nor were visualized vessel lengths[17] or percentage of uninterpretable arteries.[18]

3. The presence of an arrhythmia and breathing artifact may result in step-offs in the display of the volume.
4. Potential pitfalls also include inaccurate centerline definition of the centerline.

MIP

We believe that postprocessing with 3D MIP and VR is an essential part of every coronary CTA interpretation, potentially disclosing information not revealed by other interpretative methods. Each technique has its strengths and weaknesses. MIP is probably the easiest technique to master because of its simplicity. Designed to selectively demonstrate the arterial vasculature, the MIP algorithm involves selection of the highest attenuation voxels along rays projected through the volume, displayed as a 2D image. Accordingly, MIP enables creation of a vascular map quickly without modification of several parameters (**Fig. 8**). In addition, MIP is better for displaying small-caliber segments. Zhang and colleagues[19] evaluated vessel visualization

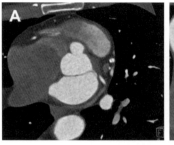
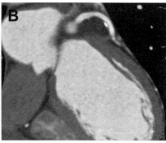

Fig. 7. A 47-year-old woman with increased Agatston score for age (44.7). Axial image (*A*) and MPR (*B*) show dense calcification in the LAD, immediately distal to the origin. Eccentric in nature, the MPR (*B*) shows that this plaque results in positive remodeling as opposed to luminal narrowing.

of 230 cases acquired with 16 × 0.75 mm detector configuration using MIP/MPR or volume-rendering technique (VRT). Results showed that the minimum vessel diameter seen with MIP was 0.7 mm versus 1.5 mm for VR. Higher percentages of smaller vessels were better visualized with MIP and MPR than with VR. However, major limitations of MIP include potential for anatomic inaccuracy because 3D relationships are not properly depicted and coronary artery calcification leads to overestimation of stenosis, even in the presence of small amounts of calcium (**Fig. 9**).

Despite its limitations, MIP renderings have been shown to be reliable compared with axial and MPRs in several MDCT studies. Choi and colleagues[20] compared the diagnostic performance of MIP renderings to axial sections using 12 × 0.75 mm detector configuration in 28 subjects.[20] Three sets of 4 × 2 mm thin-slab MIPs were created for each case: (1) horizontal long axis (4-chamber view), (2) vertical long axis (2-chamber view) and (3) short axis, and compared with 1.0 × .5 mm axial sections. Using receiver operating characteristic curve analysis, MIP images resulted in higher Az scores, but the difference was significant for only one-third of readers. Sensitivity, specificity, and accuracy were not significantly different, nor were the reading times.[20]

Thin-slab 5-mm MIPs have also been compared with 1.0-mm cross-sectional MPRs (perpendicular

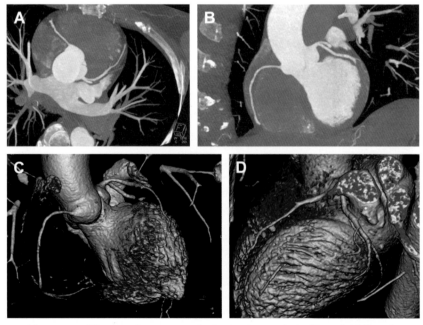

Fig. 8. A 63-year-old woman with normal coronary arteries, as demonstrated by axial (*A*) and coronal oblique (*B*) MIPs, and color-coded VRs in coronal oblique (*C*) and sagittal (*D*) orientations. This case demonstrates how MIP, which is a 2D display of the highest attenuation voxels along parallel rays projected through the volume, requires either preliminary segmentation of the volume or orientation of the volume in a plane to separate the arteries from contrast in the ventricle. VR does not require preliminary editing to generate a 3D display, and the arteries can be visualized in any orientation.

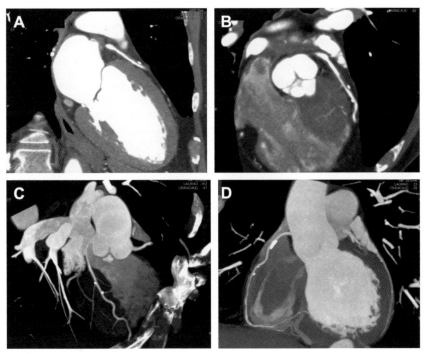

Fig. 9. A 70-year-old man with a history of cardiomyopathy. Calcified plaque is present in the LAD, left circumflex, and RCA. As shown on MPRs (*A*, *B*), the proximal one-third of the LAD contains calcified and noncalcified plaque, with a low-density noncalcified plaque several centimeters long resulting in nearly 50% diameter reduction. Both the length and attenuation of this plaque are a concern. An MIP rendering of the LAD (*C*) demonstrates only the calcified plaque. MIP renderings of the RCA (*C*, *D*) show the largest calcified plaque, in the proximal one-third of the RCA, as causing slightly greater than 50% luminal narrowing.

to the centerline) in 38 subjects imaged with 16 × 0.75 mm detector configuration.[21] Readers measured normal vessel and narrowed segments to define degree of stenosis (mean normal proximal and distal segments − maximum stenosis/mean normal segments). Results showed no significant differences in the mean measurements of vessel or stenosis, and both techniques correlated well with angiographic measurements. After categorizing stenoses as less than 40%, 41% to 70% and greater than 71%, good agreement with angiography was seen for both techniques. However, both underestimated severe stenoses greater than 71%, and MIP overestimated a few mild and moderate lesions. Further analysis showed that for both techniques, diagnostic errors for stenoses less than 50% were caused by overestimation, whereas underestimation occurred with lesions greater than 50%.[21]

More recently using 64-MDCT, Jinzaki and colleagues[14] evaluated interpretative sensitivity and accuracy using an angiographic view, which involved interactive MIP interrogation of a segmented volume, from which the

intraventricular contrast and extracardiac structures were removed. Conventional arteriography served as the gold standard in 17 patients with 44 stenoses. The segmented MIP renderings were equally sensitive (98%) and accurate (91%) to a combination of techniques, including interactive MIP and MPR as well as preset CPRs (98% sensitive, 94% accurate).[14]

In practice, MIP is usually performed interactively with a sliding slab, enabling the radiologist to adjust the window, select the optimal orientation to display each artery, and modify the slab thickness.[22] Ferencik and colleagues[23] compared 3 different methods to modify the window display settings using thin-slab MIP renderings: (1) full-width half-maximum, (2) fixed level of 100 HU, (3) adaptive windowing dictated by lumen attenuation. Thirty patients were imaged with 12 × 0.75 mm detector configuration. All 3 methods enabled close correlation with angiographic measurement; however, the full-width half-maximum and adaptive techniques slightly underestimated caliber, whereas the fixed level of 100 HU slightly overestimated diameter. The discrepancy between CTA and angiographic measurements using a fixed level was minimally greater than the other 2 techniques, and tended to increase with higher levels of luminal enhancement.[23]

Interpretative accuracy is optimized by interactive review of the volume using MIP. Choi and colleagues[20] compared interpretation of 3 sets of orthogonally oriented thin-slab MIPs with axial sections in 28 patients with clinical signs of cardiac ischemia who were imaged with 16-slice CT. Interpretative sensitivity (47% vs 54%), specificity (92% for both), and accuracy (80% vs 82%) were similar for the axial sections and the set of MIP reconstructions, respectively. However, the low sensitivity of both techniques wards against use of either in isolation.[20]

MIP is useful as an adjunct to VR. However, because of its limitations it is not advisable to use MIP in isolation, without review of axial, MPR, CPR, and/or VRT images. Even when the study looks normal, confirm by evaluating the volume with other display techniques.

Pearls

1. Because MIP selects the highest density voxels along a ray projected through the volume, adequate contrast enhancement is imperative.
2. When the arteries appear normal on axial review, MIP is often our next step to quickly generate a vascular map for display to the referring physician.
3. When you use MIP be careful not to omit pathologic conditions or "create a pseudolesion" by inappropriate selection of slab thickness.[24] In particular, be certain that the proximal portion of each artery is displayed accurately.

Pitfalls

1. Dense contrast in the ventricles can obscure visualization of the arteries with MIP, necessitating segmentation.
2. MIP images are a 2D display, such that 3D relationships cannot be determined without review of multiple MIPs rotated in real-time. Static MIP images can be misleading, by incorrect placement of arteries (see **Fig. 6**).
3. The MIP algorithm is prone to artifacts. One well-known pitfall is the "string of beads" appearance, because a normal small vessel passing obliquely through a volume is only partially represented by voxels along its length.[25]
4. The presence of even a small amount of calcification can lead to overestimation of stenosis. Heavily calcified arteries cannot be evaluated with MIP (**Fig. 10**).
5. In the patient without calcification, MIP renderings demonstrate long segments of the coronary arteries that appear as a comprehensive vascular map. However, noncalcified plaque will be overlooked unless it creates significant luminal narrowing, because of its low attenuation value (see **Figs. 5** and **9**).

VR

The ability of VRT to accurately display large volumes of data, especially with complex datasets, makes it an important component of postprocessing in cardiac CT. VRT involves the most complicated algorithm,[22,25] most often performed with a percentage classification algorithm. Every voxel is examined to determine the percentage of each tissue type present within the voxel. The most common method used to determine the

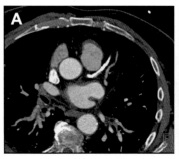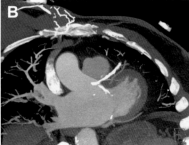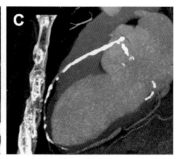

Fig. 10. An 81-year-old man with known coronary artery disease. The patient's Agatston score was markedly increased at 2690. Axial image (*A*) and axial (*B*) and sagittal (*C*) MIP renderings show extensive calcification in the proximal two-thirds of the LAD. The presence of extensive calcification as in this case can result in overestimation of the degree of diameter reduction, particularly with MIP renderings (*B*, *C*), but there is almost no opacified lumen. A critical stenosis is likely present, probably in the 70% range, but it is difficult to define accurately in the face of this degree of calcification.

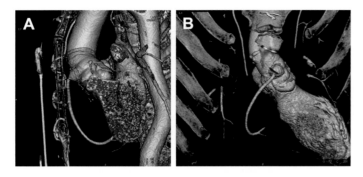

Fig. 11. A 41-year-old man with a history of Marfan syndrome, status after aortic root repair. Coronal (A) and sagittal (B) color-coded VRs show proximal dilatation of the reimplanted right coronary artery.

percentage contents is probabilistic classification involving a trapezoidal approximation, which closely models the volume averaging typical of CT voxels. A voxel composed of only 1 tissue type is assigned a value of 100%. Those made up of multiple tissue types are assigned a value between 0% and 100% of a tissue type, to reflect volume averaging. Following classification, each voxel is mapped to color and transparency. The classified and colored voxels are then displayed with 3D relationships intact, by casting simulated rays of light through the volume.[22,25] Beyond

analysis and display of the coronary arteries, VRT is used for functional assessments, including chamber motion, valve motion, or vessel motion. Volume-rendered images are ideal for explaining results to a patient and/or their family.

Pearls

1. With VRT the dataset can be viewed with spatial relationships intact without preliminary editing, quickly providing an initial overview (see **Fig. 8**). VRT can help accurately define complex anatomy of the heart and coronary

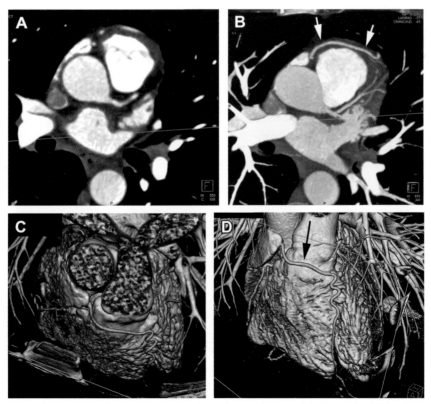

Fig. 12. A 41-year-old man participating in a research study. Axial image (A) shows the left main coronary artery giving rise to LAD. Axial MIP (B) and color-coded VRs (C, D) delineate a branch of the LAD arising from the right coronary artery (*arrows*), coursing anterior to the pulmonary artery, to perfuse a portion of the left ventricle.

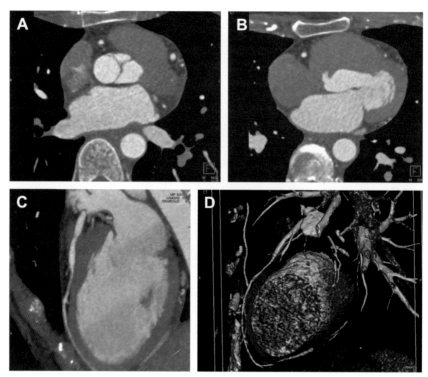

Fig. 13. A 42-year-old woman participating in a research study. Axial images (*A*, *B*), show a caliber change in the mid to distal LAD. Sagittal MPR (*C*) and color-coded VRs (*D*) confirm a long segment narrowing of the LAD.

arteries (**Fig. 11**). This is especially valuable in cases requiring delineation of relationships to the chest wall, such as operative revisions where a 3D map is necessary to guide the surgeon, pre- and postoperative complex congenital anomalies, and delineating coronary artery anomalies (**Fig. 12**). As per Zenooz and colleagues[26]: "Volume-rendered images acquired from 3D CT data sets provide an excellent overview of the cardiac and vascular anatomy and help surgeons understand the anatomic complexity before surgery."

2. VRT allows for either gray scale or color mapping; the latter is very useful in complex cases.

3. VRTs vary across vendors. Additional factors to consider in selecting a volume-rendering platform, include whether the system uses full 12-bit (−1024 to 3072 HU) input data for rendering or limits the volume size to some maximum and the quality of the video display.

Pitfalls

1. Some believe that VRT images should not be used to grade stenosis.[14] However, with a global volume-rendered overview, VRT will reveal stenoses that can be characterized using other postprocessing tools. Furthermore, the latest generation MDCT scanners and newer VR algorithms yield high-quality images that enable accurate quantification of the degree of vascular stenosis in the hands of an experienced user (**Fig. 13**). A 16-slice study of 19 patients with high Agatston scores showed that VR can be used for characterization of stenoses without compromising diagnostic accuracy. This study compared 3D VRs with arteries segmented from the volume to a combination of techniques including axial images, 2D MPRs, and CPRs and MIP renderings. Sensitivity (63% vs 74%), specificity (80% vs 76%), and accuracy (78% vs 75%) were not significantly different between the VRs and combination of techniques, respectively.[18]

2. Those with less experience may select the wrong VR parameters and this can generate a 3D display with substantial errors.

SUMMARY

As CT continues to evolve to the newest scanners with scan times for coronary CTA at less than 1 second, this only provides better datasets, not necessarily better diagnoses. It is only with tailored interpretation of the datasets that the true value of scanners, ranging from the Siemens Flash to Acquillion One to GE HCT, can be implemented. Postprocessing of data becomes even more important with these systems. Unless the user becomes skilled at analyzing CT data, the full potential of new technology will be minimized. It is to be hoped that this article provides some instruction and a few pearls to optimize your evaluation of cardiac CT data.

REFERENCES

1. Pontone G, Andreini D, Bartorelli AL, et al. Diagnostic accuracy of coronary computed tomography angiography: a comparison between prospective and retrospective electrocardiogram triggering. J Am Coll Cardiol 2009;54:346–55.

2. Pugliese F, Mollet NR, Hunink MG, et al. Diagnostic performance of coronary CT angiography by using different generations of multisection scanners: single-center experience. Radiology 2008;246: 384–93.

3. Gouya H, Varenne O, Trinquart L, et al. Coronary artery stenosis in high-risk patients: 64-section CT and coronary angiography–prospective study and analysis of discordance. Radiology 2009;252: 377–85.

4. Miller JM, Rochitte CE, Dewey M, et al. Diagnostic performance of coronary angiography by 64-row CT. N Engl J Med 2008;359:2324–36.

5. Budoff MJ, Dowe D, Jollis JG, et al. Diagnostic performance of 64-multidetector row coronary computed tomographic angiography for evaluation of coronary artery stenosis in individuals without known coronary artery disease: results from the prospective multicenter ACCURACY (Assessment by Coronary Computed Tomographic Angiography of Individuals Undergoing Invasive Coronary Angiography) trial. J Am Coll Cardiol 2008;52:1724–32.

6. Abdulla J, Abildstrom SZ, Gotzsche O, et al. 64-multislice detector computed tomography coronary angiography as potential alternative to conventional coronary angiography: a systematic review and meta-analysis. Eur Heart J 2007;28:3042–50.

7. Busch S, Johnson TR, Nikolaou K, et al. Visual and automatic grading of coronary artery stenoses with 64-slice CT angiography in reference to invasive angiography. Eur Radiol 2007;17:1445–51.

8. Khan MF, Wesarg S, Gurung J, et al. Facilitating coronary artery evaluation in MDCT using a 3D automatic vessel segmentation tool. Eur Radiol 2006;16: 1789–95.

9. Kefer J, Coche E, Legros G, et al. Head-to-head comparison of three-dimensional navigator-gated magnetic resonance imaging and 16-slice computed tomography to detect coronary artery stenosis in patients. J Am Coll Cardiol 2005;46: 92–100.

10. Dikkers R, Willems TP, de Jonge GJ, et al. Accuracy of noninvasive coronary stenosis quantification of different commercially available dedicated software packages. J Comput Assist Tomogr 2009;33:505–12.

11. Ferencik M, Ropers D, Abbara S, et al. Diagnostic accuracy of image postprocessing methods for the detection of coronary artery stenoses by using multidetector CT. Radiology 2007;243:696–702.

12. Cademartiri F, Mollet N, Alemos PA, et al. Standard versus user-interactive assessment of significant coronary stenoses with multislice computed tomography coronary angiography. Am J Cardiol 2004;94: 1590–3.

13. Cademartiri F, Marano R, Luccichenti G, et al. Image assessment with multislice CT coronary angiography. Radiol Med 2005;109:198–207.

14. Jinzaki M, Sato K, Tanami Y, et al. Diagnostic accuracy of angiographic view image for the detection of coronary artery stenoses by 64-detector row CT: a pilot study comparison with conventional post-processing methods and axial images alone. Circ J 2009;73:691–8.

15. Johnson PT, Pannu HK, Fishman EK. IV contrast infusion for coronary artery CT angiography: literature review and results of a nationwide survey. AJR Am J Roentgenol 2009;192:W214–21.

16. Husmann L, Gaemperli O, Valenta I, et al. Impact of vessel attenuation on quantitative coronary angiography with 64-slice CT. Br J Radiol 2009;82:649–53.

17. Dewey M, Schnapauff D, Laule M, et al. Multislice CT coronary angiography: evaluation of an automatic vessel detection tool. Rofo 2004;176: 478–83.

18. Cordeiro MA, Lardo AC, Brito MS, et al. CT angiography in highly calcified arteries: 2D manual vs. modified automated 3D approach to identify coronary stenoses. Int J Cardiovasc Imaging 2006;22: 507–16.

19. Zhang ZH, Jin ZY, Li DJ, et al. Non-invasive imaging of coronary artery with 16-slice spiral computed tomography. Chin Med Sci J 2004;19:174–9.

20. Choi JW, Seo JB, Do KH, et al. Comparison of transaxial source images and 3-plane, thin-slab maximal intensity projection images for the diagnosis of coronary artery stenosis with using ECG-gated cardiac CT. Korean J Radiol 2006;7:20–7.

21. Cury RC, Ferencik M, Achenbach S, et al. Accuracy of 16-slice multi-detector CT to quantify the degree of coronary artery stenosis: assessment of cross-sectional and longitudinal vessel reconstructions. Eur J Radiol 2006;57:345–50.

22. Fishman EK, Ney DR, Heath DG, et al. Volume rendering versus maximum intensity projection in

CT angiography: what works best, when, and why. Radiographics 2006;26:905–22.

23. Ferencik M, Moselewski F, Ropers D, et al. Quantitative parameters of image quality in multidetector spiral computed tomographic coronary imaging with submillimeter collimation. Am J Cardiol 2003; 92:1257–62.

24. Rybicki FJ, Lu M, Fail P, et al. Utilization of thick (>3 mm) maximum intensity projection images in coronary CTA interpretation. Emerg Radiol 2006; 13:157–9.

25. Calhoun PS, Kuszyk BS, Heath DG, et al. Three-dimensional volume rendering of spiral CT data: theory and method. Radiographics 1999; 19:745–64.

26. Zenooz NA, Habibi R, Mammen L, et al. Coronary artery fistulas: CT findings. Radiographics 2009; 29:781–9.

Computed Tomographic Evaluation of the Normal Cardiac Anatomy

Jill E. Jacobs, MD

KEYWORDS

- Normal anatomy • Cardiac • Computed tomography

Accurate interpretation of cardiac computed tomography (CT) requires fundamental knowledge of the normal cardiac anatomy and its common variations. Multidetector CT technology with submillimeter collimation and gantry rotation times of less than 0.5 seconds allows motion-free isotropic imaging of the cardiac structures to a degree that was previously not possible. The ability to perform multiplanar postprocessing enables evaluation of the cardiac structures in various imaging planes, necessitating a thorough understanding of the cardiac anatomy and the structural and functional relationships of the normal cardiac structures. This article reviews the normal anatomy of the coronary arteries, cardiac chambers, and cardiac valves.

CORONARY ARTERIES

The right and left coronary arteries arise from the right and left sinuses of Valsalva, respectively, near the aortic sinotubular ridge. A short-axis view of the trileaflet aortic valve shows that the right aortic cusp is the most anterior, the noncoronary cusp is the closest to the interatrial groove, and the left coronary cusp is the most cephalad (**Fig. 1**). The size of the coronary arteries correlates strongly with the ventricular mass and body size.[1,2] Several studies have also shown that even after correcting for left ventricular (LV) mass, gender remains an independent predictor of coronary artery size.[3–5] Kucher and colleagues[4] demonstrated that after normalization for LV mass,

the coronary artery cross-sectional areas in women were significantly smaller than those in men (left coronary artery [LCA]: 7 ± 3 vs 9 ± 3 mm^2/100 g LV mass, $P<.0001$; right coronary artery [RCA]: 3 ± 1 vs 4 ± 1 mm^2/100 g LV mass, $P<.002$).

The pattern of coronary artery distribution and coronary size also vary with coronary artery dominance. As cited by Chuadhry,[6] coronary artery dominance was first reported by Bianchi in 1904. In 1940, the criteria for arterial dominance were first described by Schlesinger,[7] who stated that the dominant artery is that which gives rise to the posterior descending artery (PDA) or supplies the posterior interventricular septum and the crux cordis (the crux of the heart). The crux of the heart is located at the point of transection of the atrioventricular (AV) groove and the posterior interventricular septum. In right dominant coronary artery systems, the RCA gives rise to the PDA, which extends down the posterior interventricular groove. In addition, at least one other branch of the RCA extends laterally to the PDA in the AV groove, giving off one or more posterolateral (PL) branches to supply the inferior surface of the LV (**Fig. 2A**). In left dominant coronary artery systems, the PDA and PL branches arise from the left circumflex (CX) artery (see **Fig. 2B**). With this dominance pattern, the RCA is typically small in caliber, usually tapering and terminating near the acute margin of the heart (see **Fig. 2C**). In right and left dominant systems, the AV nodal artery also arises from the RCA and

Department of Radiology, NYU Langone Medical Center, 560 First Avenue, TCH HW205, New York, NY 10016-6497, USA
E-mail address: jill.jacobs@nyumc.org

Radiol Clin N Am 48 (2010) 701–710
doi:10.1016/j.rcl.2010.05.001
0033-8389/10/$ – see front matter © 2010 Elsevier Inc. All rights reserved.

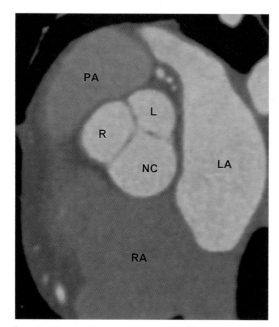

Fig. 1. Short-axis view through the aortic valve showing the 3 aortic valve cusps. The noncoronary cusp lies closest to the interatrial groove, the right cusp is the most anteriorly positioned, and the left coronary cusp is the most cephalad. L, left coronary cusp; LA, left atrium; NC, noncoronary cusp; PA, pulmonary artery; R, right coronary cusp; RA, right atrium.

LCA, respectively (see **Fig. 2**D). In codominant coronary artery systems, portions of the LV diaphragmatic wall are supplied by the RCA and the CX arteries (see **Fig. 2**E). The reported dominance rates in the literature are variable, with RCA dominance occurring in approximately 70% to 80% of the population, left dominance in approximately 8% to 10%, and codominance in the rest. The coronary arteries normally course in an epicardial position along the surface of the heart, surrounded by fat.

LCA

The left main (LM) coronary artery courses for a variable distance from the left coronary sinus before giving rise to the left anterior descending (LAD) and CX arteries (**Fig. 3**A). The length of the LM artery has been reported to vary from 5 to 20 mm.[8] In approximately 15% of cases, a third vessel, the ramus intermedius (RI) artery, arises from the LM artery between the LAD and CX arteries and courses laterally to supply the LV free wall (see **Fig. 3**B).

The LAD artery courses anterolaterally in the interventricular groove toward the apex of the heart, giving rise to lateral diagonal branches,

which supply the anterolateral LV free wall; medial septal branches, which supply the anterior two-thirds of the interventricular septum; the AV bundle; and the proximal bundle branch (**Fig. 4**). The diagonal branches and septal perforator branches are numbered sequentially from the most proximal in origin to the most distal.

The CX artery courses in the left AV groove, giving rise to obtuse marginal (OM) branches (**Fig. 5**). The OM branches are also numbered sequentially from the most proximal in origin to the most distal. The CX and OM branches supply the LV free wall and a variable portion of the anterolateral LV papillary muscle. In the majority (80%–85%) of the population, the CX branch terminates at the level of the obtuse margin of the heart, distal to the origin of the first OM branch. In left dominant coronary systems, as previously described, the CX artery continues distally to the obtuse margin of the heart to give off the PDA and PL branches that supply the inferior surface of the heart (see **Fig. 2**B).

RCA

The RCA courses from the right coronary sinus along the right AV groove and curves posteriorly at the acute margin of the right ventricle (RV) to reach the crux of the heart. In the majority of the population who are right dominant, the RCA then gives rise to the PDA and PL branches (see **Fig. 2**A). In approximately half of the population, the most proximal branch of the RCA is the conus artery, which supplies the RV outflow tract and also forms an anastomosis with the LCA via the circle of Vieussens (**Fig. 6**A). In the rest of the population, the conus artery originates directly from the aortic root (see **Fig. 6**B). The sinoatrial (SA) nodal branch arises from the RCA in approximately 60% of patients, coursing posteriorly along the anterior interatrial groove toward the superior cavoatrial junction (**Fig. 7**A). In approximately 40% of the population, the SA nodal branch originates from the proximal CX artery (see **Fig. 7**B).[9,10] Multiple ventricular branches also arise from the RCA, supplying the RV free wall. The largest of these branches is the acute marginal branch (**Fig. 8**).

Coronary Artery Segmentation

Identifying and reporting the coronary segments in a standardized fashion facilitates universal understanding of the location of coronary pathologic changes. To date, a 15-segment coronary model has most commonly been used.[11] This model has recently been adapted for coronary CT angiography (CCTA), facilitating identification of the

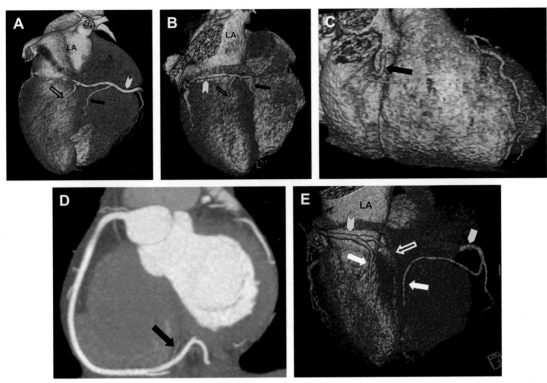

Fig. 2. (*A*) Volume-rendered posterior view of a right dominant heart shows the distal RCA (*notched arrowhead*) giving rise to the PDA (*solid black arrow*), which courses down the posterior interventricular septum, and a PL artery (*open arrow*), which courses over the LV, supplying the diaphragmatic surface of the ventricle. (*B*) Volume-rendered posterior view of a left dominant heart shows the distal circumflex artery (*notched arrowhead*) giving rise to the PDA (*solid black arrow*) and a PL artery (*open arrow*). (*C*) Volume-rendered view of the RCA (*arrow*) in the left dominant patient shown in panel *B* shows the RCA to be small in caliber, tapering and terminating just beyond the acute margin of the heart. (*D*) Maximum intensity projection reformat of the RCA in a right dominant patient shows the AV nodal artery arising from the distal RCA (*arrow*). (*E*) Volume-rendered posterior view of a codominant heart shows the distal RCA (*arrowhead*) and distal circumflex artery (*notched arrowhead*), both giving rise to PL arteries (*arrows*), which supply the diaphragmatic surface of the ventricle. The structure in the posterior interventricular septum (*open arrow*) is the middle cardiac vein. There is no PDA. LA, left atrium.

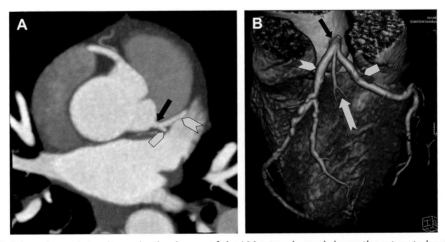

Fig. 3. (*A*) Axial maximum intensity projection image of the LM artery (*arrow*) shows the artery to be short before bifurcating into the LAD (*notched arrowhead*) and CX (*arrowhead*) arteries. (*B*) Volume-rendered image of the anterior heart in a different patient shows the LM artery (*arrow*) trifurcating into the LAD (*notched arrowhead*), CX (*arrowhead*), and ramus intermedius (RI) (*notched arrow*) arteries. The RI is located in the crotch between the LAD and CX arteries and bifurcates at its distal aspect.

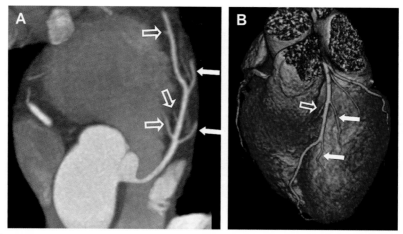

Fig. 4. (*A*) Maximum intensity projection image of the LAD artery shows the diagonal branches (*arrows*) extending laterally toward the LV free wall and the septal perforator branches (*open arrows*) extending medially into the anterior interventricular septum. (*B*) Volume-rendered image of the anterior heart shows the diagonal branches (*arrows*) and a septal perforator branch (*open arrows*).

coronary segments on standard CCTA multiplanar reconstructions.[12] Using this model, the LM segment of the LCA extends from the left coronary ostium to the bifurcation into the LAD and CX arteries, the proximal LAD artery extends from the end of the LM artery to the first large septal or diagonal branch (whichever is most proximal), the mid-LAD extends from the end of the proximal LAD to half the distance to the apex, and the distal LAD extends from the mid-LAD to the termination of the LAD. The proximal CX branch extends from the end of the LM artery to the origin of the first OM branch, and the mid and distal CX arteries extend from distal to the origin of the first OM branch to the end of the vessel or to the origin of the PDA (if it is a left dominant coronary artery system). The proximal RCA extends from the right coronary ostium to half the distance to the acute margin of the heart, the mid-RCA extends from the end of the proximal RCA to the acute margin of the heart, and the distal RCA extends from the end of the

mid-RCA to the origin of the PDA (assuming a right dominant coronary artery system) (**Fig. 9**).

RIGHT CARDIAC CHAMBERS AND VALVES

The right-sided cardiac chambers are seen to a variable degree on CCTA, depending on the injection protocol used. Triple-phase injection protocols, using an initial injection of intravenous contrast material, a second-phase injection of a mixture of contrast and saline, and a final-phase injection of a saline chaser, facilitate adequate opacification of the right-sided chambers to enable identification of pathology without precluding RCA assessment because of streak artifact from residual high-density contrast material in the superior vena cava and right atrium (RA) (**Fig. 10**).

RA, Atrial Appendage, and Tricuspid Valve

The RA forms the right lower heart border and receives inflowing blood from the superior vena

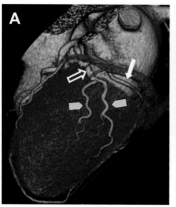
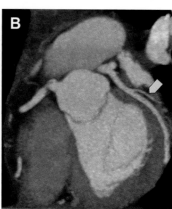

Fig. 5. (*A*) Oblique volume-rendered image of the left side of the heart shows the CX artery in the left AV groove (*arrow*) and a bifurcating OM artery (*open arrow*) with its branches extending over the lateral LV (*arrowheads*). (*B*) Multiplanar reconstruction of the CX artery shows an OM branch (*arrowhead*) extending laterally over the LV free wall.

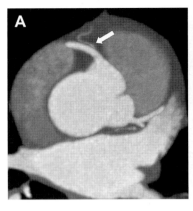
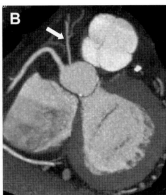

Fig. 6. (A) Axial maximum intensity projection (MIP) image shows the conus artery (arrow) arising as the first branch of the RCA, heading anteriorly toward the RV outflow tract. (B) MIP image of the RCA in a different patient shows the conus artery (arrow) arising directly from the aorta.

cava, inferior vena cava, and coronary sinus. The sinus venosus, the smooth-walled portion of the RA, is located between the superior and inferior vena caval orifices, mainly involving the PL wall of the atrium. The terminal groove, a lipomatous groove on the epicardial side of the atrium, corresponds internally to the crista terminalis and contains the sinus node and the terminal segment of the SA nodal artery.[13] The crista terminalis, a variably sized fibromuscular ridge formed by the junction of the sinus venosus and the primitive RA, separates the sinus venosus portion of the RA from the atrial appendage and gives rise to the pectinate muscles, the largest of which anteriorly is the septum spurium (Fig. 11). Superiorly, the crista terminalis extends to the anterior interatrial groove and merges with the Bachmann bundle, the largest anatomic interatrial electric connection structure (see Fig. 11A).[14] By facilitating rapid interatrial conduction, the Bachmann bundle helps

to maintain synchronous contraction of the right and left atria. The right atrial appendage typically is pyramidal, has a wider base than the left atrial appendage (LAA), and has slightly larger pectinate muscles than the LAA (Fig. 12).

The eustachian valve, located between the RA and the inferior vena cava, serves to direct inflowing blood toward the foramen ovale in utero.[15] The valve typically inserts medially into the eustachian ridge, which represents the border between the coronary sinus and oval fossa. The thebesian valve is located at the entrance of the coronary sinus into the RA and prevents reflux of blood into the coronary sinus (Fig. 13).

The RA vestibule is a smooth muscular rim surrounding the orifice of the tricuspid valve (TV). The TV separates the RA from the RV and is composed of anterior, posterior, and septal leaflets, which are connected to the RV papillary muscles by chordae tendineae. Unlike the mitral

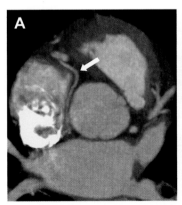
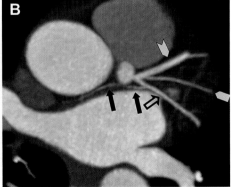

Fig. 7. (A) Axial maximum intensity projection (MIP) image of the RCA shows the SA nodal branch (arrow) coursing posteriorly toward the superior cavoatrial junction. (B) Axial MIP image of the LCA in a different patient shows the SA nodal branch (arrows) arising from the proximal CX artery (open arrow). Also note the RI branch in this patient (arrowhead) between the CX and the LAD arteries (notched arrowhead).

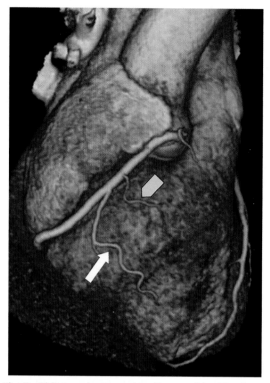

Fig. 8. Oblique volume-rendered image of the RCA shows the acute marginal branch (*arrow*) and a smaller right ventricular branch (*arrowhead*) coursing over the RV.

valve (MV), which is in direct continuity with the aortic valve, the TV is separated from the pulmonary valve (PV) by a muscular ridge, the crista supraventricularis. Also, unlike the MV, the TV has a direct connection to the interventricular septum. These characteristics help to differentiate the TV from the MV in complex congenital heart disease cases.

RV and PV

The RV is the most anterior cardiac chamber and is characterized by a heavily trabeculated apex and the presence of septomarginal bands. The moderator band, also known as the septomarginal trabeculation or trabecula septomarginalis, extends from the interventricular septum to the base of the anterior papillary muscle, contributing to its perfusion (**Fig. 14**). The moderator band contains the right bundle of the AV bundle, also known as His bundle, along with one or more arteries supplied by the LCA system. Reig and colleagues[16] demonstrated that the moderator band artery most commonly originates from the second anterior septal artery from the left coronary system. In addition, these investigators consistently found anastomoses between the moderator band artery and the right marginal artery or right ventricular branches, both of which originate from the RCA.[16] Therefore,

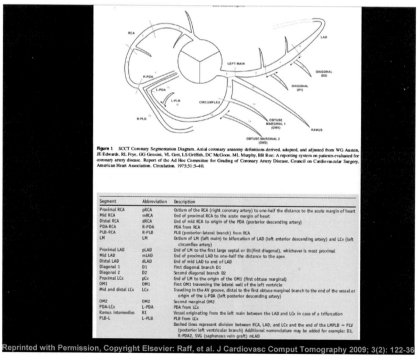

Fig. 9. Society of Cardiovascular Computed Tomography coronary segmentation diagram. *From* Raff GL, Abidov A, Achenbach S, et al. SCCT guidelines for the interpretation and reporting of coronary computed tomographic angiography. J Cardiovasc Comput Tomogr 2009;3(2):127, copyright 2009, Elsevier; with permission.

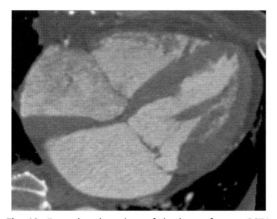

Fig. 10. Four-chamber view of the heart from a CCTA performed with a 3-phase injection protocol shows optimal opacification of the left and right sides of the heart. Opacifying the right and left atria and ventricles improves conspicuity and aids accurate identification of the interatrial and interventricular septum, respectively.

the moderator band serves as a potential anastomotic connection between the right and left coronary arteries, theoretically protecting the right ventricular myocardium in case of a proximal RCA occlusion. The smooth, muscular infundibulum (conus) of the RV is located immediately inferior to the PV and is the outflow tract for blood from the RV through the PV and into the pulmonary artery (**Fig. 15**).

The PV divides the RV outflow tract from the main pulmonary artery, but, as previously stated, it is separated from the TV by the crista supraventricularis. The PV, like the TV, is trileaflet, composed of right, left, and pulmonary leaflets.

LEFT CARDIAC CHAMBERS AND VALVES
Left Atrium, Atrial Appendage, and MV

Similar to the RA, the left atrium (LA) has a venous portion, a vestibule, and an appendage. The superior and inferior right and left pulmonary veins typically drain into its posteriorly located venous component (**Fig. 16**), but many common variants of pulmonary venous anatomy exist. Most of the LA is smooth walled, although the LAA, which arises from the superolateral LA, is tubularly shaped and trabeculated (**Fig. 17**). The pectinate muscles in the LAA are typically smaller than those in the right atrial appendage.[15]

Assessment of the left atrial size can be easily performed by calculating the left atrial area, exclusive of the LAA and pulmonary veins. An area of less than 20 cm^2 is normal, 20 to 29 cm^2 is mildly enlarged, 30 to 40 cm^2 is moderately enlarged, and greater than 40 cm^2 is severely enlarged.[17]

The vestibular component of the LA surrounds the orifice of the MV. The MV separates the LA and LV, and its apparatus is composed of 5 parts: an annulus, 2 leaflets, 2 commissures, 2 papillary muscles, and chordae tendineae. The annulus, a saddle-shaped fibrous ring embedded in the myocardium, functions to anchor the MV leaflets and is structurally continuous with the aortic annulus via 3 fibrous trigones. The MV is the only bileaflet cardiac valve, containing an anterior and a posterior leaflet (**Fig. 18**). Because of its position, the anterior leaflet functions to separate the inflow and outflow tracts of the LV. Chordae tendineae are fibrous connections between the mitral leaflets and the anterolateral and posteromedial LV papillary muscles (**Fig. 19**).

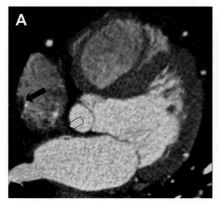
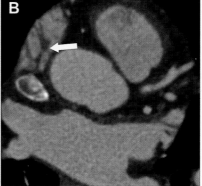

Fig. 11. (*A*) Axial CCTA image of the heart shows the crista terminalis (*arrow*) in the RA and the Bachmann bundle (*arrowhead*). (*B*) The septum spurium (*arrow*) is the largest of the pectinate muscles originating from the crista terminalis.

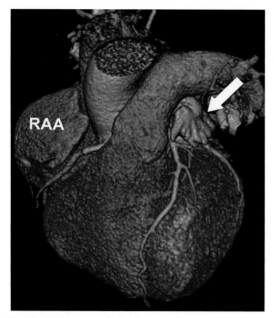

Fig. 12. Volume-rendered image of the anterior heart demonstrates the pyramidal shape of the right atrial appendage (RAA) and the narrower, more fingerlike appearance of the LAA (*arrow*).

LV and Aortic Valve

The normal LV is thick walled and lies posterior to the RV. In contradistinction to the heavily trabeculated RV, the LV contains fine trabeculations. The LV has 2 papillary muscles, anterior and posterior, which connect directly to the ventricular myocardium and function as part of the MV annulus to

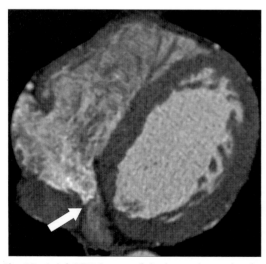

Fig. 13. Axial CCTA image of the heart shows the thebesian valve (*arrow*) at the entrance of the coronary sinus into the RA.

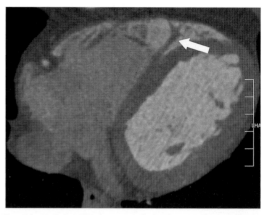

Fig. 14. Axial CCTA image of the heart shows the RV moderator band (*arrow*) extending from the right side of the interventricular septum toward the anterior papillary muscle.

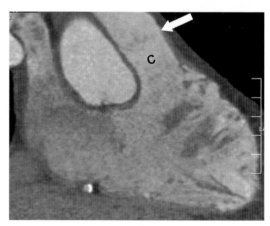

Fig. 15. Multiplanar reconstruction of the right side of the heart shows the outflow tract of the RV. The RV conus (C) is located inferior to the PV (*arrow*).

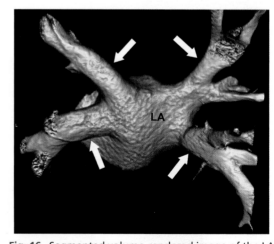

Fig. 16. Segmented volume-rendered image of the LA shows the superior and inferior right and left pulmonary veins (*arrows*) each entering the atrium via a separate ostium.

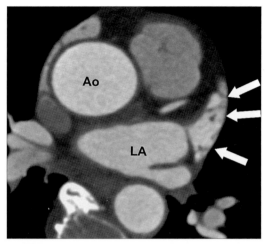

Fig. 17. Axial CCTA image through the LA and LAA shows the curvilinear, low-density pectinate muscles within the LAA (*arrows*). Ao, ascending aorta.

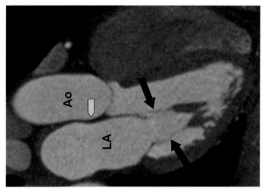

Fig. 19. Three-chamber view through left heart and the left ventricular outflow tract shows the thin fibrous chordae tendineae (*arrows*) attaching the MV leaflets to the papillary muscles. Also note the fibrous continuity between the mitral and aortic valves (*arrowhead*). Ao, ascending aorta.

ensure proper function of the MV leaflets (see **Fig. 19**).

The outflow of the LV is into the aorta via the aortic valve. The aortic valve is tricuspid and composed of the right, left, and noncoronary cusps (see **Fig. 1**). The 3 aortic cusps are half moon shaped; hence, the aortic valve is commonly referred to as a semilunar valve. In the closed position, each cusp forms a pocket that opens into the ascending aorta. Behind each cusp is a dilation of the aorta known as the sinus of Valsalva. The right and left coronary arteries arise from the sinuses of

the right and left cusps, respectively. The posterior cusp lacks a corresponding coronary artery and is therefore called the noncoronary cusp. Three aortic commissures are roughly equally spaced around the valve annulus and separate the 3 aortic cusps (**Fig. 20**). Unlike the MV, the aortic valve lacks chordae tendineae and papillary muscles. As previously described, the MV and aortic valve have fibrous continuity (see **Fig. 19**). This feature helps to distinguish the cardiac chambers and valves of the left side from those of the right side in complex congenital heart disease cases.

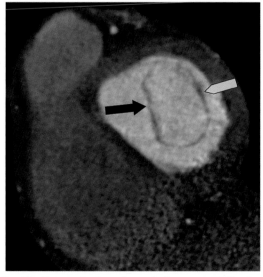

Fig. 18. Short-axis view through the open MV in diastole shows the anterior (*arrow*) and posterior (*arrowhead*) leaflets.

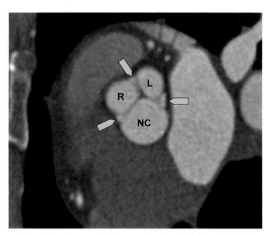

Fig. 20. Short-axis view through the aortic valve shows the 3 commissures (*arrowheads*) adjacent to the aortic cusps. L, left coronary cusp; R, right coronary cusp; NC, noncoronary cusp.

SUMMARY

Knowledge of the normal cardiac anatomy and its common variations is fundamental for accurate assessment of the heart on CCTA. Using standardized terminology to describe and localize the coronary segments and cardiac structures facilitates accurate communication of cardiac CT examination results.

REFERENCES

1. Gardin JM, Savage DD, Ware JH, et al. Effect of age, sex, and body surface area on echocardiographic left ventricular wall mass in normal subjects. Hypertension 1978;9(Suppl II):1136–9.

2. Gutsell HP, Rembold CM. Growth of the human heart relative to body surface area. Am J Cardiol 1990;65: 662–8.

3. Kim SG, Apple A, Mintz GS, et al. The importance of gender on coronary artery size: in-vivo assessment by intravascular ultrasound. Clin Cardiol 2004;27: 291–4.

4. Kucher N, Lipp E, Schwerzmann M, et al. Gender differences in coronary artery size per 100 g of left ventricular mass in a population without cardiac disease. Swiss Med Wkly 2001;131:610–5.

5. Yang F, Minutello RM, Bhagan S, et al. The impact of gender on vessel size in patients with angiographically normal coronary arteries. J Interv Cardiol 2006;19:340–4.

6. Chuadhry MS. Some observation on the coronary artery pattern and inter-coronary anastomoses in human hearts. Medicus 1965;30:160–72.

7. Schlesinger MI. Relation of anatomic pattern to pathologic condition of the coronary arteries. Arch Pathol 1940;30:403–15.

8. Miller SW. Cardiac angiography. Boston: Little, Brown; 1984, xii. p. 430.

9. Berdajs D, Patonay L, Turina MI. The clinical anatomy of the sinus node artery. Ann Thorac Surg 2003;76:732–5.

10. Sow ML, Ndoye JM, Lo EA. The artery of the sinuatrial node: anatomic considerations based on 45 injection-dissections of the heart. Surg Radiol Anat 1996;18:103–9.

11. Austen WG, Edwards JE, Frye RL, et al. A reporting system on patients evaluated for coronary artery disease. Circulation 1975;51(Suppl 4):3–40.

12. Raff GL, Abidov A, Achenbach S, et al. SCCT guidelines for the interpretation and reporting of coronary computed tomographic angiography. J Cardiovasc Comput Tomogr 2009;3(2):122–36.

13. Saremi F, Krishnan S. Cardiac conduction system: anatomic landmarks relevant to interventional electrophysiologic techniques demonstrated with 64-detector CT. Radiographics 2007;27:1539–67.

14. Saremi F, Channual S, Krishnan S, et al. Bahman bundle and its arterial supply: imaging with multidetector CT—implications for interatrial conduction abnormalities and arrhythmias. Radiology 2008; 248(2):447–57.

15. Malouf JF, Edwards WD, Tajik AJ, et al. Functional anatomy of the heart. In: Fuster V, Alexander RW, O'Rourke RA, et al, editors. Hurst's the heart. 11th edition. New York: McGraw-Hill; 2005. p. 45–82.

16. Reig J, Alberti N, Petit M. Arterial vascularization of the human moderator band: an analysis of this structure's role as a collateral circulation route. Clin Anat 2000;13:244–50.

17. Lang RM, Bierig M, Devereux RB, et al. Recommendations for chamber quantification: a report from the American Society of Echocardiography's Guidelines and Standards Committee and the Chamber Quantification Writing Group, developed in conjunction with the European Association of Echocardiography, a branch of the European Society of Cardiology. J Am Soc Echocardiogr 2005;18(12):1440–63.

Imaging of Coronary Artery Anomalies

Baskaran Sundaram, MD[a],*, Renee Kreml, MD[b],
Smita Patel, MD[b]

KEYWORDS

- Coronary anomalies • Coronary artery
- Coronary computed tomography • Coronary anatomy

Coronary artery anomalies (CAA) are rarely encountered in the general population. CAA may be either an isolated finding or associated with major congenital cardiac anomalies.[1–3] Only 20% of CAA are potentially clinically significant, and may present with life-threatening symptoms of myocardial ischemia, malignant ventricular arrhythmias, and sudden cardiac death.[4] CAA are most commonly found incidentally during catheter coronary angiography and, more recently, computed tomography (CT). Symptomatic CAA have predominantly been reported in young adults, and even in children.[5] In the United States, CAA are the second most common cause of death in young athletes, after hypertrophic obstructive cardiomyopathy.[6]

There are several types of anomalies. A single coronary artery or both coronary arteries may arise from either the systemic (aorta) or venous (pulmonary artery) circulation. Even when they originate from the systemic circulation, they may arise, course, or terminate in an anomalous fashion. The clinical presentation ranges from no symptoms to symptoms of myocardial ischemia and even sudden cardiac death. Whereas some anomalies are associated with debilitating or life-threatening cardiovascular complications, many are completely innocuous.

Catheter angiography, echocardiography, electron beam CT, and magnetic resonance imaging (MRI) have been used to diagnose and evaluate CAA.[4,7–11] More recently, electrocardiography-gated multidetector coronary CT angiography (CCTA), with isotropic spatial and temporal resolution and omnidimensional capabilities, has become the test of choice for evaluating patients with a known or suspected CAA, due to the exquisitely and highly reproducible display of coronary artery origin, course, and termination, and relationship to adjacent organs.[12]

NORMAL VERSUS ANOMALOUS CORONARY ARTERY ANATOMY

Standard coronary artery anatomy begins with the origin of the right and left coronary arteries arising from the aortic root, from the right and left aortic sinuses of Valsalva, respectively, located adjacent to the main pulmonary trunk (**Fig. 1**). The third aortic sinus, located posterior to the other sinuses, is referred to as the noncoronary sinus. On an axial cross-sectional image through the aortic root, the ostium of the right coronary artery (RCA) arises at approximately the 10- to 12-o'clock position and the left main coronary artery (LMA) at the 3- to 5-o'clock position. The RCA then courses in the right atrioventricular groove to the acute margin of the heart, where it then courses on the inferior surface of the heart in the posterior atrioventricular groove. The LMA divides into the left

The authors have nothing to disclose.
[a] Division of Cardiothoracic Radiology, Department of Radiology, Cardiovascular Center, University of Michigan Medical School, University of Michigan Health System, Room 5481, 1500 East Medical Center Drive, Ann Arbor, MI 48109-5868, USA
[b] Division of Cardiothoracic Radiology, Department of Radiology, Cardiovascular Center, University of Michigan Medical School, University of Michigan Health System, Room 5388, 1500 East Medical Center Drive, Ann Arbor, MI 48109-5868, USA
* Corresponding author.
E-mail address: sundbask@umich.edu

Radiol Clin N Am 48 (2010) 711–727
doi:10.1016/j.rcl.2010.04.006

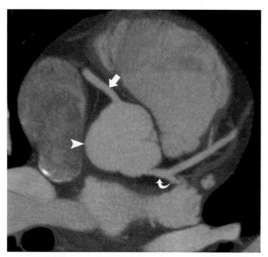

Fig. 1. Axial CT image shows that the right coronary artery (RCA) (*arrow*) arises from the right coronary sinus, and the left main coronary artery (LMA) (*curved arrow*) arises from the left coronary sinus. The arrowhead points to noncoronary sinus.

anterior descending coronary artery (LAD) and the left circumflex coronary artery (LCX). The LAD courses in the anterior interventricular groove to reach the apex of the heart, and the LCX courses in the left atrioventricular groove along the obtuse margin of the heart before passing into the posterior atrioventricular groove. The characteristics of normal coronary artery anatomy as described by Angelini are shown in **Table 1**.

The definition of a coronary artery anomaly versus a normal variant is not well defined. CAA may be described as a coronary artery pattern with a morphology that is rarely encountered in the general population. Angelini and colleagues[13]

proposed the following definitions to clarify the variability of the coronary arterial tree as (1) any morphologic feature seen in greater than 1% of the unselected population as normal, (2) normal variant as a relatively unusual morphologic feature seen in greater than 1% of the same population, and (3) anomaly as a morphologic feature rarely encountered in the same population and seen in less than 1% of the population.

EMBRYOLOGY OF CAA

The embryology of the coronary vascular circulation is complex and carefully regulated, with many unexplainable sequences and results.[14–16] Aberrations in coronary embryonic cell lineage commitment, diversification, cell migration, transition and cell differentiation, vasculogenesis, neural crest cells, and the peripheral conduction system, as well as alterations in growth factors and genes, can each result in a CAA. The coronary arteries do not grow out of aorta, as previously thought, but grow into the aorta from a peritruncal ring of coronary arterial vasculature, as shown by a monoclonal antiendothelium antibody study by Bogers and colleagues[17] that enabled detailed evaluation of the endothelium-lined vascular structures in 15 quail embryos. The coronary artery network itself is well established before establishing contact with the aortic root.

EPIDEMIOLOGY AND DETECTABILITY OF CORONARY ARTERY ANOMALIES

A variable incidence of CAA has been reported at autopsy,[3,18] catheter coronary angiography,[4,7,11] surgery,[19] and cross-sectional imaging.[8,10,20–22] For example, Alexander and Griffith[18] reported

Table 1 Normal features of human coronary artery anatomy	
Feature	**Range**
Number of ostia	2–4
Location	Right and left anterior sinuses (upper midsection)
Proximal orientation	45° to 90° off the aortic wall
Proximal common stem or trunk	Only left (LAD and LCX)
Proximal course	Direct, from ostium to destination
Mid-course	Extramural (subepicardial)
Branches	Adequate for the dependent myocardium
Essential territories supplied	RCA (RV free wall), LAD (anteroseptal), OM (LV free wall)
Termination	Capillary bed

Abbreviations: LAD, left anterior descending coronary artery; LCX, left circumflex coronary artery; LV, left ventricle; OM, obtuse marginal; RCA, right coronary artery; RV, right ventricle.

Data from Angelini P. Coronary artery anomalies: an entity in search of an identity. Circulation 2007;115(10):1296–305; with permission.

an incidence of 0.3% or 52 cases among 18,950 autopsies, the Multicenter Coronary Artery Surgery Study (CASS) reported an incidence of 0.3% among 24,959 patients,[19] and a coronary catheter angiography study of 10,661 consecutive patients found 95 cases for an incidence of 0.9%.[11] Two other catheter angiography studies reported an incidence of 1.3% among 1686 consecutive patients[4] and 7694 patients each.[7] A study on congenital heart disease specimens reported a higher incidence of 2.2% (27 of 1200), indicating a higher frequency among patients with congenital heart disease.[3]

The reported incidence of CAA on CT examinations ranges from 0.7% to 6.6%; the range is generally due to selection bias in the reports with a higher incidence.[21,22] With advancements in multidetector CT, it is possible to detect subtle CAA that may have otherwise remained undiagnosed. For example, when comparing 16-slice multidetector CT with catheter angiography in 242 patients, catheter angiography only identified 53% of the CAA identified on CT.[23]

In the majority of angiography studies, the CAA reported were predominantly anomalous origin or proximal course of the coronary arteries, and rarely fistulous terminations. CAA may involve any of the 3 major coronary arteries, and involve the LCX more commonly than the LMA, LAD, or RCA. In the Multicenter Coronary Artery Surgery Study, 60% of all CAA involved the LCX; in just over two-thirds of these, the LCX arose from a separate ostium off the right coronary sinus, and in the remainder it originated off the RCA.[19]

CLASSIFICATION OF CORONARY ARTERY ANOMALIES

Various attempts have been made to standardize the CAA classification system, with systems that are anatomic or are based primarily on clinical and functional significance. Along the lines of the latter, CAA may be classified as hemodynamically significant or insignificant, also referred to as malignant or benign, respectively. Classifying by coronary artery morphology, CAA have been classified as major or minor,[24,25] or as critical, severe, relevant, or benign,[26,27] or anatomically as anomalies of origin, intrinsic anatomy, or termination (refer also to **Box 1**).[28] The Society of Thoracic Surgery and the European Association of Cardiothoracic Surgery also reported a detailed nomenclature with multilevel hierarchy for basic categories of CAA of pulmonary/aortic origins, atresia, fistula, bridging, aneurysms, and stenosis.[29]

ANOMALIES OF ORIGIN AND COURSE
Coronary Artery Origin from the Opposite Sinus/Coronary Artery or Noncoronary Sinus

In this anomaly, the coronary artery arises from the opposite aortic sinus or coronary artery directly, rarely from the noncoronary sinus. The artery may then take 1 of 4 courses before it perfuses its usual myocardial territory: (1) course between the aorta and pulmonary artery at the level of pulmonary valve or right ventricular outflow (interarterial course), (2) traverse the upper interventricular septum (transeptal course), (3) course anterior to the pulmonary artery or right ventricular outflow tract (prepulmonic course), or (4) course between aortic root and left atrium (retroaortic course). The transeptal, prepulmonic, and retroaortic courses are considered benign or clinically insignificant, and also referred to as nonmalignant anomalies, while an interarterial course is considered clinically significant, is also referred to as malignant anomaly, is potentially lethal, and can lead to sudden cardiac death in young adults.

The LMA arises from the right sinus of Valsalva (RSV), RCA, or as a common trunk with the RCA in 0.10% of patients, and in 75% of these patients the LMA has an interarterial course (**Fig. 2**).[30] The RCA arises from the left coronary sinus in 0.03% to 0.17% of patients,[4,31,32] and takes an interarterial course. The RCA may also directly arise from a single coronary artery off the left sinus of Valsalva (LSV), and take either an interarterial or retroaortic course.

A transeptal course (**Fig. 3**) is seen when the LMA or LAD arises from the RSV or proximal RCA and courses between the aortic root and pulmonary artery, taking a subpulmonic course and entering the proximal intraventricular septum over a varying distance of the upper third of the septum, and often giving rise to a septal perforator before coursing to the epicardial surface of the heart. Although considered a benign anomaly, it has been associated with ventricular arrhythmias.[33,34]

An LMA or LAD that arises from the RSV or the proximal RCA may take a prepulmonic course (**Fig. 4**), anterior to the pulmonary artery or right ventricular outflow tract. This segment of the coronary artery is long, is not compressed or stretched, and is considered a benign or clinically insignificant anomaly. A prepulmonic LMA is also a long vessel that often branches into the LAD and LCX in the region of the mid interventricular groove. A prepulmonic LAD enters the anterior interventricular groove in its mid portion.

The retroaortic course (**Fig. 5**) is the most commonly encountered pattern, in which the

---

Box 1
Classification of coronary anomalies

A. Anomalies of origin and course

  1. Absent left main trunk (split origin of LCA)
  2. Anomalous location of coronary ostium within aortic root or near proper aortic sinus of Valsalva (for each artery)

    a. High
    b. Low
    c. Commissural

  3. Anomalous location of coronary ostium outside normal "coronary" aortic sinuses

    a. Right posterior aortic sinus
    b. Ascending aorta
    c. Left ventricle
    d. Right ventricle
    e. Pulmonary artery

      (1) LCA that arises from posterior facing sinus
      (2) LCX that arises from posterior facing sinus
      (3) LAD that arises from posterior facing sinus
      (4) RCA that arises from anterior right facing sinus
      (5) Ectopic location (outside facing sinuses) of any coronary artery from pulmonary artery

        (a) From anterior left sinus
        (b) From pulmonary trunk
        (c) From pulmonary branch

    f. Aortic arch
    g. Innominate artery
    h. Right carotid artery
    i. Internal mammary artery
    j. Bronchial artery
    k. Subclavian artery
    l. Descending thoracic aorta

  4. Anomalous location of coronary ostium at improper sinus (which may involve joint origination or "single" coronary pattern)

    a. RCA that arises from left anterior sinus, with anomalous course

      (1) Posterior atrioventricular groove or retrocardiac
      (2) Retroaortic
      (3) Between aorta and pulmonary artery (intramural)
      (4) Intraseptal
      (5) Anterior to pulmonary outflow
      (6) Posteroanterior interventricular groove (wraparound)

    b. LAD that arises from right anterior sinus, with anomalous course

      (1) Between aorta and pulmonary artery (intramural)
      (2) Intraseptal
      (3) Anterior to pulmonary outflow
      (4) Posteroanterior interventricular groove (wraparound)

    c. LCX that arises from right anterior sinus, with anomalous course

      (1) Posterior atrioventricular groove
      (2) Retroaortic

    d. LCA that arises from right anterior sinus, with anomalous course

      (1) Posterior atrioventricular groove
      (2) Retroaortic
      (3) Between aorta and pulmonary artery
      (4) Intraseptal
      (5) Anterior to pulmonary outflow
      (6) Posteroanterior interventricular groove

5. Single coronary artery (see A4)

B. Anomalies of intrinsic coronary arterial anatomy

   1. Congenital ostial stenosis or atresia (LCA, LAD, RCA, LCX)
   2. Coronary ostial dimple
   3. Coronary ectasia or aneurysm
   4. Absent coronary artery
   5. Coronary hypoplasia
   6. Intramural coronary artery (muscular bridge)
   7. Subendocardial coronary course
   8. Coronary crossing
   9. Anomalous origination of posterior descending artery from the anterior descending branch or a septal penetrating branch
  10. Split RCA

     a. Proximal + distal PDs that both arise from RCA
     b. Proximal PD that arises from RCA, distal PD that arises from LAD
     c. Parallel PDs × 2 (arising from RCA, LCX) or "codominant"

  11. Split LAD

     a. LAD + first large septal branch
     b. LAD, double (parallel LADs)

  12. Ectopic origination of first septal branch

     a. RCA
     b. Right sinus
     c. Diagonal
     d. Ramus
     e. LCX

C. Anomalies of coronary termination

   1. Inadequate arteriolar/capillary ramifications
   2. Fistulas from RCA, LCA, or infundibular artery to:

     a. Right ventricle
     b. Right atrium
     c. Coronary sinus
     d. Superior vena cava
     e. Pulmonary artery
     f. Pulmonary vein
     g. Left atrium
     h. Left ventricle
     i. Multiple, right + left ventricles

D. Anomalous anastomotic vessels

Abbreviations: LAD, left anterior descending artery; LCA, left main coronary artery; LCX, left circumflex artery; PD, posterior descending artery; RCA, right coronary artery.
Reprinted from Angelini P. Coronary artery anomalies: an entity in search of an identity. Circulation 2007;115(10):1296–305; with permission from Wolters Kluwer Health Publishers.

coronary artery courses to the right or left and posterior to the aortic root, traversing between the aortic root and left atrium. This course is seen when an LMA or LCX arises from the RSV/proximal RCA or the RCA arises from the LMA as a single artery. A retroaortic LCX is seen in 0.1% to 0.9% of the population.

An anomalous origin of a coronary artery from the noncoronary sinus is a rare anomaly, and may be seen with transposition of the great arteries or tetralogy of Fallot.[35]

Anomalous Origin from the Pulmonary Artery

Any of the coronary branches may arise from pulmonary trunk (**Fig. 6**). The most common type is when the LMA arises from the pulmonary artery (ALCAPA—Anomalous Left Coronary Artery from the Pulmonary Artery) and the RCA arises as usual from the right aortic sinus.[36,37] The reported incidence of ALCAPA is 1 in 300,000 live births.[38] In these patients, CCTA demonstrates the innumerable epicardial collateral vessels between the

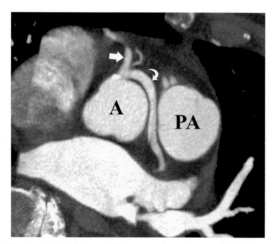

Fig. 2. Axial oblique CT image of aortic root illustrates that both the RCA (*arrow*) and the LMA (*curved arrow*) originate together from a single coronary ostium from the right coronary sinus. Subsequently, the RCA courses in a normal fashion in the right atrioventricular groove while the LMA courses in between aortic root (A) and pulmonary artery (PA).

anomalous artery that arises from the pulmonary artery and the normal coronary artery that arises from the systemic circulation.[39]

Coronary Ostial Location

RCA and LMA ostia are located in the middle of their respective sinuses of the corresponding aortic sinus, and rarely in the anterior or posterior thirds of the sinus or upper portion of the sinus. A high coronary artery origin (**Fig. 7**) refers to an ostium located

approximately 10 mm or more above the sinotubular junction, while a low coronary artery origin refers to an ostium located at the lower end of the aortic sinus. A high origin of coronary artery has been reported in 6% of random adult hearts.[40] Lastly, a commissural ostium refers to a coronary artery ostium located within 5 mm of the aortic valve apposition at the aortic annulus.

Coronary Ostial Number

While there are usually individual coronary ostia, for the RCA and LMA there are several variations. For example, instead of one LMA ostium, the LAD and LCX may have separate ostia arising from the LSV, reported in 0.4% of individuals.[41] There may be two ostia off the RSV, one for the RCA and the second for the conus branch directly arising from aorta, noted in 11.6% of 543 consecutive CCTAs (**Fig. 8**).[20]

Single Coronary Artery

A single coronary artery ostium occurs with an incidence of 0.06%, as reported on 33 of 50,000 consecutive catheter angiograms,[42] and may arise from any aortic sinus. The single artery course can be variable, with the proximal RCA or LMA dividing into branches following the distributions of the RCA, LMA, LAD, and LCX to their respective myocardial territory (see **Fig. 9**). Ogden and Goodyer[25] report 5 patterns of distribution: (1) a single coronary artery supplying the entire myocardium, (2) a single artery with 2 major branches, 1 of which has a retroaortic course, (3) 2 major branches, 1 of which has an interarterial course, (4) 2 major branches, 1 of which has a prepulmonic course, and (5) 3 equally dominant major branches.

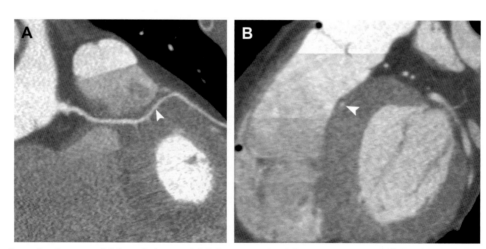

Fig. 3. Curved reformatted (*A*) and short axial left ventricular (*B*) images show the LAD arising from RSV and coursing through the upper portions of the interventricular septal course. Note small-caliber LAD in septum, giving rise to septal perforator and more distally coming to the epicardial surface of the heart where it is of normal caliber.

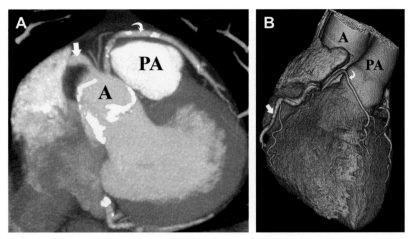

Fig. 4. Curved reformatted (*A*) and volume-rendered (*B*) images of heart show that both RCA (*arrow*) and LAD (*curved arrow*) originate from the right coronary sinus of the aortic root (A). RCA courses normally in the right atrioventricular (AV) groove, while the LAD courses anterior to the pulmonary trunk (PA) in a prepulmonic course before reaching its usual location of anterior interventricular groove. The LCX (*arrowhead*) arises from the left coronary sinus and courses normally in the left AV groove.

ANOMALIES OF INTRINSIC CORONARY ARTERY ANATOMY
Ostial Atresia and Intramural Coronary Artery Anomaly

Congenital ostial atresia is characterized by an ostial dimple in a coronary sinus without a patent arterial lumen. A fibrotic ostial ridge may be seen on pathologic studies at the atretic ostium, resulting in obstruction. Congenital atresia of the LMA is rare, and presents in early childhood with cardiac morbidity or very late in adult life.[43] The proximal LMA ends blindly with blood flowing from the RCA to the left coronary circulation via collateral arteries.

The normal angle between the ostium and coronary artery is 90° or less. If the angle is 0°, the artery usually has an intramural course within the aortic wall.[44,45] An acute angle take-off of an anomalous vessel may result in a slit-like orifice opening that may collapse during exercise in a valve-like manner. The proximal portion of the anomalous artery can be intramural, with the artery taking a tangential course in the aortic wall for a variable distance. When using intravascular ultrasound (IVUS) to document functional anatomy, Angelini describes the intramural coronary artery to be slit-like, and to undergo a phasic increase in lateral compression between the inner and outer aortic wall layers.[13,46,47] On cross-sectional imaging, the ostium and intramural portion has a characteristic "slit" or narrowing from side to side, and becomes progressively oval and then round once it exits the aortic wall **(Fig. 10)**.

Congenital Coronary Artery Aneurysms and Ectasia

Coronary artery aneurysms of congenital etiology are rare, and are more commonly associated with Kawasaki disease, lupus, and atherosclerotic coronary artery disease.[48] A coronary artery aneurysm is defined as a focal saccular or fusiform dilatation of the coronary artery that is 1.5 times or more the

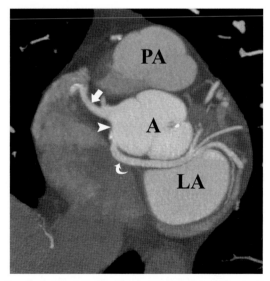

Fig. 5. Axial oblique reformatted image of the aortic root (*A*) shows LMA (*curved arrow*) arises from the RSV (*arrow head*) and courses between the aortic root and the left atrium (LA). RCA (*arrow*) arises normally from the RSV. PA, main pulmonary artery.

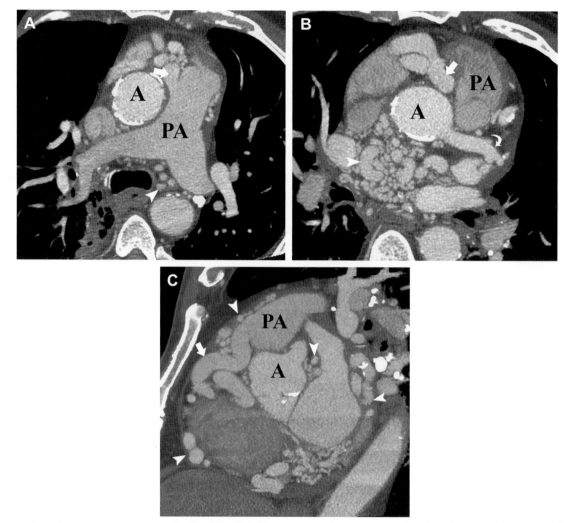

Fig. 6. Axial image at the level of mid ascending aorta (*A*), aortic root (*B*), and sagittal image of the heart (*C*) show RCA (*arrow*) originating from the right wall of main pulmonary trunk (PA). The LMA (*curved arrow*) arises normally from the left coronary sinus at the aortic root (A). There are innumerable tortuous blood vessels connecting both right and left coronary circulation (*arrowheads*).

diameter of the adjacent normal arterial segment. Focal dilatation is termed aneurysm, while diffuse dilation of an entire artery is termed "ectasia" (**Fig. 11**). Congenital coronary artery aneurysms are most common in the RCA.[49] The pathophysiology of congenital aneurysms is poorly understood, and may be the result of an inherent congenital weakening of the artery wall.[49,50] These aneurysms have been reported to be a component of rare inherited genetic syndromes.[51,52]

Congenital coronary artery aneurysms may be classified by size as small (<5 mm), medium (5–8 mm), and giant (>8 mm), by morphology as saccular and fusiform, or by the extent of disease, involving one or both coronary arteries.[53]

Myocardial Bridging

The coronary arteries run on the epicardial surface of the heart surrounded by fat, before entering the myocardium distally. Myocardial bridging is defined as a coronary artery segment that has a tunneled, intramuscular course (**Fig. 12**). The reported incidence varies with the way in which bridging is detected. For example, an incidence of 1.5% to 16% has been reported using conventional catheter angiography versus a range of 15% to 85% at pathology,[54,55] and 18% to 30% on CT.[56,57] Given the high occurrence of myocardial bridging in the general population, this entity is considered a coronary artery variant and may not be a true CAA.

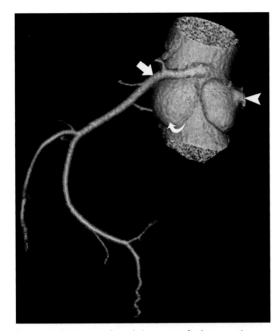

Fig. 7. Volume-rendered image of the aortic root shows the anomalous origin of the RCA (*arrow*), 1.5 cm above and anteromedial to the right coronary sinus (*curved arrow*). The LMA (*arrowhead*) arises normally from the left coronary sinus.

Myocardial bridging can be described as incomplete or superficial, and complete or deep. With incomplete bridging the affected arterial segment extends superficially into but is not completely surrounded by myocardium, whereas in complete bridging the arterial segment is completely surrounded by myocardium.[58] The middle segment of the LAD is most commonly involved, although any coronary artery segment may be involved.[59]

Coronary Artery Duplication

Duplication of the coronary arteries can be seen with the LAD, LCX, or RCA. Duplication of the LAD is more commonly reported, and LCX duplication is the least common.[60–71] The duplicated artery may arise from the corresponding coronary artery of the same name, directly from the same aortic sinus, ectopically from another aortic sinus or coronary artery, or from a pulmonary artery.[60–67,69–72]

A dual LAD entity usually consists of a short and a long LAD. Spindola-Franco and colleagues[69] report 4 subtypes (**Box 2**) of LAD duplication. In all 4 types, the short LAD terminates in the mid to distal anterior interventricular groove before reaching the apex of the heart (**Fig. 13**). A dual RCA occurs with either a single or double ostia. The paired arteries run in the right atrioventricular (AV) groove, or may have a separate course, with one in the right AV groove and the other over the epicardial surface of the right ventricle coursing inferiorly to the inferior intraventricular groove.[54,55]

ANOMALIES OF CORONARY TERMINATION
Coronary Artery Fistula

A coronary artery fistula (CAF) is defined as an abnormal termination of the coronary artery into

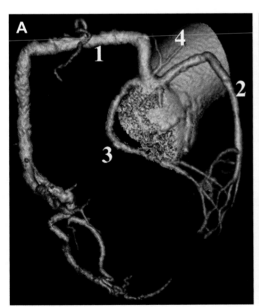
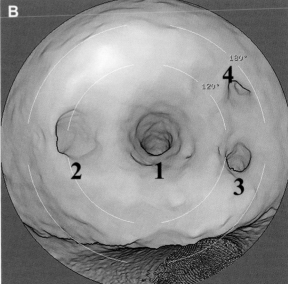

Fig. 8. Volume-rendered image of the aortic root (*A*) and endoluminal view (*B*) of the right coronary sinus. Independent coronary ostium for RCA (**1**), LAD (**2**), LCX (**3**), and conus branch (**4**) at the right coronary sinus (*arrow*). The LCX courses in a retroaortic fashion before reaching its usual location of the left atrioventricular groove.

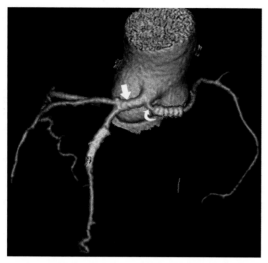

Fig. 9. Volume-rendered image of the aortic root shows combined origin of both RCA (*arrow*) and LMA (*curved arrow*) from the left coronary sinus.

a cardiac chamber, artery, or vein, with an incidence of 0.05% to 0.25% based on catheter coronary angiography.[73,74] The majority of the CAFs are congenital, with 50% arising from the RCA, 42% from the LCA, and 5% from both RCA and LCA.[75]

The fistulous connection from the coronary artery usually terminates in a cardiac chamber, less often a vessel, with distribution as follows: 41% right ventricle, 26% right atrium, 5% left atrium, 3% left ventricle, 17% into the pulmonary artery, 7% the coronary sinus, and 1% the superior vena cava (**Fig. 14**) or pulmonary veins.[76] A fistulous communication between a coronary artery and cardiac chamber is specifically known as "coronary arterio-cameral fistula."

Most fistulas have single connections, some have multiple connections. The involved coronary artery is often dilated and tortuous, due to increased blood flow and shunting.

Coronary Arcade

A coronary arcade is a short, straight, small-diameter arterial branch vessel that communicates between the major coronary arteries in the absence of significant coronary artery stenosis. Coronary arcades differ from the collateral vasculature by virtue of their nontortuous morphology and the absence of coronary artery stenosis,[77–79] and are generally difficult to visualize on imaging due to their small size.

Extracardiac Termination

Congenital communications between the coronary arteries and extracardiac vascular structures have been reported, and include various structures including the bronchial, internal mammary and phrenic arteries, intercostals and esophageal arteries, and vessels around the pulmonary venous ostia.[80–82]

CLINICAL SIGNIFICANCE OF CORONARY ARTERY ANOMALIES
Interarterial Course

An anomalous origin of a coronary artery from the opposite sinus with an interarterial course is the primary CAA associated with sudden cardiac death in young athletes.[83,84] A comprehensive review of sudden cardiac death in athletes who died during exercise suggests an anomalous LCA arising from the opposite sinus is significantly more frequent than that of the RCA arising from the opposite sinus.[85] Taylor and colleagues[86] report a 57% mortality for an anomalous coronary artery arising from the opposite sinus involving the LCA, versus 25% for the RCA. A 25-year review of autopsies on young military recruits who had sudden, nontraumatic death revealed one-third of the study cohort (21 of 64 recruits) with an identifiable cardiac abnormality, who had an interarterial course of LAD.[84] In a postmortem study of congenital cardiac disease specimens, 74% of

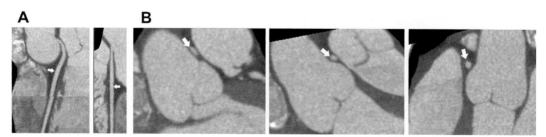

Fig. 10. Curved reformatted (*A*) and true axial (*B*) images of RCA. Note narrow caliber of RCA as it arises from the left LSV. Lumen view shows a short segment of the RCA to be narrow. On true axial image, slit-like RCA contour gradually becomes oval and then round.

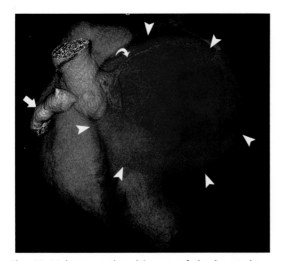

Fig. 11. Volume-rendered image of the heart shows diffusely dilated (2 cm diameter) RCA (*arrow*) and a 10-cm diameter aneurysm (*arrowheads*) arising from the LAD (*curved arrow*). This 35-year-old previously asymptomatic patient had no risk factors for atherosclerotic coronary artery disease or vasculitis or any significant childhood illness such as Kawasaki disease. Hence, these abnormalities are presumed to be congenital in origin.

27 deaths were attributed to a CAA.[3] In a retrospective review of the mode of death in 242 patients with an isolated CAA, 59% were cardiac deaths; 32% were sudden deaths, nearly half of which were exercise induced.[86] In this review, younger patients (<30 years old) died suddenly

---

Box 2
Four types of dual left anterior descending coronary artery

1. Long LAD arises from the LMA/LAD proper and descends to the left of the interventricular groove over the anterior left ventricular wall. The short LAD gives rise to all major septal perforators and the long LAD to the diagonals.
2. Long LAD descends to the right of inter ventricular groove.
3. Long LAD takes an intramyocardial course. In this subtype, the septal perforators arise from the long LAD and the diagonals from the short LAD.
4. Short LAD arises from the LMA and the long LAD from the RCA, anterior to the right ventricular outflow tract, with both arteries contributing many perforators to the upper portion of the interventricular septum.

Abbreviations: LAD, left anterior descending artery; LMA, left main coronary artery; RCA, right coronary artery.

---

compared with older patients (62% vs 12%; P = .0001), specifically during intense exercise (40% vs 2%; P = .0001).[86] Following systematic tracking of 158 young (<35 years old; median age 17 years) competitive team sport athletes for 10 years, an American Heart Association (AHA) statement reported that CAA were the second leading cause (19%) of sudden cardiac death next to hypertrophic cardiomyopathy (36%).[87] A more recent 2007 AHA statement published on preparticipation screening for competitive athletes reported similar figures, with CAA being the second leading cause of sudden cardiac death in 17%.[88] Coronary artery with an interarterial course may require major prophylactic or therapeutic interventions to prevent sudden cardiac death in young individuals taking part in strenuous activities.[83,86,89,90]

Pulmonary Artery Origin

ALCAPA is a serious CAA often presenting in infancy, with 90% mortality if untreated in the first year of life.[91] In comparison, ARCAPA is associated with relatively less incidence of sudden death and myocardial ischemia, which may be due to the development of extensive collaterals.[92] Both infantile and adult forms of ALCAPA have been described. The infantile form presents soon after birth with myocardial infarction; when diagnosed in infancy or early childhood, the majority of untreated patients die within the first year of life due to myocardial ischemia. Bland-White-Garland syndrome refers to a clinical entity in children with ALCAPA who present with failure to thrive, dyspnea, pallor, and chest pain on eating or crying.[93] The adult form presents later in life due to failing collateral coronary circulation that is unable to maintain myocardial perfusion. Following prompt diagnosis and surgical restoration of the coronary artery to the systemic circulation, long-term survival in these patients may considerably improve.[38]

Single Coronary Artery

The clinical significance of a single coronary artery is the risk of sudden cardiac death with an interarterial course or significant proximal critical stenosis before branching with the inability to develop collateral pathways, which results in high morbidity and mortality.[41]

Ostial Atresia and Intramural Course

Sudden death may also be the result of ostial atresia in young patients. Progressive hardening of the aortic wall with age may limit distortion of the coronary ostium, which may result in lesser

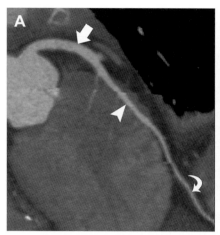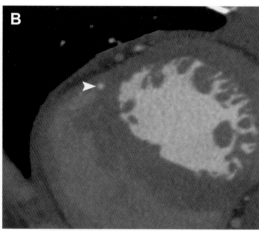

Fig. 12. Curved reformatted (*A*) and true short axial (*B*) images of LAD show that the proximal (*arrow*) and distal (*curved arrow*) portions of the LAD course along the surface of the myocardium. Approximately 4 cm of its mid portion (*arrowhead*) courses 0.3 cm beneath the epicardial surface of the myocardium. The mid portion of LAD is surrounded 360 degrees by myocardium and the remainder of the LAD is surrounded by epicardial adipose tissue.

morbidity in adults in comparison with children.[94] However, it may be difficult to cannulate these ostiae during catheter angiography, and cross-clamping during aortic root or ascending aortic surgeries may also be problematic.

When the proximal coronary artery is intramural and courses tangential to the aortic wall, it may have fixed lateral compression that becomes more severe with exercise, and leads to collapse of the intramural segment with expansion of the aorta, resulting in myocardial ischemia.[46] This anomaly can lead to severe myocardial ischemia, depressed left ventricular function, and mitral regurgitation, and is treated by surgical deroofing or revascularization.[43]

Congenital Aneurysm and Ectasia

Similar to acquired coronary aneurysms, congenital aneurysms are also at risk for thrombosis, myocardial ischemia, rupture, and fistulous communication with adjacent structures.[95–97]

Myocardial Bridging

The majority of myocardial bridges are not clinically significant. However, a small proportion may be significant, resulting in angina, myocardial ischemia, arrhythmias, or death as a result of vessel spasm and compression. Systolic compression of the tunneled segment may persist into diastole. The tunneled artery may be protected from atherosclerosis, while the segment proximal to bridged segment may have higher incidence of atherosclerosis, as Konen and colleagues[58] reported atherosclerotic plaque in the coronary artery segments that are proximal to the myocardial bridging in 19% (7 of 36) of patients.

Coronary Artery Duplication

Duplicated coronary arteries may be of significant consideration during coronary intervention and surgical revascularization procedures, as the culprit stenotic lesion producing myocardial

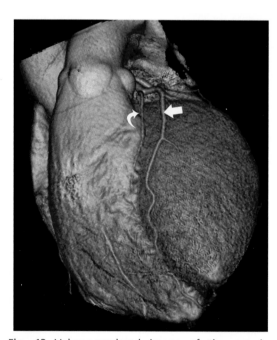

Fig. 13. Volume-rendered image of the anterior surface of the heart shows dominant (*arrow*) and nondominant (*curved arrow*) LADs. The dominant LAD courses in the caudal portions of the anterior interventricular groove to reach the left ventricular apex, while the nondominant LAD courses in the cranial portion of the anterior interventricular groove and terminates prematurely.

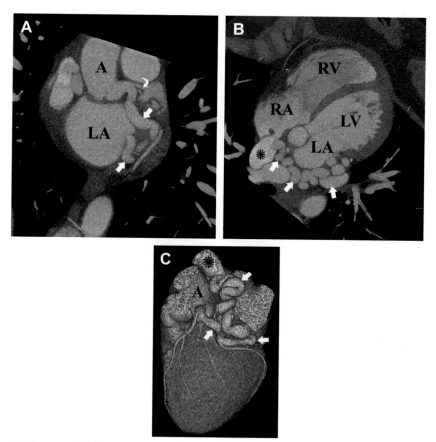

Fig. 14. Coronal reformatted (*A*), 4-chamber view (*B*), and volume-rendered (*C*) images of the left ventricle. The LCX (*arrows*) is markedly dilated and tortuous. It courses normally in the left AV groove, extends beyond the crux along the posterior surface of the heart, and terminates by draining into the superior vena cava (*asterisk*) just above the right atrium. Curved arrow points to LAD. A, aorta; RV, right ventricle; LA, left atrium; LV, left ventricle.

ischemia may be present in the duplicated artery while the conventional artery may misleadingly be normal.

Coronary Artery Fistula

The majority of adult patients with CAF, particularly those with small CAF, are asymptomatic.[73] Small CAF that drain into left-sided heart chambers or the pulmonary artery are more common and relatively benign. Larger CAF draining into a left heart chamber can lead to left ventricular overload and may clinically mimic aortic insufficiency. When a CAF drains into a right-sided chamber, the clinical presentation is a left-to-right shunt, with dilatation of right heart chambers and right ventricular overload, depending on the shunt severity. Coronary steal phenomenon can occur with larger fistulas. Other complications include endocarditis and the development of mural thrombus in the dilated coronary artery due to aneurysm formation, with potential for rupture or side branch obstruction. The drainage site of the CAF, size of the fistula, and quantity of anomalous blood flow may have prognostic implications.

Other Considerations

Coronary artery ectasia, CAF, ALCAPA, and ectopic origin of a coronary artery may lead to increased risk of coronary atherosclerotic disease (CAD) or ischemic cardiomyopathy. The association between coronary artery disease and CAA is debated to have either positive or negative impact on development of atherosclerosis.[19,98,99] In a catheter angiography study in patients with CAA (73 of 24,959 patients), anomalous arteries had a significantly ($P = .02$) higher degree of luminal stenosis than nonanomalous arteries of age- and gender-matched controls.[19] A 12-year review of catheter angiograms found that 71% (27 of 38) of patients with LCX originating from RCA/right aortic sinus had significant CAD in the proximal segment and 11% had severe atherosclerosis in that vessel alone.[11] Hence, they concluded that in patients with CAA, there is predilection of CAD in the posteriorly coursing LCX.[11] Earlier work by Page and colleagues[100] suggests there is no increased risk of CAD with the anomalous LCX. Of note, prior to CCTA of the coronary arteries many of the CAA were diagnosed on catheter angiography. Patients undergoing catheter angiography for cardiac symptoms are more likely to have coronary atherosclerosis, as it is widely prevalent in the general population. Hence, there may or may not be higher risk of coronary atherosclerosis due to the presence of a CAA, as these 2 conditions may simply coexist.

CAA have been reported with bicuspid aortic valves, suggesting the embryology of both may be related.[101,102] Using hamsters, Fernandez and colleagues[102] showed that that the probability of occurrence of CAA increases continuously according to the degree of deviation of the aortic valve from its normal (tricuspid) design when analyzed using a logistic regression model. CAA in the context of abnormal aortic valves may be a significant consideration because many of these patients may eventually undergo aortic root surgery.

SUMMARY

While CAA are rare, a small proportion can result in potentially significant myocardial ischemia and its complications, particularly in young adults. CCTA has proven to be an excellent imaging tool for the diagnosis and characterization of CAA. It is important for the interpreting and referring physicians to be familiar with the CT appearance of the complex cardiac vascular anatomy relating to CAA and their clinical significance, as correct diagnosis aids in medical, interventional, and surgical management of patients with CAA.

ACKNOWLEDGMENTS

The authors sincerely thank Dr Ella Annabelle Kazerooni, MD, MS, Division of Cardiothoracic Radiology, Department of Radiology, University of Michigan, Ann Arbor, MI, for her help in excellent edits and comments.

REFERENCES

1. Dabizzi RP, Barletta GA, Caprioli G, et al. Coronary artery anatomy in corrected transposition of the great arteries. J Am Coll Cardiol 1988; 12(2):486–91.

2. Tuzcu EM, Moodie DS, Chambers JL, et al. Congenital heart diseases associated with coronary artery anomalies. Cleve Clin J Med 1990; 57(2):147–52.

3. Frescura C, Basso C, Thiene G, et al. Anomalous origin of coronary arteries and risk of sudden death: a study based on an autopsy population of congenital heart disease. Hum Pathol 1998; 29(7):689–95.

4. Yamanaka O, Hobbs RE. Coronary artery anomalies in 126,595 patients undergoing coronary arteriography. Cathet Cardiovasc Diagn 1990; 21(1):28–40.

5. Frommelt PC, Frommelt MA. Congenital coronary artery anomalies. Pediatr Clin North Am 2004; 51(5):1273–88.

6. Maron BJ, Thompson PD, Puffer JC, et al. Cardiovascular preparticipation screening of competitive athletes. A statement for health professionals from the Sudden Death Committee (clinical cardiology) and Congenital Cardiac Defects Committee (cardiovascular disease in the young), American Heart Association. Circulation 1996;94(4):850–6.

7. Kardos A, Babai L, Rudas L, et al. Epidemiology of congenital coronary artery anomalies: a coronary arteriography study on a central European population. Cathet Cardiovasc Diagn 1997;42(3):270–5.

8. McConnell MV, Ganz P, Selwyn AP, et al. Identification of anomalous coronary arteries and their anatomic course by magnetic resonance coronary angiography. Circulation 1995;92(11):3158–62.

9. Post JC, van Rossum AC, Bronzwaer JG, et al. Magnetic resonance angiography of anomalous coronary arteries. A new gold standard for delineating the proximal course? Circulation 1995; 92(11):3163–71.

10. Ropers D, Moshage W, Daniel WG, et al. Visualization of coronary artery anomalies and their anatomic course by contrast-enhanced electron beam tomography and three-dimensional reconstruction. Am J Cardiol 2001;87(2):193–7.

11. Wilkins CE, Betancourt B, Mathur VS, et al. Coronary artery anomalies: a review of more than 10,000 patients from the Clayton Cardiovascular Laboratories. Tex Heart Inst J 1988;15(3):166–73.

12. Schoepf UJ, Becker CR, Ohnesorge BM, et al. CT of coronary artery disease. Radiology 2004; 232(1):18–37.

13. Angelini P, Velasco JA, Flamm S. Coronary anomalies: incidence, pathophysiology, and clinical relevance. Circulation 2002;105(20):2449–54.

14. Reese DE, Mikawa T, Bader DM. Development of the coronary vessel system. Circ Res 2002;91(9):761–8.

15. von Kodolitsch Y, Ito WD, Franzen O, et al. Coronary artery anomalies. Part I: recent insights from molecular embryology. Z Kardiol 2004;93(12):929–37.

16. von Kodolitsch Y, Franzen O, Lund GK, et al. Coronary artery anomalies Part II: recent insights from clinical investigations. Z Kardiol 2005;94(1):1–13.

17. Bogers AJ, Gittenberger-de Groot AC, Poelmann RE, et al. Development of the origin of the coronary

arteries, a matter of ingrowth or outgrowth? Anat Embryol (Berl) 1989;180(5):437–41.

18. Alexander RW, Griffith GC. Anomalies of the coronary arteries and their clinical significance. Circulation 1956;14(5):800–5.

19. Click RL, Holmes DR Jr, Vlietstra RE, et al. Anomalous coronary arteries: location, degree of atherosclerosis and effect on survival—a report from the Coronary Artery Surgery Study. J Am Coll Cardiol 1989;13(3):531–7.

20. Lytrivi ID, Wong AH, Ko HH, et al. Echocardiographic diagnosis of clinically silent congenital coronary artery anomalies. Int J Cardiol 2008; 126(3):386–93.

21. Budoff MJ, Ahmed V, Gul KM, et al. Coronary anomalies by cardiac computed tomographic angiography. Clin Cardiol 2006;29(11):489–93.

22. Cademartiri F, La Grutta L, Malago R, et al. Prevalence of anatomical variants and coronary anomalies in 543 consecutive patients studied with 64-slice CT coronary angiography. Eur Radiol 2008;18(4):781–91.

23. Shi H, Aschoff AJ, Brambs HJ, et al. Multislice CT imaging of anomalous coronary arteries. Eur Radiol 2004;14(12):2172–81.

24. Ogden JA. Congenital anomalies of the coronary arteries. Am J Cardiol 1970;25(4):474–9.

25. Ogden JA, Goodyer AV. Patterns of distribution of the single coronary artery. Yale J Biol Med 1970; 43(1):11–21.

26. Rigatelli G. Congenital coronary artery anomalies in the adult: a new practical viewpoint. Clin Cardiol 2005;28(2):61–5.

27. Rigatelli G, Docali G, Rossi P, et al. Validation of a clinical-significance-based classification of coronary artery anomalies. Angiology 2005;56(1): 25–34.

28. Angelini P. Coronary artery anomalies: an entity in search of an identity. Circulation 2007;115(10): 1296–305.

29. Dodge-Khatami A, Mavroudis C, Backer CL. Congenital Heart Surgery Nomenclature and Database Project: anomalies of the coronary arteries. Ann Thorac Surg 2000;69(Suppl 4):S270–97.

30. Chaitman BR, Lesperance J, Saltiel J, et al. Clinical, angiographic, and hemodynamic findings in patients with anomalous origin of the coronary arteries. Circulation 1976;53(1):122–31.

31. Kimbiris D, Iskandrian AS, Segal BL, et al. Anomalous aortic origin of coronary arteries. Circulation 1978;58(4):606–15.

32. Donaldson RM, Raphael M, Radley-Smith R, et al. Angiographic identification of primary coronary anomalies causing impaired myocardial perfusion. Cathet Cardiovasc Diagn 1983;9(3):237–49.

33. Kothari SS, Talwar KK, Venugopal P. Septal course of the left main coronary artery from right aortic sinus and ventricular tachycardia. Int J Cardiol 1998;66(2):207–9.

34. Roberts WC, Dicicco BS, Waller BF, et al. Origin of the left main from the right coronary artery or from the right aortic sinus with intramyocardial tunneling to the left side of the heart via the ventricular septum. The case against clinical significance of myocardial bridge or coronary tunnel. Am Heart J 1982;104(2 Pt 1):303–5.

35. Greenberg MA, Fish BG, Spindola-Franco H. Congenital anomalies of the coronary arteries. Classification and significance. Radiol Clin North Am 1989;27(6):1127–46.

36. Fernandes ED, Kadivar H, Hallman GL, et al. Congenital malformations of the coronary arteries: the Texas Heart Institute experience. Ann Thorac Surg 1992;54(4):732–40.

37. Fernandes J, Rutkowski M, Sanger JJ. Anomalous origin of the left coronary artery. Use of thallium perfusion scans in the evaluation of successful revascularization. Clin Nucl Med 1992;17(3):177–9.

38. Dodge-Khatami A, Mavroudis C, Backer CL. Anomalous origin of the left coronary artery from the pulmonary artery: collective review of surgical therapy. Ann Thorac Surg 2002;74(3):946–55.

39. Pena E, Nguyen ET, Merchant N, et al. ALCAPA syndrome: not just a pediatric disease. Radiographics 2009;29(2):553–65.

40. Vlodaver Z, Neufeld HN, Edwards JE. Pathology of coronary disease. Semin Roentgenol 1972;7(4): 376–94.

41. Kim SY, Seo JB, Do KH, et al. Coronary artery anomalies: classification and ECG-gated multidetector row CT findings with angiographic correlation. Radiographics 2006;26(2):317–33 [discussion: 333–4].

42. Desmet W, Vanhaecke J, Vrolix M, et al. Isolated single coronary artery: a review of 50,000 consecutive coronary angiographies. Eur Heart J 1992; 13(12):1637–40.

43. Musiani A, Cernigliaro C, Sansa M, et al. Left main coronary artery atresia: literature review and therapeutic considerations. Eur J Cardiothorac Surg 1997;11(3):505–14.

44. Sacks JH, Londe SP, Rosenbluth A, et al. Left main coronary bypass for aberrant (aortic) intramural left coronary artery. J Thorac Cardiovasc Surg 1977; 73(5):733–7.

45. Gittenberger-de Groot AC, Sauer U, Quaegebeur J. Aortic intramural coronary artery in three hearts with transposition of the great arteries. J Thorac Cardiovasc Surg 1986;91(4):566–71.

46. Angelini P. Coronary artery anomalies—current clinical issues: definitions, classification, incidence, clinical relevance, and treatment guidelines. Tex Heart Inst J 2002;29(4):271–8.

47. Angelini P, Velasco JA, Ott D, et al. Anomalous coronary artery arising from the opposite sinus: descriptive features and pathophysiologic mechanisms, as documented by intravascular ultrasonography. J Invasive Cardiol 2003;15(9):507–14.

48. Grob M, Kolb E. Congenital aneurysm of the coronary artery. Arch Dis Child 1959;34(173):8–13.

49. Chakrabarti S, Thomas E, Wright JG, et al. Congenital coronary artery dilatation. Heart 2003;89(6):595–6.

50. Ghahramani A, Iyengar R, Cunha D, et al. Myocardial infarction due to congenital coronary arterial aneurysm (with successful saphenous vein bypass graft). Am J Cardiol 1972;29(6):863–7.

51. Iwasaki Y, Horigome H, Takahashi-Igari M, et al. Coronary artery dilatation in LEOPARD syndrome. A child case and literature review. Congenit Heart Dis 2009;4(1):38–41.

52. Olgar S, Nisli K, Dindar A, et al. Can cystinosis cause coronary artery dilatation? Pediatr Cardiol 2006;27(2):263–8.

53. Antoniadis AP, Chatzizisis YS, Giannoglou GD. Pathogenetic mechanisms of coronary ectasia. Int J Cardiol 2008;130(3):335–43.

54. Egred M, Shakespeare CF, Pennell D, et al. Magnetic resonance angiography in the assessment of a first reported case of duplicate right coronary artery. Int J Cardiol 2005;101(2):329–31.

55. Resatoglu AG, Elnur EE, Yener N, et al. Double right coronary artery; fistula and atherosclerosis: rare combination. Jpn J Thorac Cardiovasc Surg 2005;53(5):283–5.

56. De Rosa R, Sacco M, Tedeschi C, et al. Prevalence of coronary artery intramyocardial course in a large population of clinical patients detected by multislice computed tomography coronary angiography. Acta Radiol 2008;49(8):895–901.

57. Leschka S, Koepfli P, Husmann L, et al. Myocardial bridging: depiction rate and morphology at CT coronary angiography—comparison with conventional coronary angiography. Radiology 2008;246(3):754–62.

58. Konen E, Goitein O, Sternik L, et al. The prevalence and anatomical patterns of intramuscular coronary arteries: a coronary computed tomography angiographic study. J Am Coll Cardiol 2007;49(5):587–93.

59. Zeina AR, Odeh M, Blinder J, et al. Myocardial bridge: evaluation on MDCT. AJR Am J Roentgenol 2007;188(4):1069–73.

60. Attar MN, Moore RK, Khan S. Twin circumflex arteries: a rare coronary artery anomaly. J Invasive Cardiol 2008;20(2):E54–5.

61. Bittner V, Nath HP, Cohen M, et al. Dual connection of the left anterior descending coronary artery to the left and right coronary arteries. Cathet Cardiovasc Diagn 1989;16(3):168–72.

62. Chang CJ, Cheng NJ, Ko YS, et al. Dual left anterior descending coronary artery and anomalous aortic origin of the left circumflex coronary artery: a rare and complicated anomaly. Am Heart J 1997;133(5):598–601.

63. Formica F, Corti F, Colombo V, et al. Dual left anterior descending coronary artery from right aortic sinus: report of a case of recurrent unstable angina after CABG. Heart Surg Forum 2005;8(5):E386–8.

64. Greenberg MA, Spindola-Franco H. Dual left anterior descending coronary artery (dual LAD). Cathet Cardiovasc Diagn 1994;31(3):250–3.

65. Harikrishnan S, Bhat A, Tharakan JM. Double right coronary artery. Int J Cardiol 2001;77(2-3):315–6.

66. Huang ZQ, Chen SJ, Chen J. Dual right coronary artery associated coronary artery fistula. Eur Heart J 2008;29(8):968.

67. Lemburg SP, Peters SA, Scheeler M, et al. Detection of a double right coronary artery with 16-row multidetector computed tomography. Int J Cardiovasc Imaging 2007;23(2):293–7.

68. Ozeren A, Aydin M, Bilge M, et al. Atherosclerotic double right coronary artery and ectasia of left coronary arteries in a patient with presented acute coronary syndrome and ventricular tachycardia. Int J Cardiol 2005;102(2):341–3.

69. Spindola-Franco H, Grose R, Solomon N. Dual left anterior descending coronary artery: angiographic description of important variants and surgical implications. Am Heart J 1983;105(3):445–55.

70. Timurkaynak T, Ciftci H, Cengel A. Double right coronary artery with atherosclerosis: a rare coronary artery anomaly. J Invasive Cardiol 2002;14(6):337–9.

71. Turhan H, Atak R, Erbay AR, et al. Double left anterior descending coronary artery arising from the left and right coronary arteries: a rare congenital coronary artery anomaly. Heart Vessels 2004;19(4):196–8.

72. Ozeren A, Aydin M, Bilge M, et al. Anomalous left coronary artery arising from the right sinus of Valsalva: a case report. Int J Cardiol 2005;101(3):491–3.

73. Gillebert C, Van Hoof R, Van de Werf F, et al. Coronary artery fistulas in an adult population. Eur Heart J 1986;7(5):437–43.

74. Vavuranakis M, Bush CA, Boudoulas H. Coronary artery fistulas in adults: incidence, angiographic characteristics, natural history. Cathet Cardiovasc Diagn 1995;35(2):116–20.

75. Nakamura M, Matsuoka H, Kawakami H, et al. Giant congenital coronary artery fistula to left brachial vein clearly detected by multidetector computed tomography. Circ J 2006;70(6):796–9.

76. Lin FC, Chang HJ, Chern MS, et al. Multiplane transesophageal echocardiography in the diagnosis of congenital coronary artery fistula. Am Heart J 1995;130(6):1236–44.

77. Voci G, Diego JN, Shafia H, et al. Type Ia tricuspid atresia with extensive coronary artery abnormalities in a living 22-year-old woman. J Am Coll Cardiol 1987;10(5):1100–4.

78. Linsenmeyer GJ 3rd, Schneider JF. Angiographically visible intercoronary collateral circulation in the absence of obstructive coronary artery disease. Am J Cardiol 1984;53(7):954–6.

79. Hines BA, Brandt PW, Agnew TM. Unusual intercoronary artery communication: a case report. Cardiovasc Intervent Radiol 1981;4(4):259–63.

80. Hudson CL, Moritz AR, Wearn JT. The extracardiac anastomoses of the coronary arteries. J Exp Med 1932;56(6):919–25.

81. St John Sutton MG, Miller GA, Kerr IH, et al. Coronary artery steal via large coronary artery to bronchial artery anastomosis successfully treated by operation. Br Heart J 1980;44(4):460–3.

82. Moritz AR, Hudson CL, Orgain ES. Augmentation of the extracardiac anastomoses of the coronary arteries through pericardial adhesions. J Exp Med 1932;56(6):927–31.

83. Basso C, Maron BJ, Corrado D, et al. Clinical profile of congenital coronary artery anomalies with origin from the wrong aortic sinus leading to sudden death in young competitive athletes. J Am Coll Cardiol 2000;35(6):1493–501.

84. Eckart RE, Scoville SL, Campbell CL, et al. Sudden death in young adults: a 25-year review of autopsies in military recruits. Ann Intern Med 2004; 141(11):829–34.

85. Virmani R, Burke AP, Farb A. The pathology of sudden cardiac death in athletes. chapter 15. In: Williams RA, editor. The athlete and heart disease: diagnosis, evaluation & management. Philadelphia: Lippincott Williams & Wilkins; 1999. p. 249–72.

86. Taylor AJ, Rogan KM, Virmani R. Sudden cardiac death associated with isolated congenital coronary artery anomalies. J Am Coll Cardiol 1992;20(3): 640–7.

87. Maron BJ, Shirani J, Poliac LC, et al. Sudden death in young competitive athletes. Clinical, demographic, and pathological profiles. JAMA 1996; 276(3):199–204.

88. Maron BJ, Thompson PD, Ackerman MJ, et al. Recommendations and considerations related to preparticipation screening for cardiovascular abnormalities in competitive athletes: 2007 update: a scientific statement from the American Heart Association Council on Nutrition, Physical Activity, and Metabolism: endorsed by the American College of Cardiology Foundation. Circulation 2007;115(12):1643–55.

89. Frommelt PC, Frommelt MA, Tweddell JS, et al. Prospective echocardiographic diagnosis and surgical repair of anomalous origin of a coronary artery from the opposite sinus with an interarterial course. J Am Coll Cardiol 2003;42(1):148–54.

90. Karagoz HY, Zorlutuna YI, Babacan KM, et al. Congenital coronary artery fistulas. Diagnostic and surgical considerations. Jpn Heart J 1989; 30(5):685–94.

91. Wesselhoeft H, Fawcett JS, Johnson AL. Anomalous origin of the left coronary artery from the pulmonary trunk. Its clinical spectrum, pathology, and pathophysiology, based on a review of 140 cases with seven further cases. Circulation 1968; 38(2):403–25.

92. Williams IA, Gersony WM, Hellenbrand WE. Anomalous right coronary artery arising from the pulmonary artery: a report of 7 cases and a review of the literature. Am Heart J 2006;152(5):1004. e1009–17.

93. Bland EF, White PD, Garland J. Congenital anomalies of the coronary arteries: report of an unusual case associated with cardiac hypertrophy. Am Heart J 1933;8:787–801.

94. Cheitlin MD, MacGregor J. Congenital anomalies of coronary arteries: role in the pathogenesis of sudden cardiac death. Herz 2009;34(4):268–79.

95. Syed M, Lesch M. Coronary artery aneurysm: a review. Prog Cardiovasc Dis 1997;40(1):77–84.

96. Cafferky EA, Crawford DW, Turner AF, et al. Congenital aneurysm of the coronary artery with myocardial infarction. Am J Med Sci 1969;257(5):320–7.

97. Kelley MP, Carver JR. Coronary artery aneurysms. J Invasive Cardiol 2002;14(8):461–2.

98. Rigatelli G. Coronary artery anomalies and superimposed coronary artery disease: intimate or simply coexisting? Minerva Cardioangiol 2004; 52(3):233–5.

99. Rigatelli G, Gemelli M, Zamboni A, et al. Are coronary artery anomalies an accelerating factor for coronary atherosclerosis development? Angiology 2004;55(1):29–35.

100. Page HL Jr, Engel HJ, Campbell WB, et al. Anomalous origin of the left circumflex coronary artery. Recognition, angiographic demonstration and clinical significance. Circulation 1974;50(4):768–73.

101. Sans-Coma V, Arque JM, Duran AC, et al. Coronary artery anomalies and bicuspid aortic valves in the Syrian hamster. Basic Res Cardiol 1991;86(2): 148–53.

102. Fernandez MC, Duran AC, Real R, et al. Coronary artery anomalies and aortic valve morphology in the Syrian hamster. Lab Anim 2000;34(2):145–54.

Evaluation of Plaques and Stenosis

Elisabeth Arnoldi, MD[a,b], Thomas Henzler, MD[a,c],
Gorka Bastarrika, MD, PhD[a,d], Christian Thilo, MD[a,e],
Konstantin Nikolaou, MD[b], U. Joseph Schoepf, MD[a,e],*

KEYWORDS
- Plaques • Stenosis • Coronary CT angiography
- Coronary artery disease

The evaluation of atherosclerotic plaques and stenosis in coronary arteries is the central element in the diagnosis of known or suspected coronary artery disease (CAD), and findings significantly influence the therapeutic management of the disease. Over the last decades, coronary CT angiography (cCTA) has advanced from research application to a widely used clinical tool in the detection of atherosclerotic lesions and grading of stenosis and, in certain clinical scenarios, is considered as a potential alternative to invasive methods in this respect. In this article, cCTA is discussed with regard to technical aspects on plaque imaging and stenosis grading, its relationship to myocardial perfusion imaging, its performance in comparison with invasive coronary angiography and intravascular ultrasound (IVUS), and, finally, its implications for patient management and outcome.

STENOSIS DETECTION AT CCTA—TECHNICAL ASPECTS
Basic Diagnostic Strategies

Owing to continuous advances in CT scanner technology, but also to technical refinements in image display and analysis tools of the acquired scans, coronary cCTA has evolved to a fast, robust, and accurate method of diagnosing CAD in clinical routine.[1–6] Despite the increased availability of computer-based visualization tools and the usefulness of automated postprocessed images, evaluation of the individual unprocessed source images in the transverse plane in each case remains indispensable. Review of the original transverse sections may yield the richest information on atherosclerotic plaque formation within the vessel wall of the coronary arteries, so that findings on these images are fundamental for a solid diagnosis.

As a first step in the diagnostic process of a cCTA study for suspected coronary artery stenosis, therefore, it is recommended to display the coronary arteries in the transverse source images and to examine the four main vessels (LM, LAD, RCA, and LCX) and their side branches individually for presence, location, and composition (calcified, noncalcified or mixed) of atherosclerotic lesions (**Fig. 1**).[7] From these images, additionally, valuable information can be obtained on the consequences of ischemic disease on the

UJS is a medical consultant for and receives research support from Bayer-Schering, Bracco, General Electric, Medrad, and Siemens.

a Department of Radiology and Radiological Science, Medical University of South Carolina, Ashley River Tower, 25 Courtenay Drive, Charleston, SC 29401, USA
b Department of Clinical Radiology, University Hospitals Munich—Grosshadern Campus, Ludwig-Maximilians University, Marchioninistrasse 15, 81377 Munich, Germany
c Department of Clinical Radiology and Nuclear Medicine, University Medical Center Mannheim, Medical Faculty Mannheim-Heidelberg University, Theodor-Kutzer-Ufer 1-3, 68167 Mannheim, Germany
d Department of Radiology, University of Navarra, Avenida Pío XII 36, 31008 Pamplona, Spain
e Division of Cardiology, Department of Medicine, Medical University of South Carolina, 25 Courtenay Drive, Charleston, SC 29401, USA
* Corresponding author. Department of Radiology and Radiological Science, Medical University of South Carolina, Ashley River Tower, 25 Courtenay Drive, MSC 226, Charleston, SC 29401.
E-mail address: schoepf@musc.edu

Radiol Clin N Am 48 (2010) 729–744
doi:10.1016/j.rcl.2010.05.002

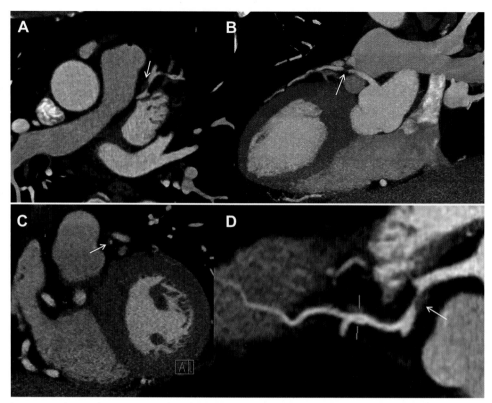

Fig. 1. Contrast-enhanced retrospectively ECG-gated cCTA study of a 52-year-old man with acute chest pain. Display as transverse images (*A*), coronal (*B*) and sagittal (*C*) MPR, and MIP (*D*), show stenosis (*arrow*) in the proximal LAD caused by exclusively non-calcified plaque.

myocardium, such as myocardial perfusion deficits or thinning of the ventricular wall subsequent to myocardial infarction.

As a secondary tool for data viewing and estimation of stenosis severity of detected lesions, maximum intensity projections (MIPs)[8] and multiplanar reformations (MPRs) are widely used and easy-to-perform visualization tools, both being available on most CT scanners.[9–12] MIPs and MPRs enable views of the coronary arteries from different angles and perspectives, and thus help to correctly assess the degree of luminal narrowing in atherosclerotic vessels. With the use of MIPs a more comprehensive and condensed display of the data in a few relevant sections or views can be achieved, so that CT data is presented to the reader in a more intuitive fashion. For routine visualization of large-volume cCTA data sets, many centers perform three dedicated MIP reconstructions to create views of the left and right coronary arteries and of the entire coronary arterial tree from a cranio-oblique perspective ("spider view").[9,10] With the application of MPR as another basic tool for secondary data visualization, image data can be rearranged in arbitrary imaging planes, for instance from a coronal or sagittal view.[12] Based on the high spatial resolution of current scanner generations allowing image acquisitions with isotropic or near isotropic voxels, these reconstructions offer similar image quality as the transverse source images. In addition to the computer-generated MPRs, the manual creation of curved MPRs following the course of the individual vessel can be opted for. However, the utility of this application in clinical routine is limited because its performance is rather cumbersome and operator-dependent.

In contrast to MIPs and MPRs, three-dimensional (3D) volume rendering display of the CT data[13,14] has little diagnostic value in the assessment of atherosclerotic lesions because individual plaques are frequently obscured or overestimated. On the other hand, 3D display of the coronary arteries may depict the anatomy of tortuous vessels or provide evidence on the overall presence of heavy calcifications and vessel remodeling. Yet, in practice, 3D postprocessing is mainly used to intuitively communicate findings to nonradiologists and does not play an essential role in the actual diagnostic process.

Advanced Visualization and Automated Stenosis Detection Tools

With increased availability and user-friendliness of advanced software tools, viewing and analysis of large-volume CT angiography data has been facilitated to a great extent. Dedicated software algorithms allow automated extraction and segmentation of the coronary artery tree from the contrast-enhanced CT data set, and help to enhance diagnosis, particularly in more complicated cases, for instance, with presence of extensive vessel calcifications. With the help of an automatically generated MPR, the entire artery can be visualized in an intuitive fashion as an unraveled and stretched reformation of the vessel or as cross-sectional reconstructions.

Additionally, on most software platforms, computer-based stenosis-grading tools for the quantitative evaluation of stenosis severity are available. This application allows the measurement of the cross-sectional diameter or area of the residual perfused lumen of the diseased vessel segment, and the grading of stenosis by calculating luminal reduction of the diseased vessel segment in comparison to a nondiseased part of the vessel proximally and distally to the stenosis (**Fig. 2**). Although this approach of computer-based evaluation may offer a more standardized estimation, the validity of the results based on automated assessment algorithms is subject to image quality and spatial resolution of the original scan acquisition, as well as to general limitations

of CT angiography in assessing stenosis severity. Therefore, measurements obtained with vessel analysis tools cannot be trusted blindly and have to be evaluated by experienced cardiac radiologists in context with the findings on the original data sets and the patient's clinical presentation.

A recent investigation reported on the initial experience of a computer-aided algorithm for fully automated, without human interaction software tool in a clinical setting.[15] In a study population of 47 patients, the algorithm showed overall good performance with 74%/100% sensitivity and 83%/65% specificity for diagnosing greater than or equal to 50% stenosis on a per vessel/per patient analysis, respectively, with quantitative coronary angiography as the reference standard (**Fig. 3**). The remarkably high negative predictive value of 94%/100% in this initial study suggests that the algorithm may be suitable for aiding the exclusion of significant coronary artery stenosis based on a normal or near-normal study. Future studies are warranted to further evaluate the potential usefulness of the algorithm, for instance, as a second reader in a learning process to confidently rule out significant stenosis, particularly in a patient population with low likelihood of disease.

STENOSIS AT CCTA—RELATIONSHIP WITH MYOCARDIAL PERFUSION IMAGING

Myocardial perfusion imaging using single photon emission CT (SPECT) scanning holds a key position in the risk stratification of patients with known

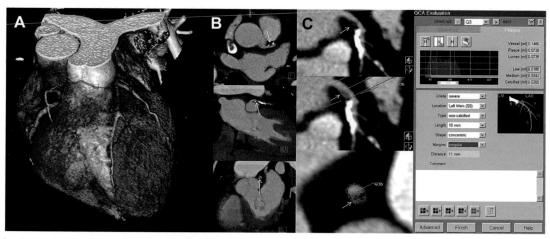

Fig. 2. Contrast-enhanced prospectively ECG-triggered cCTA study of a 64-year-old man with atypical chest pain. (*A*) Automated removing of the chest wall enables an unobstructed view of the heart as a 3D volume rendering, from the extraction of the coronary arteries can be performed individually. (*B*) The extracted coronary artery is depicted on an automatically generated MPR, which facilitates intuitive visualization of the entire vessel. (*C*) With the use of stenosis-grading tools, stenosis severity can be quantitatively evaluated. The measurement is performed by calculation of the luminal area of the diseased vessel segment in comparison to the areas of a nondiseased part of the vessel proximally and distally to the stenosis.

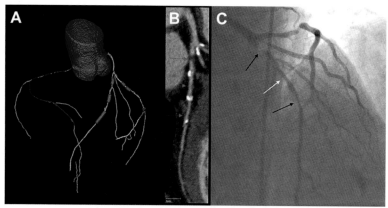

Fig. 3. Contrast-enhanced dual source cCTA study of a 46-year-old man. (*A*) In the automated 3D depiction of the coronary artery three red detection marks in LAD and LCX indicate sites of significant stenosis. (*B*) The stretched reconstruction of the LAD by the algorithm indicates significant stenoses in proximal LAD (1) and mid-LAD (2) (*red arrows*). (*C*) Invasive coronary angiography (LAO view) confirms high-grade stenosis in proximal LAD and significant stenosis in mid-LAD (*black arrows*). The proximal lesion in mid-LAD is nonsignificant (*white arrow*).

or suspected CAD.[16–20] Whereas patients with limiting angina are usually directly referred to invasive angiography for potential revascularization, in asymptomatic patients or patients with mild symptoms, nuclear perfusion imaging can be used to identify those patients who may benefit from further invasive assessment by classifying them according to their estimated risk for cardiac mortality.[18,19]

With ongoing developments in CT technology and more wide-spread use of cardiac CT, many clinicians and imagers believe that in certain clinical scenarios cCTA may replace nuclear perfusion imaging and has the potential to become the gatekeeper to the catheterization laboratory.[21] In this context, efforts are underway to correlate information on the presence of stenosis and perfusion deficits in CT and SPECT. Several studies evaluated the relationship between stenosis at cCTA and myocardial perfusion defects at nuclear imaging, and their results showed poor correlation between the findings of the two modalities.[22–24] For comparison of cCTA findings of significant stenosis defined as 50% or greater luminal narrowing with myocardial perfusion deficits seen on SPECT, the investigators report sensitivity values in the range of 85% to 95% and specificity values between 53% and 79%.[22,23] In the study by Nicol and colleagues,[24] the investigators found that the agreement between the two modalities increased to 96% on the basis of a threshold of 70% or greater stenosis on cCTA.

Taking into account the different nature of the two tests and the known variability in the hemodynamic effect of stenotic lesions on myocardial perfusion,[25] however, a valid direct comparison between the findings of the two modalities is a priori precluded. Whereas nuclear perfusion studies aim at evaluating the myocardial blood supply and thus provide information on physiologic conditions, cCTA as a foremost morphologic test enables the evaluation of anatomy by depicting the coronary vessel lumen and vessel wall. In this sense, cCTA serves to detect coronary artery stenosis, whereas nuclear perfusion imaging assesses their hemodynamic effect. However, there is evidence of an incremental diagnostic value of image fusion of nuclear imaging and cCTA over either method alone,[26,27] which shows that clearly the combination of morphologic evaluation and physiologic assessment is needed in the integrative diagnostic work-up of CAD.

With the ultimate goal of an integrative assessment of ischemic heart disease with regard to morphology and function in a single imaging modality, recently, investigators have renewed their research on CT for its potential in detection of myocardial ischemia. Whereas few early studies on human application using single-source CT suggest that analysis of ischemia and infarct generally is feasible with CT,[28,29] current research focuses on investigating dual-energy CT for its usefulness in myocardial perfusion imaging. Early evidence of a recent study on this matter suggests that dual-energy CT may allow analysis of iodine distribution as a surrogate for the myocardial blood pool and may be able to detect myocardial perfusion deficits in good correlation with [99m]-Tc-Sestamibi-SPECT as the reference standard (**Fig. 4**).[30]

Few studies have explored the use of arterial-phase stress adenosine multislice spiral CT for

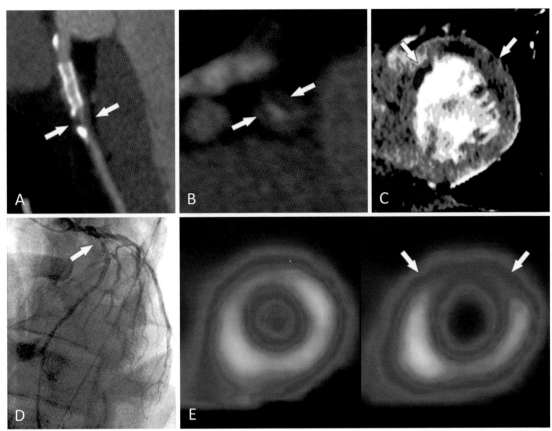

Fig. 4. Contrast-enhanced retrospectively ECG-study in a 58-year-old man with prior history of stenting in the proximal LAD and atypical chest pain. (*A, B*) Curved multiplanar and cross-sectional reconstructions of the CT scan show a patent stent in the proximal LAD with a high-grade stenosis distally to the stent due to a noncalcified plaque. (*C*) Dual-energy mode reveals an area lacking iodine in the anterior wall of the left ventricle suggestive of myocardial perfusion deficit. (*D*) Invasive angiography (RAO view) confirms significant stenosis in the proximal LAD. (*E*) Nuclear perfusion imaging during rest (*left*) and stress (*right*) shows a reversible perfusion deficit in the anterior wall during stress, which correlates well to finding in CT scan.

detection of reversible myocardial perfusion deficits.[31–33] Although early results are promising, further investigations in human application and standardization of measurements is needed to confirm the validity and reproducibility of this method. Recently, in a clinical setting, George and colleagues[34] performed cCTA scans on 40 patients with abnormal SPECT findings and correlated CT angiography and rest-stress CT myocardial perfusion imaging for detection of hemodynamically significant stenosis. In this initial experience, the investigators report sensitivity and specificity values of 86% and 92%, respectively, with 92% positive predictive value and 85% negative predictive value on a per patient level. In the analysis on a per vessel basis similar results were found with sensitivity and specificity values of 79% and 91%, respectively, and 75% PPV and 92% NPV. However, radiation exposure was relatively high with 17 and 21 mSv for stress and

combined rest and stress imaging, respectively. Further testing is warranted to verify the validity of these early results and evaluate the benefit of this method over established procedures.

STENOSIS DETECTION WITH CCTA—COMPARISON WITH INVASIVE CORONARY ANGIOGRAPHY

In the early 2000s, initial studies using 4- and 16-slice CT scanners demonstrated the potential usefulness of cCTA for the noninvasive diagnosis of CAD.[1,2,35,36] Early evidence of these studies suggested that cCTA may allow the visualization of the coronary artery lumen and the vessel wall, and thus may be able to detect significant stenosis of the coronary arteries in patients suspected of having CAD. Results of these early investigations showed values of sensitivity, specificity, positive predictive value, and negative predictive value of

75% to 90%, 90% to 95%, 70% to 90%, and 80% to 90%, respectively, for the detection of hemodynamically relevant stenosis, indicating overall good correlation with the reference standard invasive coronary angiography.[10,36–38] However, these analyses did not adequately reflect the true diagnostic performance of cCTA using 4- and 16-slice CT scanners, as they were restricted to assessable portions of vessels.[11,36] Other coronary artery segments, vessels, and patients needed to be excluded from evaluation due to motion artifacts and blooming artifacts of heavy calcifications. More systematic meta-analyses reported a pooled sensitivity in the range of 85% to 92% for the performance of cCTA for the detection of any stenosis, concluding that cCTA performed with the present scanner generations may not be sufficient to reliably rule out significant stenosis.[39,40]

The subsequent introduction of 64-slice CT with its markedly improved spatial and temporal resolution over preceding scanner generations hallmarked the advance of cCTA to a robust and accurate tool for the assessment of CAD in clinical routine. Numerous studies have evaluated 64-slice cCTA for the detection of coronary artery stenosis in comparison with invasive coronary angiography and consistently report high accuracy (**Table 1**).[3,6,41–52] With the exception of a single recent study that showed lower sensitivity than specificity (85% sensitivity, 90% specificity, 91% positive predictive value, 83% negative predictive value),[53] all investigations report high values of sensitivity and specificity in the range of 86% to 99% and 92% to 98%, respectively (**Figs. 5 and 6**). Most important for clinical practice is the high negative predictive value of this test of up to 100%, indicating that cCTA can reliably exclude significant stenosis. Accordingly, current guidelines

consider the appropriate use of cCTA in excluding significant coronary artery stenosis based on a normal or near-normal CT study in low and intermediate likelihood patients.[54] Based on this application, cCTA has become a important cornerstone in the decision-making of further management of symptomatic patients suspected of CAD.

Despite considerable advances in CT technology, two major problems remain significant drawbacks of cCTA compared with invasive catheter angiography in the diagnosis of coronary artery stenosis. First, the assessment of small distal vessels is still limited owing to motion-related blurring and partial-volume effects and, second, dense calcifications in atherosclerotic vessels hinder the exact grading of stenosis.[6] In this respect, more recently, studies using dual-energy CT technology reported promising results.[55,56] In ex vivo studies, Boll and colleagues[55,56] succeeded in reducing blooming artifacts from extensively calcified plaques and metallic stent struts with the use of dual-energy CT. In an in vivo study using dual-energy CT, Johnson and colleagues[3] reported a decreased share of nonassessable coronary artery segments of only 2%, compared with 3% to 17% of segments rated as nondiagnostic in 64-slice CT studies. Additionally, with its high temporal resolution dual-energy CT proved diagnostic image quality in smaller, distal vessels, and showed robustness in the examination of patients with higher heart rates and controlled atrial fibrillation.

However, accuracy of cCTA remains limited with the presence of heavy vessel calcifications and in patients with high and irregular heart rates or obese patients, leading to inconclusive results of the examination.[6,41] In these patients, further evaluation with noninvasive testing is necessary

Table 1
Coronary artery stenosis compared with invasive coronary angiography studies

Author	Scanner Type	Number of Patients	Sensitivity (%)	Specificity (%)	Positive Predictive Value (%)	Negative Predictive Value (%)
Raff et al[6]	64-MDCT	70	86	95	66	98
Leschka et al[45]	64-MDCT	67	94	97	87	99
Mollet et al[47]	64-MDCT	51	99	95	76	99
Fine et al[43]	64-MDCT	66	95	96	97	92
Ropers et al[50]	64-MDCT	81	93	97	56	100
Ehara et al[42]	64-MDCT	69	90	94	89	95
Ong et al[49]	64-MDCT	134	82	96	79	96
Oncel et al[48]	64-MDCT	80	96	98	91	99
Meijboom et al[46]	64-MDCT	360	88	90	47	99

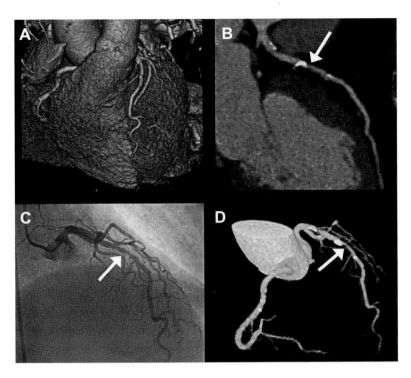

Fig. 5. Contrast-enhanced cCTA study using dual-source CT in a 65-year-old woman with stress angina. (*A*) Volume-rendered image allows 3D visualization of the heart and the coronary vessel course. (*B*) Curved multiplanar reformation of the left anterior descending artery shows moderate stenosis (*arrow*) due to soft plaque. (*C*) Invasive coronary angiography (RAO view) confirms stenotic lesion (*arrow*). (*D*) Corresponding reconstruction of the coronary artery tree in volume rendering technique allows 3D visualization of location and volume of the atherosclerotic lesion (*arrow*). (*From* Johnson TR, Nikolaou K, Busch S, et al. Diagnostic accuracy of dual-source computed tomography in the diagnosis of coronary artery disease. Invest Radiol 2007;42:684–91; with permission.)

to assess potential atherosclerotic lesions for their hemodynamic significance. On the other hand, cCTA has been shown to tend to overestimate the degree of coronary stenosis compared with invasive coronary angiography, which means that invasive angiography can be performed with a solid indication and the option to treat significant lesions.[3] With ongoing developments in CT technology, such as further improvements in temporal resolution and detector materials, as well as more refined postprocessing techniques and innovative computer-aided tools for stenosis detection and assessment, cCTA can be expected to further advance in robustness and accuracy with an even wider scope of clinical utility in future.

CT IMAGING OF CORONARY PLAQUES—TECHNICAL ASPECTS

For adequate visualization of the coronary arterial vessel wall in CT, the two major technical challenges are sufficient spatial and temporal resolution. The diameter of the coronary arteries varies between 1 to 5 mm, and the pathologic changes along the vessel course can be subtle. Therefore, to visualize the small, tortuous, and complex anatomy of the coronary arteries, isotropic, or near isotropic in-plane and through-plane resolutions are necessary (**Fig. 7**). Given the spatial resolution of 64-slice to 256-slice detectors of

0.3 to 0.35 mm voxel sizes, limitations in resolution are inevitable. Thus, important plaque components, such as the fibrous cap which may measure less than 0.07 mm thickness in vulnerable plaque, will not be clearly identified. However, two specific features of vulnerable plaques illustrate some of the analysis problems. First, they are typically located in proximal, larger-sized coronary arteries[57] and, second, they usually fill more than 50% of the vascular cross-sectional area and are often associated with positive remodeling.[58]

With regard to temporal resolution, for most practical purposes a heart rate independent temporal resolution of 100 ms or less allows elimination of cardiac motion, if images are acquired (prospective triggering) or reconstructed (retrospective gating) during mid-diastole as a time point with the least cardiac motion. In high heart rates or for improved visualization of the right coronary artery, it has been shown that a reconstruction window in systole may be more advantageous.[59,60] In addition to the factors mentioned above, contrast enhancement,[61] presence of heavy calcifications, or metal stents causing blooming artifacts[36] may influence accessibility of the coronary vessels.

As will be discussed, cCTA permits the visualization of nonstenotic plaque, both noncalcified and calcified. However, to date, the ability of CT

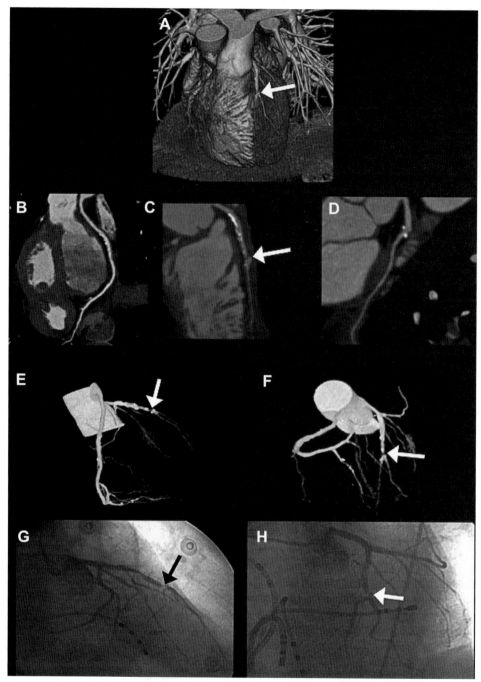

Fig. 6. Contrast-enhanced cCTA study using dual-source CT scan in a 68-year-old man with typical angina. (*A*) Volume-rendered image suggests eccentric plaque in the LAD. Curved multiplanar reformation of the RCA (*B*), the LAD (*C*), and the LCx (*D*) show focal calcifications and a high-grade, noncalcified stenosis (*arrows*) of the LAD. Corresponding reconstruction of the coronary artery tree in volume rendering technique in RAO (*E*) and LAO (*F*) show high-grade stenosis of the LAD. Corresponding projections of the invasive coronary angiography (RAO [*G*] and LAO [*H*] view) confirm stenotic lesion (*arrows*). (*From* Johnson TR, Nikolaou K, Busch S, et al. Diagnostic accuracy of dual-source computed tomography in the diagnosis of coronary artery disease. Invest Radiol 2007;42:684–91; with permission.)

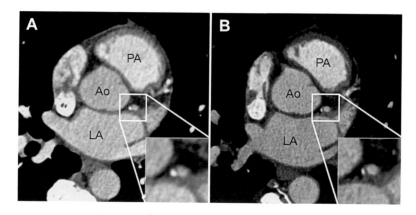

Fig. 7. Contrast-enhanced cCTA study shows mixed plaque in the proximal LAD. Compared with study performed on a 4-slice CT scanner with a spatial resolution of 1 mm (*A*), image quality and visualization of the atherosclerotic lesion is improved using dual-source CT scan (*B*) offering a spatial resolution of 0.4 mm.

scanning to quantify the size and volume of plaque is limited, with noncalcified and mixed plaques showing a tendency of being systematically underestimated; whereas calcified plaques tend to be overestimated.[62] The evaluation of plaque size or, rather, the degree of luminal narrowing caused by the atherosclerotic lesion can be performed visually, semiquantitatively (**Fig. 8**), or with the use of software tools that allow a computer-based quantification of stenosis (see **Fig. 2**). Busch and colleagues[63] performed cCTA on 23 patients and evaluated the data set for significant stenosis with the help of a software tool. They found 89% sensitivity, 100% specificity, and 89% positive predictive value, and 100% negative predictive value of significant area stenosis greater than 75%, indicating that automated quantitative assessment of stenosis is feasible with good correlation with invasive quantitative angiography. Technically, quantitative coronary angiography is

based on an automated segmentation of the coronary tree, which can be assisted manually if necessary. Each main and side vessel is than examined on curved MPRs in longitudinal rotation for stenosis. Stenosis is quantified by calculation of the diameter or area (the latter allows easier comparison with invasive angiography) and comparison of the measurement to the diameter or area distally and proximally of the stenosis in the closest healthy vessel segment. Subsequently, a threshold of attenuation value for the perfused lumen is set. Despite the evidence of practical usefulness and increased objectivity of this approach in comparison to sole visual assessment, the method has limitations. With presence of diffuse ischemic disease, healthy vessel segments of comparable luminal size may not be available. Moreover, future studies in clinical settings to improve standardization with regard to the adequate threshold of attenuation value

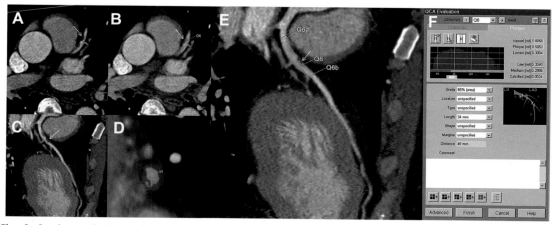

Fig. 8. Semi-quantitative volumetry of non-calcified plaques (*arrows*) detected on axial images of contrast-enhanced CT study (*A* and *B*) and visualized on MIP (*C*) can be performed on offline workstations (Leonardo, Siemens Medical Solutions, Germany). The soft plaque borders are segmented by hand (*D*), while the software measures plaque volume automatically according to predefined thresholds (*E*).

are warranted to improve robustness and reproducibility of these findings.

CT IMAGING OF CORONARY
PLAQUES—COMPARISON WITH IVUS

Detection, characterization, and quantification of
coronary artery atherosclerotic plaque may be
useful in individualized risk stratification as well as
to monitor the course of disease and to illustrate
the effect of drug therapies. Of several invasive
and noninvasive diagnostic techniques for the evaluation of the coronary artery vessel wall, IVUS
remains the standard of reference in this respect.[64]
The advantages of IVUS originate principally from
two key features, its tomographic perspective
and its ability to directly image the vessel wall,
which allows precise measurement of lumen area
and plaque size, distribution, and, to some extent,
composition. However, in clinical practice, the
application of IVUS is limited due to its invasive
and cost-intensive nature. Furthermore, although
IVUS is accurate in determining the thickness and
echogenicity of vessel wall structures, it is not
consistently able to provide histology.[64] Finally,
artifacts may adversely affect ultrasound images
and may hamper correct visual interpretation.

Although MR coronary angiography has shown
potential for accurate noninvasive characterization
of tissue composition and vessel wall structure,[65]
its application is limited in spatial resolution and, to
date, remains reserved for research applications.

With the early multidetector computed tomography (MDCT) scanner generations (4- and
16-slice) contrast-enhanced cCTA has been investigated for its potential in the detection and classification of coronary plaques and assessment of
vessel remodeling.[66–68] In these studies, the ability
of MDCT to visualize the coronary artery wall and
to delineate calcified and noncalcified plaques
has been demonstrated (**Fig. 9**). In an early study
using 4-slice MDCT, Kopp and colleagues[67]
showed that MDCT may allow one to clearly differentiate and classify plaque morphology according
to the IVUS results by determining tissue density
within the lesions. Based on 16-slice MDCT,
Achenbach and colleagues[69] reported sensitivity
and specificity values of 82% and 88% for the
detection of segments with any plaque, and sensitivity and specificity values of 78% and 87% for the
detection of segments containing noncalcified plaques. In comparison to IVUS, the investigators
found that in CT the plaque burden was underestimated and detection rate was lower for smaller
plaques. A more recent report suggests that 64-
slice MDCT with improved spatial and temporal
resolution offers more accurate evaluation of the

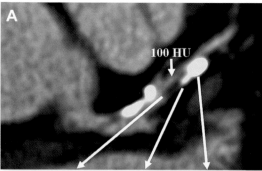
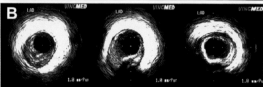

Fig. 9. (*A*) MDCT using MIP reconstruction shows
mixed fibrocalcified plaque in the proximal LAD
with fibrous plaque area (*arrow*, 100 HU) next to
significant calcifications. (*B*) IVUS images in cross-
sectional views along the course of the plaque,
moving from the noncalcified, fibrous plaque area
(*left*) toward the calcifications (*middle* and *right*).
(*From* Nikolaou K, Becker C, Fayad Z. Multidetector-
row CT vs magnetic resonance imaging for coronary
plaque characterization. In: Schoepf UJ, ed. CT of
the heart. New York: Humana Press; 2005. p. 389–98;
with permission.[91])

coronary atherosclerotic plaque burden.[70] Leber
and colleagues[70] reported sensitivity values of
90% for detection of any plaque and 83% for noncalcified plaques. However, the investigators
admit that exact plaque quantification remains
challenging as technical restrictions and influ-
ences of contrast-enhancement[71] still prevent an
exact separation of lumen, plaque, and vessel
wall. It currently seems difficult to define thresholds that would allow accurate automated or semi-
automated edge detection, which results in high
interobserver variability for 64-slice CT measurements and an only moderate concordance to
IVUS measurements.

With the use of a plaque analysis algorithm in
cCTA studies, Sun and colleagues[72] found sensitivity and specificity values of 97% and 90% for
detection of coronary plaques in comparison
with IVUS. The investigators conclude that this
software tool may be able to more reliably depict
contrast-enhanced lumen, vessel wall, and plaque
composition, and thus may allow a more accurate
detection, quantification, and morphologic analysis of plaques, whereas they admit that the
reliable differentiation of the composition of individual noncalcified plaques is still limited.

Beyond the detection of coronary atherosclerotic lesions, the accurate characterization of plaques is important to identify atheromas at risk of rupture. Plaques with high lipid content and a thin fibrous cap have been shown to be more vulnerable and associated with acute coronary syndromes. Likewise, positive remodeling has been associated with an unstable clinical presentation, whereas calcified plaques and negative remodeling are thought to be associated with more stable clinical conditions. In this context, Galonska and colleagues[73] evaluated atherosclerotic plaques of coronary arteries of isolated hearts ex vivo and compared the plaque attenuation profiles with the corresponding histopathologic sections of the vessels. Calcified plaques showed attenuation values between 333 Hounsfield Units (HU) to 1944 HU, whereas noncalcified plaques had attenuation values between 26 HU and 124 HU (see **Fig. 9**). In a further evaluation of the noncalcified plaques, the investigators found attenuation values of 26 HU to 67 HU for lipid-rich plaques with a necrotic core and 37 HU to 124 HU for fibrous plaques. However, limited spatial resolution of MDCT scanners still prohibits reliable analysis of all atherosclerotic plaque components and significant overlap may be found between different tissues, especially between lipid and fibrous components. Leber and colleagues[62] found that MDCT enabled the visualization of lipid pools in 7 of 10 (70%) sections in comparison with IVUS, yet admit limitations to these encouraging results: as the sensitivity of IVUS to detect lipid pools is limited to 50% to 75% and all lipid pools were located in large proximal segments, it has to be assumed that the true accuracy is lower than observed in their study. On the other hand, because of high CT attenuation of calcified lesions, their differentiation from fibrous and lipid-rich lesions is easy.

Whereas ongoing advances in MDCT technology and development of software tools seem to hold promise for more accurate detection, quantification, and characterization of atherosclerotic plaques using cCTA, the clinical application of plaque imaging needs to be kept in mind. Rather than the identification of the vulnerable plaque, which may lead to preemptive stenting, the identification of the vulnerable patient who might benefit from more aggressive risk modification should be the foremost goal.

ATHEROSCLEROTIC PLAQUES AND STENOSIS AT CCTA—IMPLICATIONS FOR PATIENT MANAGEMENT AND OUTCOMES
Role of cCTA in CAD Management

According to the current recommendations for the appropriate use of cardiac CT, the performance of

cCTA is indicated in symptomatic patients with low-to-intermediate likelihood of CAD.[54] Thus cCTA may replace invasive angiography as a diagnostic tool in selected patient populations. In the therapeutic management of patients with CAD, however, until recently interventional or surgical revascularization have been considered as the core treatment to improve patient outcome. Numerous studies have attempted to assess which of the two revascularization procedures should be chosen with regard to patient outcome with controversy results.[74–78] Based on these studies, apparently, the aspired benefits in terms of improved symptoms and prognosis need to be outweighed against the associated risks of the procedure in each individual case.

However, with the availability of more refined and potent pharmaceutical agents, the paradigm of medical therapy as the basis of optimal CAD management is increasingly gaining support. In a large trial, Clinical Outcomes Utilizing Revascularization and Aggressive Drug Evaluation (COURAGE),[79] and preceding studies[80–82] there is growing evidence that the outcome of patients with stable angina does not differ with optimal medical treatment compared with percutaneous coronary intervention. Although the design and conclusions of these investigations have been queried,[83,84] there is evidence that the notion of medical therapy as the central component in the management of CAD becomes more appreciated. There are ongoing investigations on successful primary and secondary prevention and improvements in screening and risk stratification with optimal medical therapy. Furthermore, the development of new markers for CAD as well as the reevaluation of calcium scoring as a disease predictor has become a focus of recent research. Lastly, the trend toward less invasive disease management is reflected in current statistics showing a slower growth or, even, decline of coronary artery stent-placement procedures.[85] In this context, in future, the role of cCTA as the only noninvasive modality for assessment of the entire coronary atherosclerotic plaque burden and plaque classification may need to be redefined with regard to a comprehensive risk stratification and modulation of disease management in the individual patient.

However, it needs to be emphasized that on the basis of current evidence, cCTA is not applicable in asymptomatic subjects for screening or risk management.[54] Even if these patients would be considered at high risk for disease on the basis of other, for example clinical factors, contrast administration and radiation exposure associated with cCTA can hardly be justified in asymptomatic individuals. Whether further advances in CT technology may make scanning in asymptomatic patients amenable will need to be determined.

Implication of cCTA on Patient Outcome

Recently, based on the evidence of the clinical utility of cCTA as a robust, noninvasive, and accurate tool in diagnosing CAD and its increasingly widespread use, numerous investigations have focused on the evaluation of patient outcomes and the prognostic value of this test. Results of these studies suggest that extent and severity of CAD defined at cCTA is associated with an higher risk for a worse outcome. In a consecutive study of more than 1000 symptomatic patients, individuals could be classified as patients with increased all-cause mortality based on CT markers for CAD on cCTA in contrast to patients with excellent prognosis based on a normal cCTA study.[86] However, similar findings in a smaller study population of 100 patients have been reported by Pundziute and colleagues.[87] They found that presence of disease markers in CT were closely related to the occurrence of major cardiac events, whereas negative test results confirmed low risk.

The clinical value of the high negative predictive value of cCTA for the safety of ruling out significant stenosis was confirmed in two studies proving safe patient management based solely on the findings of cCTA with reduction of invasive angiography procedures.[88,89] Also, in another study comparing CT with other noninvasive modalities such as SPECT, clinical outcomes of patients did not differ in a 9-month follow-up.[90] However, the available studies show substantial heterogeneity in study design, populations, and the limited number of outcome events is partly associated with imprecision of the individual risk estimates. Therefore, a more systematic data analysis is strongly warranted to correctly estimate the predictive value of cCTA. Furthermore, with respect to comparability and pooling of outcome data, further research is needed to find a reliable and simple approach to quantify the presence and extent and composition of CAD burden by cCTA. Also, the relationship of calcium scoring to disease markers in cCTA needs to be re-evaluated, to determine whether the risk estimate for significant stenosis depends on calcium score.

REFERENCES

1. Achenbach S, Ulzheimer S, Baum U, et al. Noninvasive coronary angiography by retrospectively ECG-gated multislice spiral CT. Circulation 2000;102:2823–8.

2. Hoffmann MH, Shi H, Schmitz BL, et al. Noninvasive coronary angiography with multislice computed tomography. JAMA 2005;293:2471–8.

3. Johnson TR, Nikolaou K, Busch S, et al. Diagnostic accuracy of dual-source computed tomography in the diagnosis of coronary artery disease. Invest Radiol 2007;42:684–91.

4. Kuettner A, Beck T, Drosch T, et al. Diagnostic accuracy of noninvasive coronary imaging using 16-detector slice spiral computed tomography with 188 ms temporal resolution. J Am Coll Cardiol 2005;45:123–7.

5. Ohnesorge B, Flohr T, Becker C, et al. Cardiac imaging by means of electrocardiographically gated multisection spiral CT: initial experience. Radiology 2000;217:564–71.

6. Raff GL, Gallagher MJ, O'Neill WW, et al. Diagnostic accuracy of noninvasive coronary angiography using 64-slice spiral computed tomography. J Am Coll Cardiol 2005;46:552–7.

7. Vogl TJ, Abolmaali ND, Diebold T, et al. Techniques for the detection of coronary atherosclerosis: multidetector row CT coronary angiography. Radiology 2002;223:212–20.

8. Napel S, Marks MP, Rubin GD, et al. CT angiography with spiral CT and maximum intensity projection. Radiology 1992;185:607–10.

9. Becker CR, Knez A, Leber A, et al. Detection of coronary artery stenoses with multislice helical CT angiography. J Comput Assist Tomogr 2002;26:750–5.

10. Becker CR, Ohnesorge BM, Schoepf UJ, et al. Current development of cardiac imaging with multidetector-row CT. Eur J Radiol 2000;36:97–103.

11. Nieman K, Cademartiri F, Lemos PA, et al. Reliable noninvasive coronary angiography with fast submillimeter multislice spiral computed tomography. Circulation 2002;106:2051–4.

12. Ropers D, Baum U, Pohle K, et al. Detection of coronary artery stenoses with thin-slice multi-detector row spiral computed tomography and multiplanar reconstruction. Circulation 2003;107:664–6.

13. Lawler LP, Fishman EK. Multi-detector row CT of thoracic disease with emphasis on 3D volume rendering and CT angiography. Radiographics 2001;21:1257–73.

14. van Ooijen PM, van Geuns RJ, Rensing BJ, et al. Noninvasive coronary imaging using electron beam CT: surface rendering versus volume rendering. AJR Am J Roentgenol 2003;180:223–6.

15. Arnoldi E, Gebregziabher M, Schoepf UJ, et al. Automated computer-aided stenosis detection at coronary CT angiography: initial experience. Eur Radiol 2010;20(5):1160–7.

16. Berman DS, Hachamovitch R, Kiat H, et al. Incremental value of prognostic testing in patients with known or suspected ischemic heart disease: a basis

for optimal utilization of exercise technetium-99m sestamibi myocardial perfusion single-photon emission computed tomography. J Am Coll Cardiol 1995; 26:639–47.

17. Hachamovitch R, Berman DS, Kiat H, et al. Exercise myocardial perfusion SPECT in patients without known coronary artery disease: incremental prognostic value and use in risk stratification. Circulation 1996;93:905–14.

18. Klocke FJ, Baird MG, Lorell BH, et al. ACC/AHA/ASNC guidelines for the clinical use of cardiac radionuclide imaging—executive summary: a report of the American College of Cardiology/American Heart Association Task Force on Practice Guidelines (ACC/AHA/ASNC Committee to Revise the 1995 Guidelines for the Clinical Use of Cardiac Radionuclide Imaging). J Am Coll Cardiol 2003; 42:1318–33.

19. Klocke FJ, Baird MG, Lorell BH, et al. ACC/AHA/ASNC guidelines for the clinical use of cardiac radionuclide imaging—executive summary: a report of the American College of Cardiology/American Heart Association Task Force on Practice Guidelines (ACC/AHA/ASNC Committee to Revise the 1995 Guidelines for the Clinical Use of Cardiac Radionuclide Imaging). Circulation 2003;108:1404–18.

20. Marcassa C, Bax JJ, Bengel F, et al. Clinical value, cost-effectiveness, and safety of myocardial perfusion scintigraphy: a position statement. Eur Heart J 2008;29:557–63.

21. Hachamovitch R, Di Carli MF. Nuclear cardiology will remain the "gatekeeper" over CT angiography. J Nucl Cardiol 2007;14:634–44.

22. Gaemperli O, Schepis T, Valenta I, et al. Functionally relevant coronary artery disease: comparison of 64-section CT angiography with myocardial perfusion SPECT. Radiology 2008;248:414–23.

23. Hacker M, Jakobs T, Hack N, et al. Sixty-four slice spiral CT angiography does not predict the functional relevance of coronary artery stenoses in patients with stable angina. Eur J Nucl Med Mol Imaging 2007;34:4–10.

24. Nicol ED, Stirrup J, Reyes E, et al. Sixty-four-slice computed tomography coronary angiography compared with myocardial perfusion scintigraphy for the diagnosis of functionally significant coronary stenoses in patients with a low to intermediate likelihood of coronary artery disease. J Nucl Cardiol 2008;15:311–8.

25. Gaemperli O, Schepis T, Koepfli P, et al. Accuracy of 64-slice CT angiography for the detection of functionally relevant coronary stenoses as assessed with myocardial perfusion SPECT. Eur J Nucl Med Mol Imaging 2007;34:1162–71.

26. Adams GL, Trimble MA, Brosnan RB, et al. Evaluation of combined cardiac positron emission tomography and coronary computed tomography

angiography for the detection of coronary artery disease. Nucl Med Commun 2008;29:593–8.

27. Sampson UK, Dorbala S, Limaye A, et al. Diagnostic accuracy of rubidium-82 myocardial perfusion imaging with hybrid positron emission tomography/computed tomography in the detection of coronary artery disease. J Am Coll Cardiol 2007;49:1052–8.

28. Mahnken AH, Koos R, Katoh M, et al. Assessment of myocardial viability in reperfused acute myocardial infarction using 16-slice computed tomography in comparison to magnetic resonance imaging. J Am Coll Cardiol 2005;45:2042–7.

29. Nikolaou K, Sanz J, Poon M, et al. Assessment of myocardial perfusion and viability from routine contrast-enhanced 16-detector-row computed tomography of the heart: preliminary results. Eur Radiol 2005;15:864–71.

30. Ruzsics B, Lee H, Zwerner PL, et al. Dual-energy CT of the heart for diagnosing coronary artery stenosis and myocardial ischemia-initial experience. Eur Radiol 2008;18:2414–24.

31. Kurata A, Mochizuki T, Koyama Y, et al. Myocardial perfusion imaging using adenosine triphosphate stress multi-slice spiral computed tomography: alternative to stress myocardial perfusion scintigraphy. Circ J 2005;69:550–7.

32. Ruzsics B, Lee H, Powers ER, et al. Images in cardiovascular medicine. Myocardial ischemia diagnosed by dual-energy computed tomography: correlation with single-photon emission computed tomography. Circulation 2008;117:1244–5.

33. George RT, Silva C, Cordeiro MA, et al. Multidetector computed tomography myocardial perfusion imaging during adenosine stress. J Am Coll Cardiol 2006;48:153–60.

34. George RT, Arbab-Zadeh A, Miller JM, et al. Adenosine stress 64- and 256-row detector computed tomography angiography and perfusion imaging: a pilot study evaluating the transmural extent of perfusion abnormalities to predict atherosclerosis causing myocardial ischemia. Circ Cardiovasc Imaging 2009;2:174–82.

35. Garcia MJ, Lessick J, Hoffmann MH. Accuracy of 16-row multidetector computed tomography for the assessment of coronary artery stenosis. JAMA 2006;296:403–11.

36. Nieman K, Oudkerk M, Rensing BJ, et al. Coronary angiography with multi-slice computed tomography. Lancet 2001;357:599–603.

37. Knez A, Becker C, Ohnesorge B, et al. Noninvasive detection of coronary artery stenosis by multislice helical computed tomography. Circulation 2000; 101:E221–2.

38. Kopp AF, Schroeder S, Kuettner A, et al. Non-invasive coronary angiography with high resolution multidetector-row computed tomography. Results in 102 patients. Eur Heart J 2002;23:1714–25.

39. Hamon M, Morello R, Riddell JW, et al. Coronary arteries: diagnostic performance of 16- versus 64-section spiral CT compared with invasive coronary angiography—meta-analysis. Radiology 2007; 245:720–31.

40. van der Zaag-Loonen HJ, Dikkers R, de Bock GH, et al. The clinical value of a negative multi-detector computed tomographic angiography in patients suspected of coronary artery disease: a meta-analysis. Eur Radiol 2006;16:2748–56.

41. Brodoefel H, Burgstahler C, Tsiflikas I, et al. Dual-source CT: effect of heart rate, heart rate variability, and calcification on image quality and diagnostic accuracy. Radiology 2008;247:346–55.

42. Ehara M, Surmely JF, Kawai M, et al. Diagnostic accuracy of 64-slice computed tomography for detecting angiographically significant coronary artery stenosis in an unselected consecutive patient population: comparison with conventional invasive angiography. Circ J 2006;70:564–71.

43. Fine JJ, Hopkins CB, Ruff N, et al. Comparison of accuracy of 64-slice cardiovascular computed tomography with coronary angiography in patients with suspected coronary artery disease. Am J Cardiol 2006;97:173–4.

44. Leber AW, Johnson T, Becker A, et al. Diagnostic accuracy of dual-source multi-slice CT-coronary angiography in patients with an intermediate pretest likelihood for coronary artery disease. Eur Heart J 2007;28:2354–60.

45. Leschka S, Alkadhi H, Plass A, et al. Accuracy of MSCT coronary angiography with 64-slice technology: first experience. Eur Heart J 2005;26: 1482–7.

46. Meijboom WB, Meijs MF, Schuijf JD, et al. Diagnostic accuracy of 64-slice computed tomography coronary angiography: a prospective, multicenter, multivendor study. J Am Coll Cardiol 2008;52: 2135–44.

47. Mollet NR, Cademartiri F, van Mieghem CA, et al. High-resolution spiral computed tomography coronary angiography in patients referred for diagnostic conventional coronary angiography. Circulation 2005;112:2318–23.

48. Oncel D, Oncel G, Tastan A, et al. Detection of significant coronary artery stenosis with 64-section MDCT angiography. Eur J Radiol 2007;62:394–405.

49. Ong TK, Chin SP, Liew CK, et al. Accuracy of 64-row multidetector computed tomography in detecting coronary artery disease in 134 symptomatic patients: influence of calcification. Am Heart J 2006;151:1323 e1321–6.

50. Ropers D, Rixe J, Anders K, et al. Usefulness of multidetector row spiral computed tomography with 64- x 0.6-mm collimation and 330-ms rotation for the noninvasive detection of significant coronary artery stenoses. Am J Cardiol 2006;97:343–8.

51. Ropers U, Ropers D, Pflederer T, et al. Influence of heart rate on the diagnostic accuracy of dual-source computed tomography coronary angiography. J Am Coll Cardiol 2007;50:2393–8.

52. Weustink AC, Meijboom WB, Mollet NR, et al. Reliable high-speed coronary computed tomography in symptomatic patients. J Am Coll Cardiol 2007; 50:786–94.

53. Miller JM, Rochitte CE, Dewey M, et al. Diagnostic performance of coronary angiography by 64-row CT. N Engl J Med 2008;359:2324–36.

54. Hendel RC, Patel MR, Kramer CM, et al. ACCF/ACR/SCCT/SCMR/ASNC/NASCI/SCAI/SIR 2006 appropriateness criteria for cardiac computed tomography and cardiac magnetic resonance imaging: a report of the American College of Cardiology Foundation Quality Strategic Directions Committee Appropriateness Criteria Working Group, American College of Radiology, Society of Cardiovascular Computed Tomography, Society for Cardiovascular Magnetic Resonance, American Society of Nuclear Cardiology, North American Society for Cardiac Imaging, Society for Cardiovascular Angiography and Interventions, and Society of Interventional Radiology. J Am Coll Cardiol 2006;48:1475–97.

55. Boll DT, Merkle EM, Paulson EK, et al. Coronary stent patency: dual-energy multidetector CT assessment in a pilot study with anthropomorphic phantom. Radiology 2008;247:687–95.

56. Boll DT, Merkle EM, Paulson EK, et al. Calcified vascular plaque specimens: assessment with cardiac dual-energy multidetector CT in anthropomorphically moving heart phantom. Radiology 2008;249:119–26.

57. Cheruvu PK, Finn AV, Gardner C, et al. Frequency and distribution of thin-cap fibroatheroma and ruptured plaques in human coronary arteries: a pathologic study. J Am Coll Cardiol 2007;50:940–9.

58. Farb A, Burke AP, Tang AL, et al. Coronary plaque erosion without rupture into a lipid core. A frequent cause of coronary thrombosis in sudden coronary death. Circulation 1996;93:1354–63.

59. Hong C, Becker CR, Huber A, et al. ECG-gated reconstructed multi-detector row CT coronary angiography: effect of varying trigger delay on image quality. Radiology 2001;220:712–7.

60. Kopp AF, Schroeder S, Kuettner A, et al. Coronary arteries: retrospectively ECG-gated multi-detector row CT angiography with selective optimization of the image reconstruction window. Radiology 2001; 221:683–8.

61. Becker CR, Hong C, Knez A, et al. Optimal contrast application for cardiac 4-detector-row computed tomography. Invest Radiol 2003;38:690–4.

62. Leber AW, Becker A, Knez A, et al. Accuracy of 64-slice computed tomography to classify and quantify plaque volumes in the proximal coronary

system: a comparative study using intravascular ultrasound. J Am Coll Cardiol 2006;47:672–7.

63. Busch S, Johnson TR, Nikolaou K, et al. Visual and automatic grading of coronary artery stenoses with 64-slice CT angiography in reference to invasive angiography. Eur Radiol 2007;17:1445–51.

64. Nissen SE, Yock P. Intravascular ultrasound: novel pathophysiological insights and current clinical applications. Circulation 2001;103:604–16.

65. Botnar RM, Stuber M, Kissinger KV, et al. Noninvasive coronary vessel wall and plaque imaging with magnetic resonance imaging. Circulation 2000; 102:2582–7.

66. Becker CR, Nikolaou K, Muders M, et al. Ex vivo coronary atherosclerotic plaque characterization with multi-detector-row CT. Eur Radiol 2003;13: 2094–8.

67. Kopp AF, Schroeder S, Baumbach A, et al. Noninvasive characterisation of coronary lesion morphology and composition by multislice CT: first results in comparison with intracoronary ultrasound. Eur Radiol 2001;11:1607–11.

68. Schroeder S, Kopp AF, Baumbach A, et al. Noninvasive detection and evaluation of atherosclerotic coronary plaques with multislice computed tomography. J Am Coll Cardiol 2001;37:1430–5.

69. Achenbach S, Moselewski F, Ropers D, et al. Detection of calcified and noncalcified coronary atherosclerotic plaque by contrast-enhanced, submillimeter multidetector spiral computed tomography: a segment-based comparison with intravascular ultrasound. Circulation 2004;109:14–7.

70. Leber AW, Knez A, von Ziegler F, et al. Quantification of obstructive and nonobstructive coronary lesions by 64-slice computed tomography: a comparative study with quantitative coronary angiography and intravascular ultrasound. J Am Coll Cardiol 2005; 46:147–54.

71. Cademartiri F, Mollet NR, Runza G, et al. Influence of intracoronary attenuation on coronary plaque measurements using multislice computed tomography: observations in an ex vivo model of coronary computed tomography angiography. Eur Radiol 2005;15:1426–31.

72. Sun J, Zhang Z, Lu B, et al. Identification and quantification of coronary atherosclerotic plaques: a comparison of 64-MDCT and intravascular ultrasound. AJR Am J Roentgenol 2008;190:748–54.

73. Galonska M, Ducke F, Kertesz-Zborilova T, et al. Characterization of atherosclerotic plaques in human coronary arteries with 16-slice multidetector row computed tomography by analysis of attenuation profiles. Acad Radiol 2008;15:222–30.

74. Goy JJ, Kaufmann U, Hurni M, et al. 10-year follow-up of a prospective randomized trial comparing bare-metal stenting with internal mammary artery grafting for proximal, isolated de novo left anterior

coronary artery stenosis the SIMA (Stenting versus Internal Mammary Artery grafting) trial. J Am Coll Cardiol 2008;52:815–7.

75. Hannan EL, Wu C, Walford G, et al. Drug-eluting stents vs. coronary-artery bypass grafting in multivessel coronary disease. N Engl J Med 2008;358: 331–41.

76. Javaid A, Steinberg DH, Buch AN, et al. Outcomes of coronary artery bypass grafting versus percutaneous coronary intervention with drug-eluting stents for patients with multivessel coronary artery disease. Circulation 2007;116:I200–6.

77. Park DW, Yun SC, Lee SW, et al. Long-term mortality after percutaneous coronary intervention with drug-eluting stent implantation versus coronary artery bypass surgery for the treatment of multivessel coronary artery disease. Circulation 2008;117:2079–86.

78. Seung KB, Park DW, Kim YH, et al. Stents versus coronary-artery bypass grafting for left main coronary artery disease. N Engl J Med 2008;358:1781–92.

79. Boden WE, O'Rourke RA, Teo KK, et al. Optimal medical therapy with or without PCI for stable coronary disease. N Engl J Med 2007;356:1503–16.

80. Hueb W, Soares PR, Gersh BJ, et al. The medicine, angioplasty, or surgery study (MASS-II): a randomized, controlled clinical trial of three therapeutic strategies for multivessel coronary artery disease: one-year results. J Am Coll Cardiol 2004;43:1743–51.

81. Parisi AF, Folland ED, Hartigan P. A comparison of angioplasty with medical therapy in the treatment of single-vessel coronary artery disease. Veterans Affairs ACME Investigators. N Engl J Med 1992; 326:10–6.

82. Pitt B, Waters D, Brown WV, et al. Aggressive lipid-lowering therapy compared with angioplasty in stable coronary artery disease. Atorvastatin versus Revascularization Treatment Investigators. N Engl J Med 1999;341:70–6.

83. Kereiakes DJ, Teirstein PS, Sarembock IJ, et al. The truth and consequences of the COURAGE trial. J Am Coll Cardiol 2007;50:1598–603.

84. Tommaso CL. One year perspective on COURAGE. Catheter Cardiovasc Interv 2008;72:426–9.

85. Syre S. Bleeding stent sales. Boston Globe, July 19, 2007. Available at: http://www.boston.com/bostonglobe/. Accessed May 8, 2010.

86. Min JK, Shaw LJ, Devereux RB, et al. Prognostic value of multidetector coronary computed tomographic angiography for prediction of all-cause mortality. J Am Coll Cardiol 2007;50:1161–70.

87. Pundziute G, Schuijf JD, Jukema JW, et al. Prognostic value of multislice computed tomography coronary angiography in patients with known or suspected coronary artery disease. J Am Coll Cardiol 2007;49:62–70.

88. Gilard M, Le Gal G, Cornily JC, et al. Midterm prognosis of patients with suspected coronary artery

disease and normal multislice computed tomographic findings: a prospective management outcome study. Arch Intern Med 2007;167:1686–9.

89. Lesser JR, Flygenring B, Knickelbine T, et al. Clinical utility of coronary CT angiography: coronary stenosis detection and prognosis in ambulatory patients. Catheter Cardiovasc Interv 2007;69: 64–72.

90. Min JK, Shaw LJ, Berman DS, et al. Costs and clinical outcomes in individuals without known coronary artery disease undergoing coronary computed tomographic angiography from an analysis of Medicare category III transaction codes. Am J Cardiol 2008;102:672–8.

91. Schoepf UJ. CT of the heart. Totowa (NJ): Humana Press; 2004.

Evaluation of the Patient with Acute Chest Pain

Ari Goldberg, MD, PhD*, Harold I. Litt, MD, PhD

KEYWORDS

- CT technology • Acute chest pain • MDCT • TRO-CT

Presentation of acute chest pain is commonly faced in clinical practice. It accounts for nearly 4% of all emergency room diagnoses in the United States[1] and just under 2% of all outpatient physician visits.[2] It is the single most common presenting emergency room complaint of patients older than 15 years of age.[3] The diagnostic challenge of chest pain in large part, results from its manifestation as a presenting symptom of varied pathologies, some with markedly different severity and prognoses. Origins of chest pain include diseases of the heart, aorta, pulmonary system, esophagus, upper abdomen, chest wall, and even psychiatric disorders. Although different types of chest pain are classically ascribed to different corresponding diseases ("squeezing" with myocardial ischemia, "burning" with esophageal reflux), sufficient nonspecificity means that determination of the underlying etiology is often difficult. This creates a true diagnostic need to distinguish the more serious causes of acute chest pain, as timely triage of these diseases has a pronounced effect on treatment and prognosis. This is apparent when one considers that acute coronary syndrome, defined as acute chest pain arising from acute myocardial ischemia, is estimated to be responsible for 20% of all clinical encounters of acute chest pain.[4]

Modern standard of care dictates that patients with acute chest pain are evaluated via clinical and medical history, risk factors, electrocardiogram (ECG), and serum cardiac enzyme levels. These elements have been combined into the Thrombosis in Myocardial Infarction (TIMI) score,[5] wherein patients stratified with a high-risk score are referred for intravenous (IV) heparin and usually investigated with catheterization for intervention.[6] Patients without initial enzyme level elevation or ECG changes, and a low-intermediate TIMI score, are typically admitted to an observation unit or inpatient setting to complete the evaluation process via further enzyme analysis and often myocardial perfusion (usually nuclear) stress testing.

It is this latter cohort of patients, those without definite evidence of acute coronary syndrome but with chest pain of unclear origin, that comprise a large group posing a significant diagnostic and financial challenge. Indeed, the rate of missed diagnosis of acute coronary syndrome remains in the 2% to 4% range.[7–9] In addition to this morbidity and mortality looms the expanding numbers of tests and hospitalizations related to these relatively low-risk populations.[10] Further, this description of care does not address the clinically pertinent conditions of pulmonary embolus or acute aortic syndromes. Over the past decade, the role of computed tomography (CT) has grown dramatically to fill in this diagnostic void, demonstrating an ability to lift much of the ambiguity associated with acute chest pain.

EMERGENCE OF CT IN ASSESSMENT OF ACUTE CHEST PAIN

The remainder of this article is devoted to review of the developing role of CT in evaluation of acute chest pain. We consider the technological chronology and its relevance to cardiac CT in the

Cardiovascular Imaging Section, Department of Radiology, Hospital of the University of Pennsylvania, 1 Silverstein, 3400 Spruce Street, Philadelphia, PA 19104, USA
* Corresponding author.
E-mail address: ari.goldberg@uphs.upenn.edu

Radiol Clin N Am 48 (2010) 745–755
doi:10.1016/j.rcl.2010.05.003
0033-8389/10/$ – see front matter © 2010 Elsevier Inc. All rights reserved.

radiologic.theclinics.com

emergency department (ED), while examining the approaches, results, and implications of the related literature.

Advances in CT angiography have enabled more rapid and definitive diagnoses of pulmonary emboli, acute aortic syndromes, and acute coronary syndrome associated with myocardial ischemia. At this point, exclusion of pulmonary emboli and acute aortic syndromes have primarily fallen into the domain of CT angiography, which has become the test of choice for evaluation of the pulmonary arteries and thoracic aorta, with nearly 100% sensitivity and specificity provided by modern multidetector CT (MDCT).[11–13] Because of greater technical requirements, cardiac CT angiography, as a reliable tool to exclude or confirm the presence of cardiac disease, continues to evolve rapidly.

Early research established coronary artery calcification as an indicator and quantitative marker of atherosclerosis.[14] As electron beam CT could depict and quantify calcified plaque within the coronary vessels, the role of CT as a diagnostic tool in the triage of acute chest developed,[15,16] creating the eponymous Agatston score.[17] Laudon and colleagues[18] and Georgiou and colleagues[19] conducted prospective observational studies, with follow-up, on patients in the ED undergoing workup for chest pain with serum enzymes, ECG, and other cardiac testing modalities. These studies found high (approaching 100%) negative predictive values for unenhanced electron-beam CT (EBCT) evaluation, in the emergency room setting, of patients demonstrating negative early enzyme levels and negative or indeterminate ECG changes. Accordingly, they supported the safety of discharge, without further testing, of low-intermediate risk patients with calcium score of 0; exceedingly small rates of future cardiac events were seen in the article by Georgiou and colleagues.[19]

Despite these results, it is clear from other trials that the absence of coronary calcium does not sufficiently exclude the presence of significant atherosclerosis and that CT calcium assessment is, by itself, inadequate as a triage method.[20,21] Fortunately, further advances in MDCT and ECG-gating have made reliance on unenhanced calcium scoring obsolete. Detailed visualization of the coronary vessels throughout the cardiac cycle is now possible. Qualitatively, the current feasibility of CT coronary angiography is attributable to the ability to acquire images at a high temporal and spatial resolution. This has been enabled by the evolution of fast helical scanners with multidetector capabilities and, most recently, dual x-ray sources. Although there is no theoretical requirement for a specific number of detectors, the practical limiting factor is the duration of breath hold required for scan completion. Even a 16-slice scan typically requires a breath hold of 20 to 25 seconds, resulting in motion artifacts and image degradation. In contrast, 64-multislice scanners can routinely complete a scan within 7 to 13 seconds.[22,23]

Sensitivities and specificities ranging from 90% to 100% and 92% to 98%, for calcified and noncalcified coronary artery lesions, respectively, have been widely reported[24] when compared with invasive angiography (**Fig. 1**). The widespread use of 64-slice scanners means that cardiac and coronary conditions (as well as acute disease of the great vessels) can be investigated quickly and noninvasively. A current-generation 64-slice scanner provides spatial resolution on the order of 0.4 mm and temporal resolution of 75 to 200 ms. (Note that conventional coronary angiography still achieves ~0.2 mm and also superior temporal resolution.)

Building on the high sensitivity and specificity of coronary CT angiography, attention has turned to its efficacy as a guide to treatment of acute chest pain in the ED. Investigations have demonstrated as high as 96% sensitivity of MDCT in detection of coronary plaque[25,26] in the setting of acute coronary syndrome in the emergency room. Subsequent studies have aimed to further define the role of CT as it relates to standards of risk assessment, earlier diagnosis, reduced hospitalization, and reduced cost. Hoffman and colleagues[27,28] conducted prospective trials of up to 103 patients of those patients in the ED awaiting hospital admission for evaluation of acute coronary syndrome. These patients were evaluated via usual care during hospitalization, including serial ECGs and cardiac biomarkers, with subsequent cardiac testing (exercise testing, stress perfusion imaging, or cardiac catheterization) as deemed clinically indicated. Providers were blinded to the results of MDCT. The results demonstrated exclusion of significant coronary stenosis in over 70% of patients, with a negative predictive value of 100% when correlated with lack of acute coronary syndrome in those patients. For patients in whom significant stenoses were identified or could not be excluded, the findings suggested high sensitivity for acute coronary syndrome, with quantitative added value of MDCT in the prediction of acute coronary syndrome beyond the conventional methods of evaluation. Furthermore, the data indicated reductions both in time to diagnosis as well as cost for this general cohort of intermediate-risk population.

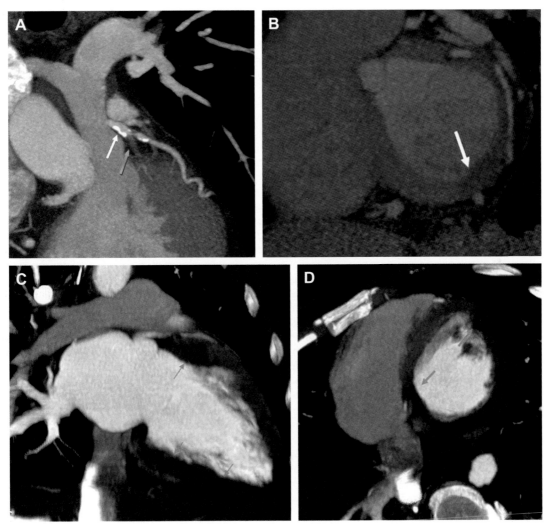

Fig. 1. Examples of stenotic coronary lesions and associated findings on CT studies of low-intermediate risk patients presenting to the emergency department with chest pain. (*A*) Mixed stenotic lesions. Calcified plaque in the distal left main causing 40% to 50% stenosis (*white arrow*). In addition, there is occlusion of a diminutive left anterior descending artery (LAD) on the basis of noncalcified plaque (*red arrow*), and a mixed lesion causing stenosis of the proximal dominant first diagonal branch artery. (*B*) Occlusion of the left circumflex artery by noncalcified plaque, with distal reconstitution. Note the perfusion defect in the left circumflex coronary artery (LCX)-territory myocardium (inferolateral wall), an inconsistent finding on CT (*arrow*). Vertical long-axis (*C*) and short-axis (*D*) images of myocardium with transmural myocardial perfusion defects in an LCX-territory distribution secondary to infarct.

Rubinshtein and colleagues[29,30] conducted prospective trials of MDCT efficacy in the ED, using 58 similarly low-intermediate risk patients undergoing rule-out of acute coronary syndrome. This also revealed very high negative predictive values for the MDCT-negative group, including no adverse events at 15-month follow-up. Sensitivity and positive predictive values were 100% and 87% respectively. In addition, they quantified the effect on the clinical course, noting that it led to "a revision of the initial ED diagnosis of ACS in 44% of cases, obviated hospitalization in 45%,

and led to a change in the planned management strategy in 43% of the patient cohort." In another, larger, prospective cohort trial, Hollander and colleagues[31] studied 568 patients in the ED with low TIMI scores. Of the 84% of patients who were discharged based on a negative coronary study, none experienced an adverse cardiac outcome in the following 30 days, with only one potential cardiac death at 1-year follow-up.[32] Goldstein and colleagues[33] randomized 99 low-intermediate risk patients in the ED with acute chest pain to immediate MDCT, and 98 patients to a control cohort that received the conventional standard of care. Of the patients who received MDCT, 66% were discharged because of minimal or no coronary stenosis, with no 6-month adverse outcomes. A small number were immediately referred for catheterization based on severe coronary disease. The remaining 25%, with indeterminate lesions or nondiagnostic scans, underwent nuclear stress testing. Overall, based on both 6-month outcomes and invasive angiography, there was equal safety and accuracy of early MDCT to the conventional workup. This result is supported by the results of Gallagher and colleagues,[34] which showed accuracy of MDCT to be as good as nuclear myocardial perfusion stress imaging in both exclusion and diagnosis of acute coronary syndrome. Furthermore, with appropriate planning, typical coronary CT radiation dose has been shown to be reducible to as low as 8 to 10 mSv. Available methods for dose reduction include tube current modulation relative to the cardiac phase (peak at end-diastole)[35,36] and use of lower kV and mAs technique when appropriate. Luaces and colleagues[37] demonstrated a 53% dose reduction using 100-kVp scanning for coronary CT studies performed on low-risk patients with chest pain in the ED. The use of prospective ECG triggering, ie, data acquisition during a single predetermined phase of the cardiac cycle without multiphasic functional data, can lead for further dose reduction.[38–40] By comparison, the dose for rest–stress ^{99m}Tc-sestamibi scintigraphy is on the order of 20 mSv, ^{201}Tl scan approximately 40 mSv, and conventional diagnostic invasive coronary catheterization is 5 to 10 mSv.[38–42] In addition, the average cost of evaluation and time required for diagnosis was reduced in the MDCT group. The principal drawback to the MDCT evaluation was noted to be the 25% of patients who required additional nuclear stress testing because of nondiagnostic or indeterminate scans.

Taken together, the literature from these trials demonstrate a growing consistency of MDCT to definitively exclude or identify hemodynamically significant lesions in most low-intermediate risk patients, with a minority requiring referral for stress testing because of indeterminate lesions or nondiagnostic scans. These studies have shown a remarkably high negative predictive value (>95%) of MDCT as a tool for acute chest pain triage, with identical outcomes to the traditional method of evaluating acute coronary syndrome. However, the data to support widespread routine use of MDCT in the ED requires further development. As noted previously, with the current technology, a group of patients is consistently present within these trials that require additional myocardial stress imaging because of indeterminate MDCT scans, and stress-perfusion imaging is certainly superior in depicting physiologic relevance of intermediate lesions. Also, elevated heart rates and arrhythmia, in particular, are sources of reduced image quality and diagnostic information. A heart rate of no more than 70, and preferably 60, has been widely recommended in the literature for high-quality studies.[43,44] In addition, extensive calcium and the presence of stents provide current limitations to interpretation. Although the administration of beta-blockers to lower heart rates is widely accepted and implemented, this is neither entirely effective nor efficient, with many contraindications also noted. Newer dual-source scanners provide improved temporal resolution (~83 msec), with recent studies[45,46] demonstrating the intuitive result that use of dual-source scanners in acute chest pain resulted in fewer nondiagnostic examinations with sensitivities and negative predictive values approaching 100%. Dedicated ED trials with these, as well as 128- and even 320-slice scanners, will likely further reduce the component of nondiagnostic examinations. Importantly, consideration must be given to the size of these trials; as low-risk patients inherently have low event rates, there are relatively few patients who have undergone invasive angiography or had adverse cardiac events in these studies. This makes it difficult to evaluate the true incidence of false positive and false negative coronary CT findings. A related concept is that the trials thus far are likely sensitive to the variability of coronary disease prevalence in the given populations studied. Budoff and colleagues[47] conducted a 230-patient multicenter trial, which revealed a negative predictive value of 99%. However, a different multicenter study by Miller and colleagues[48] demonstrated a negative predictive value of only 83%. In addition, longer-term costs incurred during any follow-up testing during the outcome periods have not been included in the cost-effectiveness considerations. Larger trials, with greater power and with more complete cost- and time-effectiveness have recently been initiated, including the Computed Tomographic Angiography for the Systematic Triage of Acute Chest Pain Patients to Treatment (CT-STAT) trial recently reported at the American Heart Association meeting.[49] Investigators included 750 low-risk patients in the ED with acute chest pain. They were randomized to a standard diagnostic workup or CT angiography (CTA). Similar to prior studies, those with minimal or no stenosis were discharged (82% of patients) and those with severe stenosis (>70%) were triaged immediately for catheterization. Patients with intermediate stenosis or uninterpretable CT images were sent for nuclear stress testing. An abnormal stress test resulted in invasive angiography, whereas patients with a normal result were sent home. Both coronary CTA and conventional care led to a similar number of patients referred for invasive coronary angiography, 6.9% and 6.2%, respectively. Diagnostic time and hospital costs were significantly reduced with CTA, noting average discharge of patients who received MDCT in approximately 3 hours compared with 7 hours for those who received standard care. The direct costs were reduced 38% among those treated with CT, reduced from roughly $3500 with standard care to $2000 for CTA. Additional, randomized, controlled trials currently under way include the multicenter Rule-out Myocardial Infarction Using Computer-Assisted Tomography (ROMI-CAT2) study with recruitment of 1250 patients, and the American College of Radiology Imaging Network (ACRIN) PA 4005 trial, which will include 1365 patients.

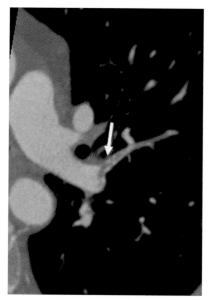

Fig. 2. Acute pulmonary emboli in the left upper lobe branch, discovered incidentally on coronary CT angiography.

COMBINED CARDIAC AND THORACIC CT EVALUATION

In parallel with the evolution of coronary CTA, the concept of both identifying and differentiating among acute coronary syndrome, pulmonary embolus, and acute aortic pathology has been increasingly considered. The triple-rule-out (TRO) has gained increased feasibility because of the proliferation of 64-slice technology, particularly dual-source innovations.[11] Whereas a 16-slice CT scan of the thorax might take 25 seconds, this can now be accomplished in approximately 15 seconds with 64-slice MDCT. The utility of TRO-CT in the ED setting appears relevant for a cohort similar to that described previously, that is patients of low-intermediate risk for acute coronary syndrome, but with symptoms possibly attributable to pulmonary embolus or acute aortic pathology. White and colleagues[11] and Johnson and colleagues[50] performed early small ED trials, the former with 69 low-intermediate risk patients with acute chest pain and short-term follow-up. Similar to the prospective trials described previously, there was immediate exclusion of acute coronary syndrome in most participants, with a minority of patients referred for catheterization. In addition, 3 causes of noncardiac pathology (pulmonary embolus, pericardial effusion, and pneumonia) (**Figs. 2–4**) were identified. In those investigations, the technically limiting factor was the coronary angiography. More recently, Johnson and colleagues[45] prospectively investigated 109

patients with acute chest pain using 64-slice dual source technology and Takakuwa and Halpern[51] prospectively evaluated TRO-CT in 201 low-intermediate risk patients with acute chest pain. These studies demonstrated exquisitely high sensitivity and negative predictive value of dual-source MDCT for differentiation of coronary and noncoronary causes of acute chest pain (**Figs. 5–7**). As expected, the distribution of cardiovascular-related pathology has overwhelmingly favored coronary artery disease, followed

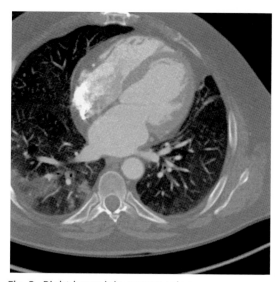

Fig. 3. Right lower lobe pneumonia seen on coronary CT angiography.

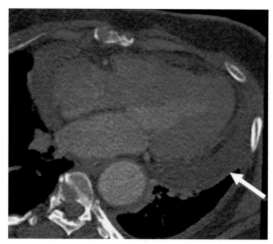

Fig. 4. Large pericardial effusion demonstrated by diffuse pericardial fluid-attenuation.

by valvular and myocardial disease, pulmonary embolism, and, finally, acute aortic syndromes. TRO was shown to obviate the necessity of further testing in up to 75% of the low-intermediate risk patients, with no adverse outcomes at 30 days. Also evident was the additional benefit of providing a noncoronary diagnosis in as many as 11% of the cases, with lower costs and fewer examinations, especially in cases of recurrent chest pain. However, as larger and randomized trials are yet to be completed, the appropriate patient cohort is, at present, incompletely defined. A patient in whom acute coronary syndrome is suspected is more appropriately sent for a dedicated coronary CT. This, in part, reflects a lower radiation dose (16–18 mSv vs 10–12 mSv), a more simple and smaller contrast profile, and

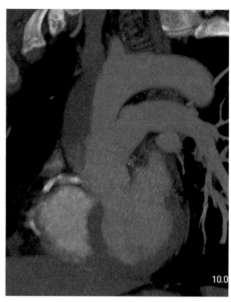

Fig. 6. Type A aortic dissection with clear hypo-enhancing false lumen extending into the brachiocephalic artery. Extension into the right coronary artery is unclear. Coronary artery extension is one of the potential cardiac complications that makes timely diagnosis essential.

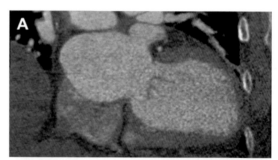

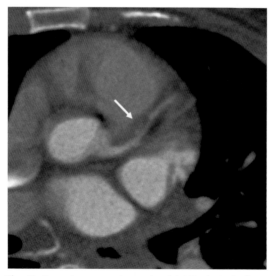

Fig. 5. Seventy percent proximal LAD stenosis from mixed, predominantly soft, plaque.

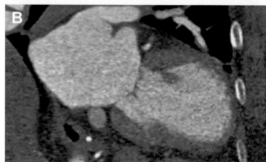

Fig. 7. Takotsubo cardiomyopathy. (*A*) Vertical long-axis orientation during diastole. Note the dilated and aneurysmal apex. (*B*) During systole, the aneurysmal dyskinetic motion is exaggerated. The patient was a 37-year-old female with recent stressful episodes and acute onset of chest pain. No coronary disease was found. The presentation and appearance is classic for Takotsubo, or "broken heart" cardiomyopathy.

a more established protocol in the dedicated coronary study, with bolus timing optimized for the coronaries.[52] Thus, patients considered relatively low risk for acute coronary syndrome but suspected for the possibility of pulmonary embolus or aortic pathology are advanced as the appropriate candidates for TRO-CT. However, although this approach is intuitively appealing, it is also clear that even the small numbers of patients with positive findings of pulmonary embolus or acute aortic syndrome would have coexisting coronary disease. This would imply further testing. Because of considerations such as these, more research, in the form of larger and more detailed trials, is required to justify TRO protocol implementation as a matter of routine.[53,54]

FURTHER CONSIDERATIONS RELATED TO CT USE IN THE ED

We have seen that demonstration and quantification of stenosis caused by atherosclerotic plaque is feasible, with high sensitivity and specificity. The intuitive assumption that such temporally and spatially detailed evaluation of the coronary arteries and great vessels is diagnostically, as well as economically, beneficial, has been developing support in the literature. However, it is also instructive to consider some specific pathologic entities and current pathophysiologic thought when evaluating the capability of CT as it relates to diagnosis of acute chest pain. For example, growing evidence suggests that many myocardial infarctions may actually occur in patients with coronary luminal narrowing of less than 50%. The morphology and biochemical structure of a hemodynamically nonsignificant plaque may render it prone to rupture. One of these characteristics is pronounced positive remodeling (**Fig. 8**). The other is fibrous versus lipid-rich content, the former being more ominous.[55–61] Although CTA is intuitively equipped to play a role in identifying concerning lesions in such a developing paradigm, conventional coronary angiography is likely less relevant.

Similarly, myocardial bridging (**Fig. 9**), in which a coronary artery tunnels through the myocardium as opposed to the epicardium, may result in vessel narrowing, particularly during systole. Such lesions may be associated with acute chest pain[62] when hemodynamically significant. Bridging is routinely evaluated via multiphase angiographic CT, but not conventional angiography.

Figs. 10 and **11** provide examples of relatively rare coronary artery abnormalities, seen in approximately 1% of coronary angiography, but in as

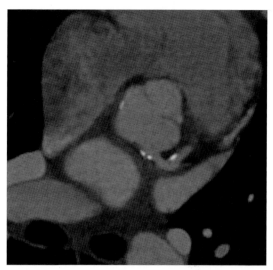

Fig. 8. Positive remodeling. Substantial mixed atherosclerotic plaque at the proximal left main and LAD coronary arteries. Note, however, that there has been remodeling of the vessel lumen, particularly in the left main, so that the stenosis is minimal and only 30% in the LAD. Conventional angiography is only able to quantify vessel stenosis.

many as 15% of young sudden death cases.[63] Both coronary artery fistulas and anomalous coronary origins can be associated with acute chest pain.[64] Coronary CTA is ideal for demonstration of such anatomic courses and depiction of vessel caliber throughout the cardiac cycle.

Finally, we note that evaluation of the cardiac valves is rarely the primary focus of a cardiac CT in the setting of acute chest pain; however, mitral valve dysfunction is a known complication of inferior wall infarcts[65] and aortic stenosis is a less common cause of acute chest pain.[66] Both of these diseases can be well evaluated using multiphase data with the temporal resolution provided

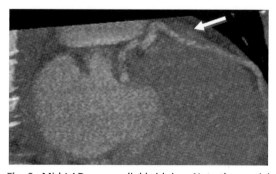

Fig. 9. Mid-LAD myocardial bridging. Note the partial intramyocardial course of the mid-LAD, with narrowing of the vessel at the distal aspect of the bridging. This finding was more pronounced during systole.

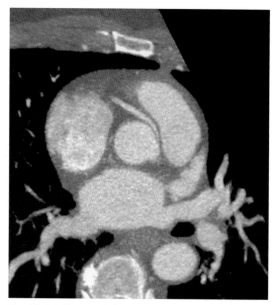

Fig. 10. Malignant right coronary artery (RCA) course, characterized by anomalous origin from the left coronary cusp, acute angulation, and intra-arterial segment between the aorta and pulmonary artery. These patients are at risk for sudden death.

by 64-slice scanners, especially dual-source technology. In addition, disorders such as Takotsubo cardiomyopathy (stress-induced myocardial dysfunction) and myocarditis may be manifest by wall motion abnormalities visible by CT. These conditions and other less common noncoronary diagnoses may not be well evaluated by a single-phase examination, and therefore careful

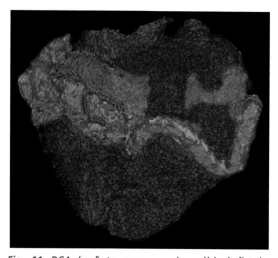

Fig. 11. RCA (*red*) to coronary sinus (*blue*) fistula, causing a dilated and tortuous RCA. Physiologic complications are attributed to vascular steal phenomenon.

consideration should be given to the trade off required when using a low-dose ECG-triggered technique.

SUMMARY

The past decade has brought rapid advances in CT technology, which allows increasingly precise application to the study of coronary arteries and acute chest pain. The literature has expanded to lend quantifiable justification to the intuitive appeal of a rapid, reproducible, 3-dimensional study of the heart and vasculature. More complete analysis of efficacy and costs on broader populations will further refine our understanding of how best to implement what may become the new gold standard. Meanwhile, evolving technology promises to further challenge radiologists and clinicians to optimize approach and diagnosis to acute chest pain.

REFERENCES

1. McCaig LF, Burt CW. National Hospital Ambulatory Medical Care Survey: 2002 emergency department summary. Adv Data 2004;340:1–34.
2. Hing E, Hall MJ, Xu J. National Hospital Ambulatory Medical Care Survey: 2006 outpatient department summary. Natl Health Stat Report 2008;4:1–32.
3. Pitts SR, Niska RW, Xu J, et al. National Hospital Ambulatory Medical Care Survey: 2006 emergency department summary. National health statistics reports; no 7. Hyattsville (MD): National Center for Health Statistics; 2008. Available at: http://www.cdc.gov/nchs. Accessed January 3, 2010.
4. Pozen MW, D'Agostino RB, Selker HP, et al. A predictive instrument to improve coronary-care-unit admission practices in acute ischemic heart disease: a prospective multicenter clinical trial. N Engl J Med 1984;310:1273–8.
5. Antman EM, Cohen M, Bernink PJ, et al. The TIMI risk score for unstable angina/non-ST elevation MI: a method for prognostication and therapeutic decision making. JAMA 2000;284:835–42.
6. Braunwald E, Antman EM, Beasley JW, et al. ACC/AHA guideline update for the management of patients with unstable angina and non-ST-segment elevation myocardial infarction—2002: summary article: a report of the American College of Cardiology/American Heart Association Task Force on Practice Guidelines (Committee on the Management of Patients With Unstable Angina). Circulation 2002; 106:1893–900.
7. Pope JH, Aufderheide TP, Ruthazer R, et al. Missed diagnoses of acute cardiac ischemia in the emergency department. N Engl J Med 2000; 342:1163–70.

8. Lee TH, Goldman L. Evaluation of the patient with acute chest pain. N Engl J Med 2000;342: 1187–95.

9. Lee TH, Rouan GW, Weisberg MC, et al. Clinical characteristics and natural history of patients with acute myocardial infarction sent home from the emergency room. Am J Cardiol 1987;60:219–24.

10. Fineberg HV, Scadden D, Goldman L. Care of patients with a low probability of acute myocardial infarction: cost effectiveness of alternatives to coronary-care-unit admission. N Engl J Med 1984;310: 1301–7.

11. White CS, Kuo D, Kelemen M, et al. Chest pain evaluation in the emergency department: can MDCT provide a comprehensive evaluation? AJR Am J Roentgenol 2005;185:533–40.

12. Manghat NE, Morgan-Hughes GJ, Roobottom CA. Multi-detector row computed tomography: imaging in acute aortic syndrome. Clin Radiol 2005;60(12): 1256–67.

13. Schoepf UJ. Computed tomography for pulmonary embolism diagnosis: the making of a reference standard. J Thromb Haemost 2005;3:1924–5.

14. Budoff MJ, Achenbach S, Blumenthal RS, et al. Assessment of coronary artery disease by cardiac computed tomography: a scientific statement from the American Heart Association Committee on Cardiovascular Imaging and Intervention, Council on Cardiovascular Radiology and Intervention, and Committee on Cardiac Imaging, Council on Clinical Cardiology. Circulation 2006;114:1761–91.

15. Tanenbaum SR, Kondos GT, Veselik KE, et al. Detection of calcific deposits in coronary arteries by ultrafast computed tomography and correlation with angiography. Am J Cardiol 1989;63:870–2.

16. McLaughlin VV, Balogh T, Rich S. Utility of electron beam computed tomography to stratify patients presenting to the emergency room with chest pain. Am J Cardiol 1999;84:327–8.

17. Agatston AS, Janowitz WR, Hildner FJ, et al. Quantification of coronary artery calcium using ultrafast computed tomography. J Am Coll Cardiol 1990;15: 827–32.

18. Laudon DA, Vukov LF, Breen JF, et al. Use of electron-beam computed tomography in the evaluation of chest pain patients in the emergency department. Ann Emerg Med 1999;33:15–21.

19. Georgiou D, Budoff MJ, Kaufer E, et al. Screening patients with chest pain in the emergency department using electron beam tomography: a follow-up study. J Am Coll Cardiol 2001;38:105–10.

20. Ohnesorge B, Flohr T, Becker C, et al. Cardiac imaging by means of electrocardiographically gated multisection spiral CT: initial experience. Radiology 2000;217:564–71.

21. Achenbach S, Ulzheimer S, Baum U, et al. Non-invasive coronary angiography by retrospectively ECG-gated multislice spiral CT. Circulation 2000;102: 2823–8.

22. White CS, Kuo D. Chest pain in the emergency department: role of multidetector CT. Radiology 2007;245:672–81.

23. Flohr T, Stierstorfer K, Raupach R, et al. Performance evaluation of a 64-slice CT system with z-flying focal spot. Rofo 2004;176:1803–10.

24. Ropers D, Baum U, Pohle K, et al. Detection of coronary artery stenoses with thin-slice multidetector row spiral computed tomography and multiplanar reconstruction. Circulation 2003;107:664–6.

25. Sato Y, Matsumoto N, Ichikawa M, et al. Efficacy of multislice computed tomography for the detection of acute coronary syndrome in the emergency department. Circ J 2005;69:1047–51.

26. Raff GL, Gallagher MJ, O'Neill WW, et al. Diagnostic accuracy of noninvasive coronary angiography using 64-slice spiral computed tomography. J Am Coll Cardiol 2005;46:552–7.

27. Hoffmann U, Pena AJ, Moselewski F, et al. MDCT in early triage of patients with acute chest pain. AJR Am J Roentgenol 2006;187:1240–7.

28. Hoffmann U, Nagurney JT, Moselewski F, et al. Coronary multidetector computed tomography in the assessment of patients with acute chest pain. Circulation 2006;114:2251–60.

29. Rubinshtein R, Halon DA, Gaspar T, et al. Usefulness of 64-slice cardiac computed tomographic angiography for diagnosing acute coronary syndromes and predicting clinical outcome in emergency department patients with chest pain of uncertain origin. Circulation 2007;115:1762–8.

30. Rubinshtein R, Halon DA, Gaspar T, et al. Impact of 64-slice cardiac computed tomographic angiography on clinical decision-making in emergency department patients with chest pain of possible myocardial ischemic origin. Am J Cardiol 2007; 100:1522–6.

31. Hollander J, Chang AM, Shofer F, et al. Coronary computed tomographic angiography for rapid discharge of low-risk patients with potential acute chest syndromes. Ann Emerg Med 2009;53:295–304.

32. Hollander JE, Chang AM, Shofer FS, et al. One year outcomes following coronary computerized tomographic angiography for evaluation of emergency department patients with potential acute coronary syndrome. Acad Emerg Med 2009;16(8):693–8.

33. Goldstein JA, Gallagher MJ, O'Neill WW, et al. A randomized controlled trial of multi-slice coronary computed tomography for evaluation of acute chest pain. J Am Coll Cardiol 2007;49:863–71.

34. Gallagher MJ, Ross MA, Raff GL, et al. The diagnostic accuracy of 64-slice computed tomography coronary angiography compared with stress nuclear imaging in emergency department low-risk chest pain patients. Ann Emerg Med 2007;49:125–36.

35. Jakobs TF, Becker CR, Ohnesorge B, et al. Multislice helical CT of the heart with retrospective ECG gating: reduction of radiation exposure by ECG-controlled tube current modulation. Eur Radiol 2002;12:1081–6.

36. Poll LW, Cohnen M, Brachten S, et al. Dose reduction in multi-slice CT of the heart by use of ECG-controlled tube current modulation ("ECG pulsing"): phantom measurements. Rofo 2002;174:1500–5.

37. Luaces M, Akers S, Litt H. Low kVp imaging for dose reduction in dual-source cardiac CT. Int J Cardiovasc Imaging 2009;25:165–75.

38. Hirai N, Horiguchi J, Fujioka C, et al. Prospective versus retrospective ECG-gated 64-detector coronary CT angiography: assessment of image quality, stenosis, and radiation dose. Radiology 2008;248:424–30.

39. Ketelsen D, Luetkhoff MH, Thomas C, et al. Estimation of the radiation exposure of a chest pain protocol with ECG-gating in dual-source computed tomography. Eur Radiol 2009;19:37–41.

40. Stolzmann P, Scheffel H, Schertler T, et al. Radiation dose estimates in dual-source computed tomography coronary angiography. Eur Radiol 2008;18:592–9.

41. Takakuwa KM, Halpern EJ, Gingold EL, et al. Radiation dose in a "triple rule-out" coronary CT angiography protocol of emergency department patients using 64-MDCT: the impact of ECG-based tube current modulation on age, sex, and body mass index. AJR Am J Roentgenol 2009;192(4):866–72.

42. Mettler FA Jr, Huda W, Yoshizumi TT, et al. Effective doses in radiology and diagnostic nuclear medicine: a catalog. Radiology 2008;248:254–63.

43. Giesler T, Baum U, Ropers D, et al. Noninvasive visualization of coronary arteries using contrast-enhanced multidetector CT: influence of heart rate on image quality and stenosis detection. AJR Am J Roentgenol 2002;179:911–6.

44. Shim SS, Kim Y, Lim SM. Improvement of image quality with beta-blocker premedication on ECG-gated 16-MDCT coronary angiography. AJR Am J Roentgenol 2005;184:649–54.

45. Johnson TR, Nikolaou K, Becker A, et al. Dual-source CT for chest pain assessment. Eur Radiol 2008;18:773–80.

46. Schertler T, Scheffel H, Frauenfelder T, et al. Dual-source computed tomography in patients with acute chest pain: feasibility and image quality. Eur Radiol 2007;17:3179–88.

47. Budoff MJ, Dowe D, Jollis JG, et al. Diagnostic performance of 64-multidetector row coronary computed tomographic angiography for evaluation of coronary artery stenosis in individuals without known coronary artery disease: results from the prospective multicenter ACCURACY (Assessment by Coronary Computed Tomographic Angiography of Individuals Undergoing Invasive Coronary Angiography) trial. J Am Coll Cardiol 2008;52(21):1724–32.

48. Miller JM, Rochitte CE, Dewey M, et al. Diagnostic performance of coronary angiography by 64-row CT. N Engl J Med 2008;359(22):2324–36.

49. Results from CT-STAT. Available at: http://directnews.americanheart.org/extras/sessions2009/. Accessed January 3, 2010.

50. Johnson TRC, Nikolaou K, Wintersperger BJ, et al. ECG gated 64 slice CT angiography for the differential diagnosis of acute chest pain. AJR Am J Roentgenol 2007;188:76–82.

51. Takakuwa KM, Halpern EJ. Evaluation of a "triple rule-out" coronary CT angiography protocol: use of 64-section CT in low-to-moderate risk emergency department patients suspected of having acute coronary syndrome. Radiology 2008;248(2):438–46.

52. Lee HY, Yoo SM, White CS. Coronary CT angiography in emergency department patients with acute chest pain: triple rule-out protocol versus dedicated coronary CT angiography. Int J Cardiovasc Imaging 2009;25:319–26.

53. Shapiro MD. Is the "triple rule-out" study an appropriate indication for cardiovascular CT? J Cardiovasc Comput Tomogr 2009;3:100–3.

54. Litt H. Are three diagnoses always better than one? Acad Radiol 2009;16(9):1037–8.

55. Burke AP, Taylor A, Farb A, et al. Coronary calcification: insights from sudden coronary death victims. Z Kardiol 2000;89(Suppl 2):49–53.

56. Wallentin L. Non-ST-elevation acute coronary syndrome: fuel for the invasive strategy. Lancet 2002;360:738–9.

57. Roe MT, Harrington RA, Prosper DM, et al. Clinical and therapeutic profile of patients presenting with acute coronary syndromes who do not have significant coronary artery disease. The Platelet Glycoprotein IIb/IIIa in Unstable Angina: Receptor Suppression Using Integrilin Therapy (PURSUIT) Trial Investigators. Circulation 2000;102:1101–6.

58. Burke AP, Kolodgie FD, Farb A, et al. Healed plaque ruptures and sudden coronary death: evidence that subclinical rupture has a role in plaque progression. Circulation 2001;103:934–40.

59. Falk E. Why do plaques rupture? Circulation 1992;86:III30–42.

60. Nakamura M, Nishikawa H, Mukai S, et al. Impact of coronary artery remodeling on clinical presentation of coronary artery disease: an intravascular ultrasound study. J Am Coll Cardiol 2001;37:63–9.

61. Maehara A, Mintz GS, Bui AB, et al. Morphologic and angiographic features of coronary plaque rupture detected by intravascular ultrasound. J Am Coll Cardiol 2002;40:904–10.

62. Ferreira AG Jr, Trotter SE, Konig B Jr, et al. Myocardial bridges: morphological and functional aspects. Br Heart J 1991;66:364–7.

63. Shirani J, Brofferio A. Isolated coronary artery anomalies. Available at: http://www.emedicine.com/med/topic445.htm. Accessed March 13, 2008.

64. Taylor AJ, Rogan KM, Virmani R. Sudden cardiac death associated with isolated congenital coronary artery anomalies. J Am Coll Cardiol 1992;20:640–7.

65. Levi GS, Bolling SF, Bach DS. Eccentric mitral regurgitation jets among patients having sustained inferior wall myocardial infarction. Echocardiography 2001;18(2):97–103.

66. Nishimura RA. Aortic valve disease. Circulation 2002;106:770.

Evaluation of Bypass Grafts and Stents

Minh Lu, MD*, Joseph Jen-Sho Chen, MD,
Omer Awan, MD, Charles S. White, MD

KEYWORDS

- CT angiography • Coronary artery bypass graft
- Coronary stent • Internal mammary artery
- Saphenous vein

Cardiovascular disease remains the number 1 cause of mortality in the United States, with coronary artery disease accounting for approximately 425,400 deaths in 2006.[1] A 2004 guideline published by an American College of Cardiology/American Heart Association task force recommended coronary artery bypass graft (CABG) surgery in the treatment of patients with advanced coronary artery disease, such as significant left main coronary artery stenosis, stenosis greater than or equal to 70% in the proximal left anterior descending (LAD) and proximal left circumflex artery, and 3-vessel coronary artery disease. Currently, well over 469,000 CABG surgeries are performed in the United States annually.[2] The goal of CABG is to restore myocardial perfusion, which not only relieves symptoms but also prolongs life. Patients often experience recurrent symptoms, however, related to the stenosis or occlusion of their coronary bypass grafts.[3] The long-term prognostic factors for survival after myocardial revascularization are dependent on the patency of the bypass graft and native coronary artery disease progression.[4–6] Conventional angiography is regarded as the gold standard in evaluating the patency of coronary bypass grafts, but in recent years, the development of sophisticated multidetector CT (MDCT) has enabled accurate visualization of grafts noninvasively. Recent published studies have explored the diagnostic potential of various scanner generations in the evaluation of CABG patency and stenosis.[7–9]

Evaluation of bypass graft patency using single-slice CT was first described in the 1980s. Improvements in technical performance with 4- and 16-slice CT using ECG gating further established a role for this technology in evaluating bypass grafts.[10–12] The introduction of 64-slice MDCT scanners with high spatial and temporal resolution enabled detection of stenoses of coronary arteries and grafts with submillimeter slice thickness within a single breath hold.[13] Interactive 3-D multiplanar applications now allow detailed evaluation of arterial and venous bypass grafts and native coronary arteries, including degree of stenosis caused by coronary plaques. To date, published studies on 64-slice CT indicate sensitivity and specificity of 93.3% to 100% and 91.4% to 100%, respectively, when assessing CABG occlusion and significant stenosis (>50%).[14–18]

A recent study by Liu and colleagues[19] evaluated diagnostic accuracy of 64-slice CT angiography (CTA) in 228 patients after CABG. The sensitivity, specificity, positive predictive value, negative predictive value, and accuracy for detecting graft stenosis were 93.3%, 98.1%, 93.3%, 98.1%, and 97.1%, respectively. For graft occlusion, the sensitivity, specificity, positive predictive value, negative predictive value, and accuracy were 96.4%, 98.1%, 96.4%, 98.1%, and 97.6%, respectively.

MDCT PROTOCOL

Many different scanning protocols are in routine clinical use for the performance of noninvasive evaluation of CABG with MDCT. The diagnostic performance of coronary CTA relies on proficient technical studies and optimized image parameters, including image timing and image reconstruction.

Department of Diagnostic Radiology, University of Maryland, 22 South Greene Street, Baltimore, MD 21201, USA
* Corresponding author.
E-mail address: mlu@umm.edu

Radiol Clin N Am 48 (2010) 757–770
doi:10.1016/j.rcl.2010.04.009
0033-8389/10/$ – see front matter. Published by Elsevier Inc.

In coronary assessment, it is important to know the nature of the prior surgical procedure to determine the level of scanning. Evaluation of saphenous vein graft (SVG) patency, for example, should extend from the mid–ascending aorta to the base of the heart, whereas imaging of the internal mammary graft includes the origin of the vessel at the subclavian artery to the cardiac apex. Patients are scanned in the supine position in the craniocaudal direction during a single breath hold. In some institutions, a caudal cranial approach is used with 64-slice CT to minimize breathing during imaging acquisition of the heart.

For coronary CTA, intravenous administration of a nonionic iodine contrast agent through an 18- or 20-gauge angiocatheter into an antecubital vein is adequate depending on the intravenous administration rate. Automated bolus timing is performed when contrast density in the descending aorta reaches a predefined threshold (usually +100 Hounsfield units) with a 5- to 10-second delay before the start of a scan, to better optimize visualization of the left ventricles, coronary arteries, and bypass grafts. Alternatively, a test bolus can be performed.

β-Blockade is administered orally or intravenously (eg, metoprolol) before scanning to achieve a heart rate of less than 70 beats per minute and to minimize cardiac motion artifacts. In addition, images are acquired with a single breath hold during midinspiration to reduce heterogeneity of contrast in the right atrium caused by inflow of unopacified blood from the *inferior vena cava*.

In MDCT angiography, ECG gating is conventionally done using retrospective gating for creating optimal images for reconstruction at various increments of the cardiac cycle. Axial slices of the heart are reconstructed using 60% to 80% of the R–R interval, with 0.9-mm–thick images reconstructed in 0.45-mm increments (depending on the scanning protocol used), 3-D volume rendering images, and multiplanar reformatted (MPR) images. CABG grafts, including the proximal and distal anastomosis and cardiac topography, are assessed using 3-D volume rendering images whereas MPR and maximum intensity projections are used to evaluate coronary artery disease.

CABG ANATOMY

Knowledge of CABG anatomy and coronary artery graft procedures is crucial in the assessment of graft patency. Left internal mammary artery (IMA) grafts and SVGs are the most common graft types. Of these, arterial grafts provide better and longer-term patency than SVGs. Other vessels, including the radial arteries, right gastroepiploic artery (RGEA), and inferior epigastric artery, are used less often. Initial CTA assessment after CABG surgery focuses on graft type, origin, course, and anastomosis. Graft morphology and patency are then evaluated with contrast media. CABG bypass grafts are divided into 3 segments: (1) origin or proximal anastomosis; (2) body of the graft; and (3) distal anastomosis.[20] The proximal anastomosis is better visualized on CTA than the distal anastomosis, which is more prone to motion artifact. Distal anastomoses that are not well visualized are considered patent when contrast is present within the graft conduit lumen.

SAPHENOUS VEIN GRAFTS

The saphenous vein was first used in CABG surgery in the late 1960s.[21] Use of the saphenous vein for revascularization of coronary arteries offers many advantages, including availability, accessibility, ease of harvest, and resistance to spasm. The saphenous vein approach is limited, however, by a higher incidence of neointimal hyperplasia and development of atherosclerosis after exposure to systemic blood pressure and deficiency of nitric oxide production when compared with arterial grafts.[4,7] In addition, varicosity and sclerotic disease limit the use of the saphenous vein as a conduit. Early occlusion of the saphenous vein can result from surgical techniques used in harvesting (endothelial injury), storage procedures, or mechanical trauma. Recent studies have reported that approximately 15% to 20% of vein grafts occlude within the first year. The graft occlusion rate thereafter is 1% to 2% between 1 and 6 years and 4% to 5% between 6 and 10 years. The patency rate after 10 years for SVGs is approximately 60%, and only 50% of these vein grafts are free of stenosis.[4,22,23] Antiplatelet therapy and lipid-lowering medications reduce the occlusion rate of saphenous vein grafts.[24,25]

SVGs are typically attached proximally on the anterior wall of the ascending aorta and distally below the stenosis or obstruction (**Figs. 1** and **2**). For grafts revascularizing the LAD territory or left circumflex, a proximal anastomosis is made on the left side of the aorta and stabilized on the main pulmonary artery.[26] In the case of right-sided grafts to the right coronary artery (RCA) territory, the saphenous vein is anastomosed to the right side of the aorta, permitting it to course toward the right arterioventricular groove. The SVG can be attached directly to the aorta with sutures or with an intraluminal anastomosis device that allows a quicker, sutureless attachment without the need to clamp target vessels. With the aortic connector system, the proximal vein graft is anastomosed at

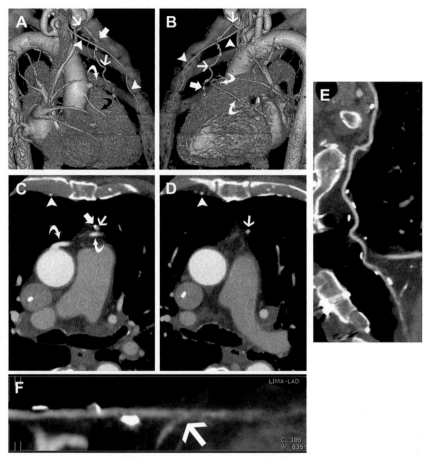

Fig. 1. An 89-year-old man who underwent cardiac CTA to evaluate for CABG patency. (*A–B*) 3-D volume-rendered images show the typical appearances of right SVG (*black curved arrow*) sutured to the right anterior ascending aorta and connected to the PDA (*not shown*) and a left SVG (*white curved arrows*) sutured to the left anterior ascending aorta and connected to an OM branch. The left IMA (LIMA) (*arrow*) is attached to the LAD artery with multiple surgical clips (*block arrows*) adjacent to the artery. The RIMA (*arrowheads*) is in normal position, lateral to the sternum. (*C, D*) Axial CTA images demonstrate a contrast-enhancing LIMA (*arrow*) with a surgical clip (*block arrow*) adjacent to the artery. The proximal portion of the SVG (*curved arrows*), including the anastomosis, is well opacified by contrast as well. The RIMA demonstrates normal enhancement and position. (*E*) Curved MPR image of the LIMA demonstrates bypass graft patency with multiple surgical clips that are used to ligate collateral branches. (*F*) Linear reformatted image of distal LIMA demonstrates end-to-side anastomosis (*arrow*) to the distal LAD artery. Although the anastomosis is not well enhanced, enhancement proximal to the anastomosis makes distal occlusion unlikely.

a 90° angle to the left side of the aorta and is stabilized on the main pulmonary artery.

SVGs usually appear larger than native coronary arteries or arterial grafts on CTA. For revascularization of the RCA, posterior descending artery (PDA), or distal LAD artery, SVG grafts are anastomosed proximally on the right side. The SVG is then attached distally to the RCA, PDA, or distal LAD in right-sided anastomosis. The distal graft may lie on the phrenic wall of the heart. In left-sided anastomosis, the SVG is usually attached distally to the LAD artery, diagonal artery, left circumflex artery, or obtuse marginal (OM) arteries. In cases where the SVG is grafted to more than two coronary arteries, a side-to-side and end-to-side anastomosis surgical technique is used. The smaller native coronary arteries distal to the anastomosis should also be evaluated for patency. In contrast to arterial grafts, fewer streak artifacts from surgical clips are seen with SVG grafts.

INTERNAL MAMMARY ARTERY GRAFTS

The IMA has become the conduit of choice for revascularization of obstructed coronary arteries. Recent studies have shown that IMA grafts have

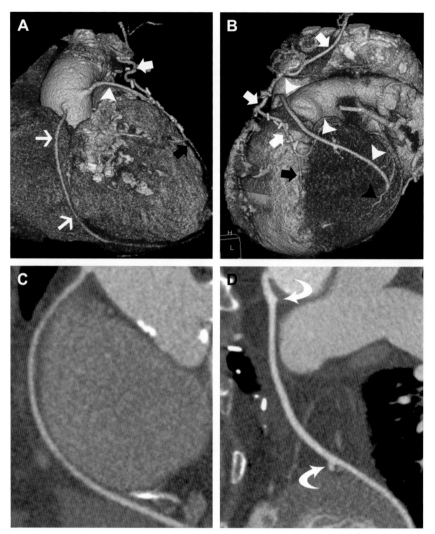

Fig. 2. A 91-year-old man who underwent cardiac CTA to evaluate for CABG patency. (*A, B*) 3-D volume-rendered images show the typical appearances of left SVG (*white arrowheads*) sutured to the left anterior ascending aorta and connected to the OM branch (*black arrowhead*) and a LIMA (*white block arrows*) sutured to the left anterior ascending aorta and connected to an LAD artery (*black block arrow*) with multiple surgical clips. The RA graft (*arrows*) is attached to the right ascending aorta and connected to the PDA (*not shown*). (*C*) Curved MPR image of the RA graft demonstrates a small caliber bypass graft. The graft appears patent. (*D*) Curved MPR image demonstrates a contrast-filled SVG with two outpouchings, one proximally and one mid to distally, concerning for pseudoaneurysms (*curved arrows*).

long-term patency rates superior to those of SVGs and are more resistant to atherosclerosis. Another advantage over SVGs is the IMA endothelium production of prostacyclin and relaxing factors (such as nitric oxide) in response to vasoactive stimuli. In addition, the biologic characteristics of the IMA, including nonfenestrated internal elastica lamina, prevent cellular migration and intimal hyperplasia.[27] The wall structure of the arterial conduit is also better suited to a high-pressure system and high flow velocity after coronary artery bypass surgery. Studies indicate that IMA

conduits are less likely to result in postoperative complications and mortality and have a long-term patency rate of greater than 90% after 10 years.[28–30] Because of its anatomic location, the left IMA is often considered the graft of choice to revascularize the LAD or diagonal artery. The graft is conventionally used in situ from its proximal origin at the left subclavian with distal anastomosis below the occluded LAD or diagonal branches (see **Figs. 1** and **2**). Sequential distal grafting with side-to-side or end-to-side anastomoses is sometimes performed between branches of the same coronary arteries, including the LAD and adjacent diagonal branches or both on LAD.[31] The IMA graft is usually seen as a vessel along the left anterior mediastinum on CTA and may be difficult to visualize distally because of artifacts from surgical clips.[32]

The right IMA is less commonly used in situ to revascularize the RCA territory or the left-sided coronary system. If the right IMA is anastomosed to the diagonal or oblique marginal branches of the circumflex artery, it is passed through the transverse sinus of the pericardium, because this technique has been associated with improved patency rates.[33] The right IMA can also be used as a free or composite graft. As a free graft, the right IMA is anastomosed proximally to the ascending aorta and distally to the occluded coronary artery. Alternatively, as a composite graft the right IMA is attached proximally to the left IMA and distally to the left circumflex artery territory in a Y configuration, resulting in total arterial myocardial revascularization. The use of the left IMA to bypass the LAD and circumflex systems in double-vessel disease avoids the harvesting of a second conduit. Another advantage of the Y-graft technique is that the graft can be attached more proximally to the LAD than with a sequential graft, resulting in an increased available length of the left IMA. Studies have demonstrated that the use of both mammary arteries results in lower rates of angina recurrence and improved 1-year patency rates when compared with the use of the left IMA combined with an SVG.[34–36]

RADIAL ARTERY

The radial artery (RA) was first introduced as an arterial conduit for coronary bypass surgery by Carpentier and colleagues[37] in the early 1970s. Early graft occlusion and development of vasospasm resulted in its abandonment as a source for revascularization. Recent advances in harvesting techniques, however, that minimize endothelial damage and the postoperative use of calcium channel blockers to decrease arterial spasm have resulted in the reintroduction of the RA as a viable arterial graft choice.[38,39] The RA is harvested from the nondominant arm and used in combination with other arterial grafts or as a free or composite graft. The RA is generally used as an alternative to a venous graft or when a third graft is required. It is most commonly used as an independent conduit to perfuse the left cardiac territory. It can be used, however, as part of a Y configuration or a conduit to perfuse the distal RCA or PDA (see **Fig. 2; Fig. 3**). Reported short-term patency rates are comparable with those associated with the left IMA, whereas the mid- to long-term patency rate is 89% after 4 years, similar to that associated with SVGs.[40] The diameter of the RA is similar to that of the IMA on CTA as it courses from the ascending aorta to the targeted occluded vessel. Because of the muscular character of the RA, assessment on

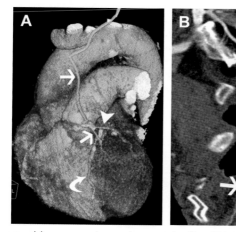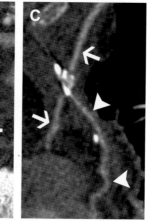

Fig. 3. A 60-year-old woman who underwent cardiac CTA 1 week after CABG surgery. (A) 3-D volume-rendered image shows total arterial revascularization of the left ventricle using the LIMA (arrows) and RA (arrowhead) to form a Y composite bypass graft. The free left RA is attached proximally to mid-LIMA and connected to an OM branch (not shown). The LIMA takes off from the left subclavian artery and anastomoses distally to LAD artery (curved arrow). (B, C) Curved planar image shows a well-opacified LIMA (arrows) with an end-to-side RA (arrowheads). The evaluation of the proximal RA anastomosis to mid-LIMA is limited because of surgical clips in the region. Tthe opacification of RA, however, with contrast is consistent with a patent graft.

CTA may be limited by the higher number of clips necessary to anastomose the collaterals compared with IMA grafts.

RIGHT GASTROEPIPLOIC ARTERY

Pym and colleagues[41] and Suma and colleagues[42] independently described the use of the RGEA as a conduit for coronary bypass surgery in 1987. The RGEA is used as a second- or third-choice conduit for total myocardial revascularization or when no viable grafts are available (**Fig. 4**).[43] The RGEA is histologically similar to the IMAs, but surgical difficulties in harvesting the vessel along with perioperative and long-term abdominal complications limit its use. Rarely, it is anastomosed in situ proximally from the greater curvature of the stomach to the PDA distally. On CTA, the RGEA is seen coursing anterior to the liver and through the diaphragm to the occluded target artery.

OTHER ARTERIES

The current trend in cardiac bypass surgery is to evaluate arterial conduits given the established long-term superiority patency rate of the IMAs over venous grafts. Various other arterial vessels, including ulnar, left gastric, splenic, thoracodorsal, and lateral femoral circumflex arteries, have been used in cases where no alternative arterial conduits exist.[44–49] The inferior epigastric artery is also considered an alternative as a conduit, with promising results reported.[50,51]

COMPLICATIONS
Graft Thrombosis and Occlusion

Complications associated with coronary bypass grafting can occur acutely or chronically. During the acute phase (within 1 month after bypass surgery), vein graft attrition from thrombosis resulting from endothelial injury during graft harvesting and anastomosis of vessels is the main cause of

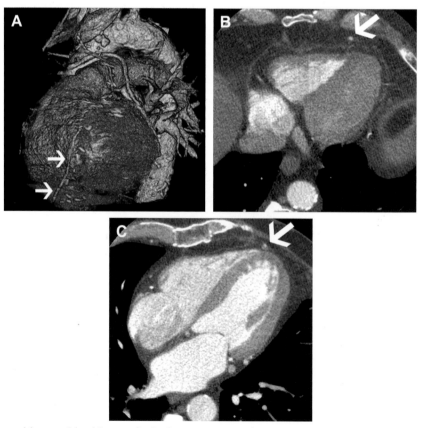

Fig. 4. A 69-year-old man with a history of prior bypass surgery who present with new high-grade proximal lesion in the LAD artery. Patient underwent another cardiac bypass surgery using a right gastroepipolic graft. (*A*) A 3-D volume-rendered image illustrates the right gastroepiploic graft extending from below the diaphragm to anastomose to the distal LAD artery anteriorly (*arrows*). (*B, C*) Axial images of the upper abdomen show a well-enhanced right gastroepiploic graft (*arrow*) traversing superiorly to the thorax.

graft failure. Patients with a hypercoaguable state or mechanical trauma from pulling and stretching of grafts that are too short, resulting in activation of the coagulation cascade, contribute to higher rates of graft occlusion during the first postoperative month. Between 3% and 12% of SVGs occlude within the first postoperative month.[31]

Neointimal hyperplasia from exposure of the venous graft to arterial circulation is the primary cause of later venous graft thrombosis. After the first postoperative month, venous grafts develop intimal thickening, causing up to 25% stenosis of the lumen.[31] Subsequent proliferation and migration of the smooth-muscle cell to the intima lead to the development of atheroma, which eventually causes late graft occlusion. In contrast, IMA conduits are remarkably resistant to development of atherosclerosis, resulting in better long-term patency rates than in SVGs. The distal site of anastomosis to the native coronary artery is a common site for atherosclerosis resulting in late IMA graft failure.

Graft stenosis and occlusion can be defined and characterized with CTA. Once the calcified or non-calcified atherosclerotic plaque is identified, the degree of lumen narrowing is analyzed using qualitative or quantitative approaches. A completely occluded graft may not be visualized on CTA or may appear as an abrupt, often proximal interruption of the contrast-enhanced lumen. In many cases, only the proximal portion of the anastomosis is visualized as it fills with contrast to form a distinctive outpouching, button, or nubbin (**Fig. 5**). Graft stenosis is characterized by an intraluminal filling defect characterized by a change in diameter of the vessel.

Graft Malposition

An early cause of myocardial revascularization failure is malpositioning or kinking of a graft that is too long.[52] A graft that is too short is often stretched, a complication often seen in patients with hyperinflated lungs, such as those with chronic obstructive pulmonary disease. Choice of anastomosis technique may also contribute to graft kinking. If an aortic connector used to attach the proximal anastomosis is not adequately supported, the conduit may kink. This kinking can often be observed on CTA.

Graft Vasospasm

A major postoperative concern with arterial grafts is vasospasm. In particular, the RA with its prominent muscular wall is prone to spasm. Reports suggest that intraoperative use of α-adrenergic blocking agents and postoperative administration of calcium channel blockers are effective in preventing graft vasospasm.[53,54] The associated finding on CTA is an extensive reduction in lumen caliber without evidence of intraluminal defects.

Graft Aneurysm

Two types of CABG aneurysms have been reported in the literature: true aneurysms and pseudoaneurysms. True aneurysms are atherosclerotic in nature and appear 5 to 7 years after CABG.[55] Pseudoaneurysms may occur early after surgery from infection or tension at the attachment site as well as at a later time. The late developing pseudoaneurysms are likely related to atherosclerotic changes. Initial CTA may reveal a mediastinal lesion exerting mass effect (**Fig. 6**). Aneurysms should be evaluated for patency, size, and mass effect on local structures.[55] Although no consensus has been reached on management of aneurysms, intervention to prevent complications may be considered based on patient presentation and aneurysm size. Complications of graft aneurysms include embolization of the bypass graft, myocardial infarction, fistula formation, rupture of the aneurysm leading to hemopericardium, hemothorax, or death.[55]

Pericardial and Pleural Effusions

The prevalence of pericardial effusion after cardiac surgery is as high as 85%. This condition, also known as postpericardiotomy syndrome, is detected clinically when patients develop heart failure, chest discomfort, and the presence of pericardial rub on physical examination. Pericardial effusions can progress to cardiac tamponade in 0.8% to 6% of patients.[56,57] Postpericardiotomy syndrome is usually a febrile illness due to an inflammatory reaction involving the pleura or pericardium. This syndrome has been reported in patients in whom the pericardium is opened as well as an unusual complication after percutaneous procedures, such as coronary stent implantation and transvenous pacemaker lead implantation.[58] Postoperative anticoagulant treatment and coagulation abnormality are risk factors. Pericardial effusion may lead to early or late postoperative cardiac tamponade and even recurrent tamponade. Fever, dyspnea, pleuritic chest pain, and emesis are typical clinical symptoms associated with the syndrome; and tachycardia with a pleural friction rub is also a classic sign. In most cases the condition is self-limiting, although anti-inflammatory drugs may be used to facilitate resolution. Approximately 89% of patients who undergo CABG surgery develop pleural effusions postoperatively.[57] The primary symptom is dyspnea with chest pain, with fever as an atypical

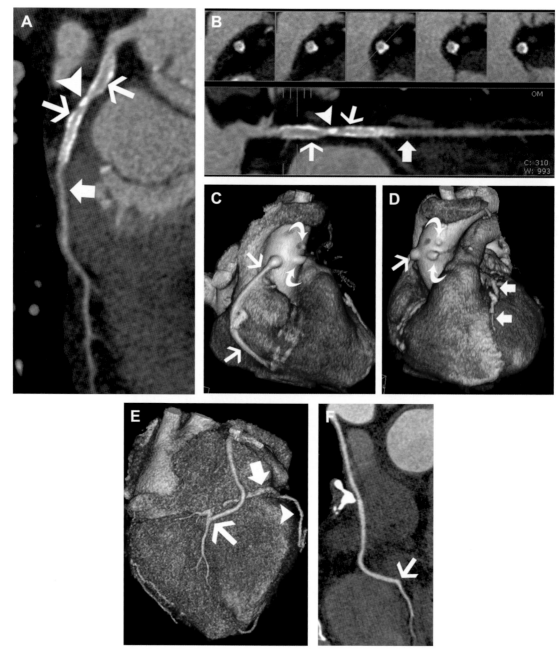

Fig. 5. A 74-year-old man status post PCI with stent placements and CABG surgery with new-onset chest pain. (*A*) Curved MPR and (*B*) linear reformatted images of the left circumflex artery with two stents in the proximal and mid vessel demonstrate areas of noncalcified intraluminal (*arrows*) and calcified extraluminal (*arrowheads*) plaques. The vessel distally is diminutive in size (*block arrows*), which can also be seen with proximal in-stent restenosis. (*C–E*) 3-D volume-rendered images demonstrate the typical appearance of SVG (*arrows*) coursing posteriorly to the right atrium and anastomosing to the PDA. There are also two occluded left SVGs originating from the left anterior ascending aorta showing the nubbin sign (*curved arrows*). Incidentally noted is an irregular-appearing LAD artery (*block arrows*) consistent with significant atherosclerotic disease. (*F*) Curved MPR image again demonstrates a contrast-filled SVG with patent end-to-side distal anastomosis to the PDA (*arrow*). Also noted is an irregular-appearing RCA (*block arrow*) with a patent acute marginal branch (*arrowhead*).

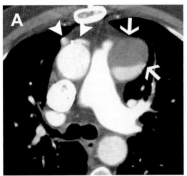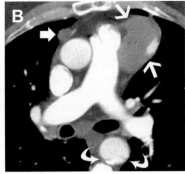

Fig. 6. A 69-year-old man with history of CABG surgery with new back pain. (*A, B*) Axial CTA images demonstrate two proximally patent SVGs at the origin of the anterior ascending aorta (*arrowheads*). The SVG to the PDA is thrombosed more distally (*block arrow*), however. Additionally, the SVG to the LAD artery has a large, partially thrombosed pseudoaneurysm (*arrows*). Intimal flaps (*curved arrows*) are incidentally noted in the descending thoracic aorta.

symptom. Most effusions are small and left-sided and resolve spontaneously.

Sternal Infection

Sternal wound infection after CABG occurs in 1% to 20% of patients.[59] Several risk factors play a role in the development of sternal wound infection, including diabetes mellitus, obesity, male gender, duration and complexity of surgery, and blood transfusions. Mediastinitis is a severe complication of deep sternal wound infection, with a mortality rate of approximately 22%.[60] CT may play an integral role in evaluating and characterizing mediastinitis after cardiac surgery. Obliteration of mediastinal fat planes and diffuse soft tissue infiltration with or without gas collections are indicative of mediastinitis.

Incidental Findings

Although the main role of CTA after CABG surgery is to evaluate graft patency, extracardiac pathology can be detected in the visualized thorax and upper abdomen. The presence of extracardiac findings on CTA is well reported in the literature. Extracardiac findings have been reported in up to 13.2% of patients undergoing cardiac CTA in the immediate postoperative period.[61] Incidental findings include pulmonary embolism, pulmonary nodules, pneumonia, mucous plugging, pneumothorax, and aortic dissection (see **Fig. 6**). Therefore, clinically significant noncardiac findings must be analyzed by radiologists to ensure that important findings are not missed.

CORONARY STENTS
Introduction

Percutaneous coronary intervention (PCI) involving the placement of stents is the main nonsurgical

procedure for myocardial revascularization, with an estimated 652,000 coronary artery stent placements in the United States in 2006.[1] It is clinically indicated in patients presenting with various symptoms of ischemia or myocardial infarction or in post-CABG patients who are poor candidates for revascularization surgery.[62] The two main types of stents used in PCI are bare-metal stents and drug-eluting stents. Although stents have a lower rate of restenosis compared with balloon angioplasty, in-stent restenosis and thrombosis remain problems. Coronary angiography is the gold standard for evaluation of coronary stents but is invasive and is associated with peri- and postoperative complications. Noninvasive assessment using MDCT may offer an alternative for detection of stent restenosis (see **Fig. 5**). The ability of MDCT, however, to accurately assess the coronary artery stent lumen may be limited by metallic stent artifacts, which can obscure the stent lumen. In addition, the blooming effect caused by radio-opaque metal stents may exaggerate the size of stent struts, resulting in a false appearance of a narrowed lumen. Newer-generation 64-slice MDCT scanners with higher temporal and spatial resolution enable higher-quality direct visualization of stent lumen and assessment of in-stent patency. A recent study to evaluate the usefulness of 64-slice CTA for assessment of coronary artery stent patency reported sensitivity and specificity of stent restenosis of 89% and 95%, respectively.[63]

Stent Imaging

The diagnostic accuracy of MDCT in evaluating stent patency is dependent on various factors, including stent diameter, material, and design.[64] Multiplanar and cross-sectional reformation images are used to visualize and accurately assess stent patency, restenosis, or neointimal hyperplasia. In addition, characterization of contrast enhancement patterns is vital in the analysis of stent patency (**Fig. 7**). Coronary stents are considered occluded if there is complete loss of contrast inside the stent lumen with decreased or absent distal runoff, indicating significant restenosis. Visualization of contrast in the vessel distal to the stent does not necessarily indicate patency because it may be due to retrograde filling of the vessels.[64]

The degree of artifacts varies with the composition and type of stent used. The majority of stents are made of stainless steel, but other materials may include tantalum, cobalt alloys, platinum, nitinol, and titanium. Stents made of tantalum create the most intense artifacts, whereas titanium and nitinol stents cause the least artifacts. The appearance of stents on CTA also depends on the design of the stent. Strut diameter can affect the magnitude of artifacts and limit accuracy in evaluation of coronary stent patency. Another factor contributing to lumen visibility is stent diameter. In general,

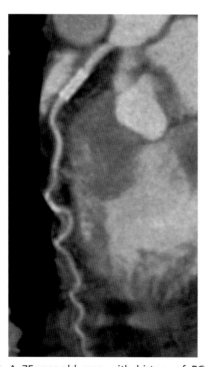

Fig. 7. A 75-year-old man with history of PCI with stent placement. Curved MPR image demonstrates a well-contrast opacified stent with in the proximal aspect of the LAD artery, consistent with a patent stent without evidence of thrombosis or in-stent restenosis.

stents with a diameter greater than or equal to 3.5 mm are better visualized.[63]

COMPLICATIONS
Restenosis

Restenosis remains a challenge for the long-term success of percutaneous transluminal coronary angioplasty and is defined as a reduction in 50% of the lumen diameter, although such stenosis is often difficult to evaluate in stents with small diameters (**Fig. 8**). The 1-year restenosis rate after percutaneous transluminal coronary angioplasty is 8.6% to 21.3% and results from a combination of elastic recoil, smooth muscle cell hyperplasia, and vascular remodeling induced by local vessel trauma.[65,66] Coronary stent placement reduces restenosis by preventing early recoil and late vascular remodeling after angioplasty but is associated with increased neointimal proliferation. The rate of in-stent restenosis ranges from less than 10% with drug-eluting stents to 40% with uncoated metallic stents.[67–70] Patients with in-stent restenosis often present with recurrent angina. Balloon angioplasty is the most common procedure for the treatment of in-stent restenosis.

Thrombosis

In-stent thrombosis is a rare but serious complication after PCIs (see **Fig. 8**). According to a recent study, the frequency of in-stent thrombosis ranges from 1.3% to 1.7% during a 9-month follow-up.[71] Acute stent thrombosis can occur during the 24 hours after intervention whereas subacute thrombosis typically occurs between 1 and 30 days after implantation of bare-metal coronary stent. Moreover, drug-eluting stents are associated with delayed in-stent thrombosis, which usually occurs after 30 days of intervention. The occurrence of this delayed thrombotic event is related to endothelization of the stent resulting from discontinuation of anticoagulation therapy. In addition to patient risk factors (renal failure, diabetes mellitus, and reduced ejection fraction),[72] increased risk factors for stent thrombosis after stent implantation include long stent lengths, with a reported 1.03 relative risk of thrombosis for each 1-mm increase in length.[71]

RECENT DEVELOPMENTS

Recent advancements in imaging technology have dramatically expanded the capabilities of CT for noninvasive coronary imaging. Emerging technologic scanners, such as 256- and 320-slice CT scanners with increased longitudinal coverage and improved temporal resolution,

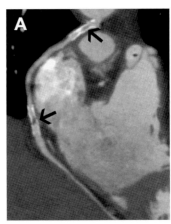
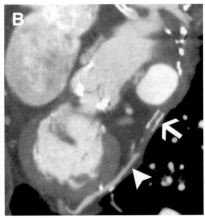

Fig. 8. A 76-year-old woman with history of CABG surgery and PCI with multiple stent placements, presenting with new onset of chest pain. (*A*) Curved MPR image demonstrates a SVG from the ascending aorta to the distal RCA with two intraluminal stents. There are hypodense areas within the stents (*arrows*) with contrast opacification distally, consistent with partial in-stent restenosis. (*B*) Curved MPR image of a thrombosed stent in the RIMA, without contrast opacification proximal to and within the stent (*arrow*). There is contrast filling in the vessel distal to the stent (*arrowhead*), likely from retrograde flow from collateral vessels.

have substantially improved cardiac imaging. Recently, dual-source CT has emerged in evaluation of coronary arteries in patients with elevated heart rates and arrhythmias while simultaneously assessing global ventricular function, regional wall motion, and cardiac valves. The use of prospective gating has led to a reduction in radiation dose in patients compared with retrospective ECG gating without compromise in the diagnostic accuracy of coronary CTA. This technique can also be applied to evaluating bypass grafts and coronary stents. The main disadvantages include the necessity for a low heart rate and the lack of functional information because only a portion of the cardiac cycle is imaged. Perfusion imaging is an emerging capability that may allow simultaneous visualization of graft and stent status and assessment of myocardial status.

SUMMARY

MDCT technology has improved substantially over the years and is often a practical alternative to invasive coronary angiography in evaluating bypass graft patency and stents. Cardiac CTA allows for simultaneous evaluation of complications poststenting and postoperative complications that manifest as chest pain. With respect to CABG, knowledge of coronary graft anatomy, type of surgical procedure performed, signs of graft stenosis, and potential extracardiac findings are necessary for appropriate interpretation.

REFERENCES

1. Lloyd-Jones D, Adams R, Brown T, et al. American Heart Association Statistics Committee and Stroke Statistics Subcommittee. Heart disease and stroke statistics—2010 update: a report from the American Heart Association Statistics Committee and Stroke Statistics Subcommittee. Circulation 2010; 121:e46–215.
2. Eagle K, Guyton R, Davidoff R, et al. ACC/AHA 2004 guideline update for coronary artery bypass graft surgery: summary article: a report of the American College of Cardiology/American Heart Association Task Force on Practice Guidelines (Committee to Update the 1999 Guidelines for Coronary Artery Bypass Graft Surgery). Circulation 2004;110(9): 1168–76.
3. Coronary artery surgery study (CASS): a randomized trial of coronary artery bypass surgery. Quality of life in patients randomly assigned to treatment groups. Circulation 1983;68(5):951–60.
4. Bourassa MG, Fisher LD, Campeau L, et al. Long-term fate of bypass grafts: the Coronary Artery Surgery Study (CASS) and Montreal Heart Institute experiences. Circulation 1985;72(6 Pt 2): V71–78.
5. Cameron A, Davis KB, Green G, et al. Coronary bypass surgery with internal-thoracic-artery grafts—effects on survival over a 15-year period. N Engl J Med 1996;334(4):216–9.
6. Campeau L, Lesperance J, Corbara F, et al. Aorto-coronary saphenous vein bypass graft changes 5 to 7 years after surgery. Circulation 1978;58(3 Pt 2):1170–5.

7. Treede H, Becker C, Reichenspurner H, et al. Multi-detector computed tomography (MDCT) in coronary surgery: first experience with a new tool for diagnosis of coronary artery disease. Ann Thorac Surg 2002;74(4):S1398–402.

8. Burgstahler C, Keuttner A, Kopp AF, et al. Non-invasive evaluation of coronary artery bypass grafts using multi-slice computed tomography: initial experience. Int J Cardiol 2003;90(2–3):275–80.

9. Nieman K, Pattynama PM, Rensing BJ, et al. Evaluation of patients after coronary artery bypass surgery: CT angiographic assessment of grafts and coronary arteries. Radiology 2003;229(3): 749–56.

10. Ropers D, Baum U, Pohle K, et al. Detection of coronary artery stenoses with thin-slice multi-detector row spiral computed tomography and multiplanar reconstruction. Circulation 2003;107(5):664–6.

11. Nieman K, Cademartiri F, Lemos PA, et al. Reliable noninvasive coronary angiography with fast submillimeter multislice spiral computed tomography. Circulation 2002;106(16):2051–4.

12. Heuschmid M, Keuttner A, Schroeder S, et al. ECG-gated 16-MDCT of the coronary arteries: assessment of image quality and accuracy in detecting stenoses. AJR Am J Roentgenol 2005;184(5): 1413–9.

13. Flohr T, Stierstorfer K, Raupach R, et al. Performance evaluation of a 64-slice CT system with z-flying focal spot. Rofo 2004;176(12):1803–10.

14. Miller J, Rochitte C, Dewey M, et al. Diagnostic performance of coronary angiography by 64-row CT. N Engl J Med 2008;359(22):2324–36.

15. Onuma Y, Tanabe K, Chihara R, et al. Evaluation of coronary artery bypass grafts and native coronary arteries using 64-slice multidetector computed tomography. Am Heart J 2007;154(3):519–26.

16. Meyer TS, Martinoff S, Hadamitzky M, et al. Improved noninvasive assessment of coronary artery bypass grafts with 64-slice computed tomographic angiography in an unselected patient population. J Am Coll Cardiol 2007;49(9):946–50.

17. Malagutti P, Nieman K, Meijboom WB, et al. Use of 64-slice CT in symptomatic patients after coronary bypass surgery: evaluation of grafts and coronary arteries. Eur Heart J 2007;28(15):1879–85.

18. Ma E, Yang Z, Wang Q, et al. Clinical application of 64-slice CT in evaluation of vessel before and after coronary artery bypass graft surgery. Sheng Wu Yi Xue Gong Cheng Xue Za Zhi 2009;26(3):491–5.

19. Liu ZY, Gao CQ, Li BJ, et al. Diagnostic study on the coronary artery bypass grafts lesions using 64 multi-slice computed tomography angiography. Zhonghua Wai Ke Za Zhi 2008;46(4):245–7.

20. von Kiedrowski H, Wiemer M, Franzke K, et al. Noninvasive coronary angiography: the clinical value of multi-slice computed tomography in the assessment of patients with prior coronary bypass surgery. Int J Cardiovasc Imaging 2009; 25(2):161–70.

21. Garrett HE, Dennis EW, DeBakey ME. Aortocoronary bypass with saphenous vein graft. Seven-year follow-up. JAMA 1973;223(7):792–4.

22. Fitzgibbon GM, Kafka HP, Leach AJ, et al. Coronary bypass fate and patient outcome: angiographic follow up of 5,065 grafts related to survival and reoperation in 1,388 patients during 25 years. J Am Coll Cardiol 1996;28(3):616–26.

23. Campeau L, Enjalbert M, Leasperance J, et al. The relation of risk factors to the development of atherosclerosis in saphenous vein bypass grafts and the progression of disease in native circulation: a study 10 years after aortocoronary bypass surgery. N Engl J Med 1984;311(21):1329–32.

24. The effect of aggressive lowering of low-density lipoprotein cholesterol levels and low-dose anticoagulation on obstructive changes in saphenous-vein coronary-artery bypass grafts. The Post Coronary Artery Bypass Graft Trial Investigators. N Engl J Med 1997;336(3):153–62.

25. Cannon CP, Mehta SR, Aranka SF. Balancing the benefit and risk of oral antiplatelet agents in coronary artery bypass surgery. Ann Thorac Surg 2005;80(2):768–79.

26. Souza DS, Johansson B, Bojö L, et al. Harvesting the saphenous vein with surrounding tissue for CABG provides long-term graft patency comparable to the left internal thoracic artery: Results of a randomized longitudinal trial. J Thorac Cardiovasc Surg 2006;132(2):373–8.

27. Eckstein FS, Bonilla LF, Englberger L, et al. Minimizing aortic manipulation during OPCAB using the Symmetry™ Aortic Connector System for proximal vein graft anastomoses. Ann Thorac Surg 2001;72(3):S995–8.

28. Marano R, Storto ML, Merlino B, et al. A pictorial review of coronary artery bypass grafts at multidetector row CT. Chest 2005;127(4):1371–7.

29. Motwani JG, Topol EJ. Aortocoronary saphenous vein graft disease: pathogenesis, predisposition, and prevention. Circulation 1998;97(9):916–31.

30. Loop FD, Lytle BW, Cosgrove DM, et al. Influence of the internal-mammary-artery graft on 10-year survival and other cardiac events. N Engl J Med 1986;314(1):1–6.

31. Sabik JH III, Lytle BW, Blackstone EH, et al. Comparison of saphenous vein and internal thoracic artery graft patency by coronary system. Ann Thorac Surg 2005;79(2):544–51.

32. Marano R, Liguori C, Rinaldi P, et al. Coronary artery bypass grafts and MDCT imaging: what to know and what to look for. Eur Radiol 2007;17(12):3166–78.

33. Ura M, Sakata R, Nakayama Y, et al. Long term patency rate of right internal thoracic artery

bypass via the transverse sinus. Circulation 1998; 98(19):2043–8.

34. Lyte BW, Blackstone EH, Loop FD, et al. Two internal thoracic artery grafts are better than one. J Thorac Cardiovasc Surg 1999;117(5):855–72.

35. Muneretto C, Negri A, Manfredi J, et al. Safety and usefulness of composite grafts for total arterial myocardial revascularization: a prospective randomized evaluation. J Thorac Cardiovasc Surg 2003;125(4):826–35.

36. Pick AW, Orszulak TA, Anderson BJ, et al. Single versus bilateral internal mammary artery grafts:10-year outcome analysis. Ann Thorac Surg 1997; 64(3):599–605.

37. Carpentier A, Guermonprez JL, Doloche A, et al. The aorta-to-coronary radial bypass graft: a technique avoiding pathological changes in grafts. Ann Thorac Surg 1973;16(2):111–21.

38. Royse AG, Royse CF, Shah P, et al. Radial artery harvest technique, use and functional outcome. Eur J Cardiothorac Surg 1999;15(2):186–93.

39. Calafiore AM, Teodori G, Di Giammarco G, et al. Coronary revascularization with the radial artery: new interest for an old conduit. J Card Surg 1995; 10(2):140–6.

40. Tatoulis J, Buxton BF, Fuller JA. Patencies of 2127 arterial to coronary conduits over 15 years. Ann Thorac Surg 2004;77(1):93–101.

41. Pym J, Brown PM, Charrette EJ. Gastroepiploic coronary anastomosis: a viable alternative bypass graft. J Thorac Cardiovasc Surg 1987;94(2):256–9.

42. Suma H, Fukumoto H, Takeuchi A. Coronary artery bypass grafting by utilizing in situ right gastroepiploic artery: basic study and clinical application. Ann Thorac Surg 1987;44(4):39.

43. Grandjean JG, Boonstra PW, den Heyer P, et al. Arterial revascularization with the right gastroepiploic artery and internal mammary arteries in 300 patients. J Thorac Cardiovasc Surg 1994;107(5):1309–15.

44. Grandjean JG, Voors AA, Boonstra PW, et al. Exclusive use of arterial grafts in coronary artery bypass operations for three-vessel disease: use of both thoracic arteries and the gastroepiploic artery in 256 consecutive patients. J Thorac Cardiovasc Surg 1996;112(4):935–42.

45. Formica F, Ferro O, Greco P, et al. Long-term follow-up of total arterial myocardial revascularization using exclusively pedicle bilateral internal thoracic artery and right gastroepiploic artery. Eur J Cardiothorac Surg 2004;26(6):1141–8.

46. Buxton BF, Chan AT, Dixit AS, et al. Ulnar artery as a coronary bypass graft. Ann Thorac Surg 1998; 65(4):1020–4.

47. Moro H, Ohzeki H, Hayashi JI, et al. Evaluation of the thoracodorsal artery as an alternative conduit for coronary bypass. Thorac Cardiovasc Surg 1997; 45(6):277–9.

48. Mueller DK, Blakeman BP, Pickleman J. Free splenic artery used in aortocoronary bypass. Ann Thorac Surg 1993;55(1):162–3.

49. Schamun CM, Duran JC, Rodriguez JM, et al. Coronary revascularization with the descending branch of the lateral femoral circumflex artery as a composite arterial graft. J Thorac Cardiovasc Surg 1998;116(5):870–1.

50. Buche M, Schroeder E, Gurne O, et al. Coronary artery bypass grafting with the inferior epigastric artery. Midterm clinical and angiographic results. J Thorac Cardiovasc Surg 1995;109(3):553–9.

51. Cremer J, Mugge A, Schulze M, et al. The inferior epigastric artery for coronary bypass grafting. Functional assessment and clinical results. Eur J Cardiothorac Surg 1993;7(8):423–7.

52. Ricci M, Karamanoukian HL, D'Ancona G, et al. Reoperative "off-pump" circumflex revascularization via left thoracotomy: How to prevent graft kinking. Ann Thorac Surg 2000;70(1):309–10.

53. Possati G, Gaudino M, Prafti F, et al. Long-term results of the radial artery used for myocardial revascularization. Circulation 2003;108(11):1350–4.

54. Locker C, Mohr R, Paz Y, et al. Pretreatment with alpha-adrenergic blockers for prevention of radial artery spasm. Ann Thorac Surg 2002;74(4): S1368–70.

55. Memon AQ, Huang RI, Marcus F, et al. Saphenous vein graft aneurysm: Case report and review. Cardiol Rev 2003;11(1):26–34.

56. Pepi M, Muratori M, Barbier P, et al. Pericardial effusion after cardiac surgery: incidence, site, size, and heamodynamic consequences. Br Heart J 1994; 72(4):327–31.

57. Vargas FS, Cukier A, Hueb W, et al. Relationship between pleural effusion and pericardial involvement after myocardial revascularization. Chest 1994;105(6):1748–52.

58. Vinit J, Sagnol P, Buttard P, et al. Recurrent delayed pericarditis after pacemaker implantation: a postpericardiotomy-like syndrome? Rev Med Interne 2007;28(2):137–40.

59. Loop FD, Lytle BW, Cosgrove DM, et al. J. Maxwell Chamberlain memorial paper. Sternal wound complications after isolated coronary artery bypass grafting: early and late mortality, morbidity, and cost of care. Ann Thorac Surg 1990;49(4):179–86 [discussion: 186–7].

60. Braxton JH, Marrin CA, McGrath PD, et al. Mediastinitis and long-term survival after coronary artery bypass graft surgery. Ann Thorac Surg 2000;70(6):2004–7.

61. Mueller J, Jeudy J, Poston R, et al. Cardiac CT angiography after coronary bypass surgery: Prevalence of incidental findings. Am J Roentgenol 2007;189(2): 414–9.

62. Smith SC, Feldman TE, Hirshfeld JW, et al. ACC/AHA/SCAI 2005 Guideline Update for Percutaneous

Coronary Intervention—summary article: a report of the American College of Cardiology/American Heart Association Task Force on Practice Guidelines (ACC/AHA/SCAI Writing Committee to Update the 2001 Guidelines for Percutaneous Coronary Intervention). Circulation 2006;113(1):156–75.

63. Antoniucci D, Valenti R, Santoro GM, et al. Restenosis after coronary stenting in current practice. Am Heart J 1998;135(3):510–8.

64. Pugliese F, Cademartiri F, van Mieghem C, et al. Multidetector CT for visualization of coronary stents. Radiographics 2006;26(3):887–904.

65. Menichelli M, Parma A, Pucci E, et al. Randomized trial of Sirolimus-Eluting Stent Versus Bare-Metal Stent in Acute Myocardial Infarction (SESAMI). J Am Coll Cardiol 2007;49(19):1924–30.

66. Stone GW, Ellis SG, Cannon L, et al. Comparison of a polymer-based paclitaxel-eluting stent with a bare metal stent in patients with complex coronary artery disease: a randomized controlled trial. JAMA 2005; 294(10):1215–23.

67. Serruys PW, de Jaegere P, Kiemeneij F, et al. A comparison of balloon-expandable-stent implantation with balloon angioplasty in patients with coronary artery disease. Benestent Study Group. N Engl J Med 1994;331(8):489–95.

68. Fischman DL, Leon MB, Baim DS, et al. A randomized comparison of coronary-stent placement and balloon angioplasty in the treatment of coronary artery disease. Stent Restenosis Study Investigators. N Engl J Med 1994;331(8):496–501.

69. Kiemeneij F, Serruys PW, Macaya C, et al. Continued benefit of coronary stenting versus balloon angioplasty: five-year clinical follow-up of Benestent-I trial. J Am Coll Cardiol 2001;37(6):1598–603.

70. Morice MC, Serruys PW, Sousa JE, et al. A randomized comparison of a sirolimus-eluting stent with a standard stent for coronary revascularization. N Engl J Med 2002;346(23):1773–80.

71. Iakovou I, Schmidt T, Bonizzoni E, et al. Incidence, predictors, and outcome of thrombosis after successful implantation of drug-eluting stents. JAMA 2005;293(17):2126–30.

72. Ong AT, Hoye A, Aoki J, et al. Thirty-day incidence and six-month clinical outcome of thrombotic stent occlusion after bare-metal, sirolimus, or paclitaxel stent implantation. J Am Coll Cardiol 2005;45(6):947–53.

Evaluation of Myocardial Abnormalities and Ischemia

Hersh Chandarana, MD[a], Monvadi B. Srichai, MD[a,b,*]

KEYWORDS

- Cardiac computed tomography • Myocardial infarction
- Myocardial ischemia • Myocardial perfusion
- Coronary artery disease • Nonischemic cardiomyopathy

Cardiac computed tomography angiography (CCTA) has emerged as a powerful noninvasive technique for anatomic evaluation of the coronary arteries. Multiple studies have demonstrated very good diagnostic accuracy for detection of coronary artery disease, particularly with 64-slice systems.[1,2] However, the presence of calcified plaques often limits the ability to distinguish obstructive from nonobstructive lesions, and the physiologic significance of stenoses can be uncertain. Additional information is obtained through invasive angiography with or without assessment of coronary artery fractional flow reserve or noninvasive imaging techniques to assess the functional significance of lesions by evaluating myocardial structure, perfusion, and/or function. There are also extensive data regarding the prognostic information provided by the amount of infarcted and ischemic myocardium that can help determine which patients benefit most from revascularization versus optimized medical treatment.[3–7]

Myocardial structure, perfusion, and function are routinely assessed with echocardiography, nuclear imaging techniques, or cardiac magnetic resonance imaging. Two-dimensional echocardiography including Doppler flow study is an established technique for assessment of left ventricular (LV) size and function. Information on myocardial structure is gained from observation of abnormalities in end-diastolic myocardial wall thickness (eg, too thin or too thick), and information on myocardial function is obtained via assessment for regional myocardial wall motion abnormalities. Further, information on myocardial states (eg, ischemia or infarction) can be obtained by observing the effect of either exercise or pharmacologic (eg, dobutamine) stress on myocardial function. Nuclear imaging techniques, including single photon emission tomography (SPECT) and positron emission tomography (PET), evaluate myocardial perfusion and viability through the use of cardiac-specific radionuclide tracers, which are administered at rest and/or stress depending on the information sought. Gated SPECT and PET acquisitions allow for assessment of myocardial function similar to echocardiography, but with limited spatial and temporal resolution. Contrast-enhanced magnetic resonance (CMR) is an established method for the evaluation of myocardial infarction and viability. The most commonly implemented technique is through the assessment of late contrast enhancement using extracellular gadolinium contrast agents, which has been shown to have an excellent correlation with the extent of acute and chronic myocardial infarction[8] and in predicting improvement of regional myocardial function.[9–11] In addition, information on myocardial ischemia can also be obtained with the use of pharmacologic

[a] Department of Radiology, NYU School of Medicine, 530 First Avenue, New York, NY 10016, USA
[b] Department of Medicine (Cardiology Division), NYU School of Medicine, 530 First Avenue, New York, NY 10016, USA
* Corresponding author.
E-mail address: srichm01@med.nyu.edu

Radiol Clin N Am 48 (2010) 771–782
doi:10.1016/j.rcl.2010.04.008

stress agents. Although widely accepted in clinical practice, not all patients are eligible for CMR given its limited availability to specialized cardiac imaging centers, and potential contraindication in patients with pacemakers, internal cardiac defibrillators, or other electronic implants.

Emerging techniques in CCTA allow for accurate assessment of myocardial structure, perfusion, and function, comparable to established techniques already discussed. CCTA has the potential to be a "one-stop shop" because it can be used to assess coronary artery anatomy and myocardial structure, perfusion, and function. In this article, established and emerging CCTA techniques for the evaluation of myocardial structure, perfusion, and function are reviewed.

COMPUTED TOMOGRAPHY TECHNIQUES FOR EVALUATION OF THE MYOCARDIUM

Advances in computed tomography (CT) hardware and software have increased cardiac imaging capabilities with improvements in spatial resolution, temporal resolution, and volume coverage. Although these developments are important for coronary artery imaging, they have also expanded the potential utility of noncoronary applications in CT imaging. In fact, evaluation of myocardial function and perfusion requires CT systems with high temporal resolution and large volume coverage to sufficiently capture the heart during the same phase of contrast opacification with adequate image quality.

CCTA for evaluation of the coronary arteries is distinguished from conventional CT techniques by the need for electrocardiographic (ECG) gating to minimize cardiac motion. ECG gating allows for the synchronization of data acquisition to the heart cycle to combine data acquired from consecutive gantry rotations in volumetric datasets with minimal blurring artifact related to cardiac motion. Similarly, accurate evaluation of the myocardium, particularly for functional assessment, requires the use of ECG gating techniques to minimize cardiac motion.

Myocardial Structure and Perfusion

Because normal myocardium is indistinguishable from the ventricular cavity on noncontrast CT, administration of iodinated contrast is frequently required to assess the myocardium (**Fig. 1**). Normal myocardium on CCTA is fairly uniform in thickness (6–11 mm in end-diastole), and enhances homogeneously over time after the intravenous administration of iodinated contrast. Noncontrast, early-phase, and late-phase perfusion imaging techniques have all been used to distinguish different myocardial structural states including normal, ischemic, and infarcted myocardium. Several studies have shown that iodinated contrast agents used in CCTA have similar kinetics to gadolinium used in CMR.[12,13] Intravenous administration of iodinated contrast produces CT attenuation numbers (Hounsfield units, HU) that are directly proportional to iodine content in tissue, and this relationship remains linear well above the concentrations required for myocardial perfusion imaging.[14] In animal studies, ischemic myocardium demonstrates delay in onset and time to peak attenuation density compared with normal

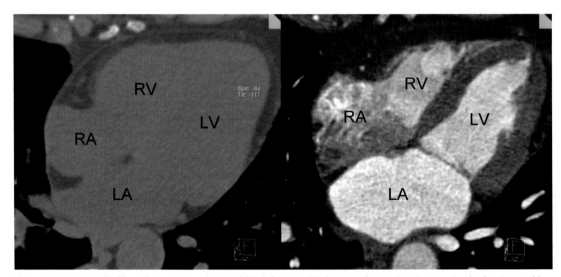

Fig. 1. Noncontrast (*left*) and contrast-enhanced (*right*) CT multiplanar reformation images in the horizontal long axis view of the heart demonstrating the appearance of normal myocardium. RA, right atrium; LA, left atrium; RV, right ventricle; LV, left ventricle.

myocardium,[14] and infarcted myocardium demonstrates significantly higher attenuation density compared with normal myocardium, starting approximately 2 minutes and lasting up to 24 minutes after iodinated contrast administration.[12]

Early-phase CCTA perfusion imaging with and without pharmacologic stress has been used in a similar manner to radionuclide imaging and CMR techniques to identify areas of abnormally decreased myocardial perfusion suggestive of either myocardial infarction or ischemia.[12,15] In addition, late-phase perfusion imaging techniques (5–15 minutes following contrast administration) have been used in a manner similar to CMR for the identification of hyperenhanced areas, suggestive of myocardial fibrosis, to distinguish viable from nonviable myocardium.[12,16–18] CCTA myocardial perfusion studies are commonly performed using static, morphologic imaging of a single perfusion phase, as opposed to time-resolved perfusion imaging. As such, contrast timing is important in

myocardial perfusion studies, and image acquisition should attempt to cover the heart during the same phase of contrast opacification to allow for accurate delineation of small or subtle perfusion defects.

Myocardial Function

Unlike anatomic evaluations in which only a single phase of the cardiac cycle is needed for assessment of structure and perfusion, myocardial functional assessment requires acquisition of information throughout the cardiac cycle, often obtained with the use of retrospective ECG-gating techniques, to visualize wall motion and wall thickening at different phases of the cardiac cycle (**Fig. 2**). At present, myocardial functional evaluation requires combining data from consecutive gantry rotations to generate a 4-dimensional moving image of the heart. Given this requirement for image reconstruction, it is important for patients to have a regular heart rhythm,

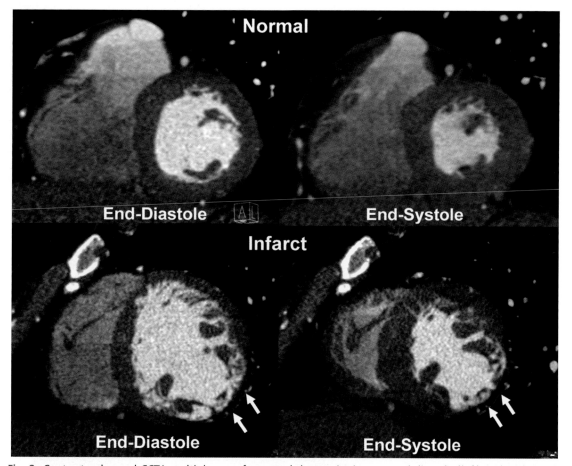

Fig. 2. Contrast-enhanced CCTA multiplanar reformatted short-axis views at end-diastole (*left*) and end-systole (*right*) from a normal patient demonstrating normal myocardium with normal wall motion (*top*), and a patient with evidence of myocardial infarction (*bottom*) with significant wall thinning and associated wall motion abnormality (decreased myocardial thickening at end-systole) in the inferolateral wall (*arrows*).

preferably normal sinus rhythm, during data acquisition for the volumetric datasets to match up phase by phase during image reconstruction.

Multiple studies have documented the diagnostic value of CCTA to evaluate LV size and global and regional LV function.[19–21] In general, when compared with CMR, CCTA demonstrates excellent agreement for assessment of LV ejection fraction and regional wall motion.[20,21] In one study multidetector CT showed better agreement with CMR than 2-dimensional echocardiography.[22] Although the postprocessing requires some manual interaction, the process has become automated, with minimal user interaction due to improvement in these algorithms.

CCTA MYOCARDIAL APPLICATIONS
Myocardial Infarction and Viability

Early animal studies demonstrated the general feasibility of conventional CT for infarction imaging,[23–25] although single-slice systems used at that time were not valuable as a clinical tool for cardiac imaging. With the advent of multidetector CT systems with improved temporal resolution capable of diagnostic coronary artery imaging, several investigators have explored the potential clinical utility of CCTA in the evaluation of myocardial infarction and viability.[12,15–18]

Infarcted myocardium often appears thinned because of loss of muscle mass, which can be easily identified on CCTA (**Fig. 2**). In some instances, there may be subendocardial fat accumulation within the infarcted myocardium (**Fig. 3**). In one study of patients with a prior history of myocardial infarction who underwent CCTA, myocardial fat was found in

approximately 20% of cases, and more commonly occurred with infarctions of older age and infarctions in the left anterior descending artery territory.[26] In addition, there is often impairment of myocardial function in the infarction segments, which is manifest on CCTA imaging as a regional wall motion abnormality (hypokinesis, akinesis, or dyskinesis) with decreased systolic wall thickening when compared with normal myocardium (**Fig. 2**). CCTA has been shown to provide an accurate method for measurement of regional and global LV function in patients with myocardial infarction.[27]

Infarcted myocardium may demonstrate relative hypoperfusion on early-phase imaging after contrast administration when compared with normal myocardium and relative hyperenhancement on late-phase imaging (**Fig. 4**). In one study, investigators demonstrated that acute myocardial infarction is detectable on contrast-enhanced chest CT as a focal decrease in LV myocardial enhancement of 20 HU or more in the coronary artery distribution of the acute myocardial infarction. This finding was visually detected in approximately 50% of the cases in that study.[28] Another study assessed the pattern of early and delayed myocardial enhancement in patients with acute and chronic myocardial infarction. An early perfusion defect was identified in all patients and in 97% of the affected myocardial territories. The attenuation of the early perfusion defects was significantly lower than that of noninfarcted areas, and these perfusion defects were subendocardial in greater than one-half of the cases and transmural in approximately 40% of cases. Delayed enhancement at 7 minutes after contrast administration was seen in 94% of cases of acute

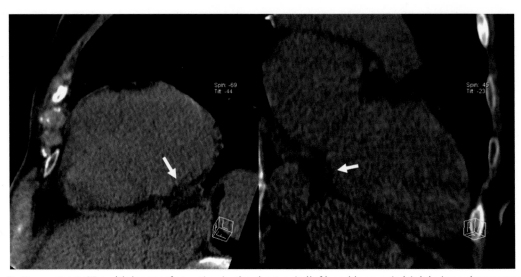

Fig. 3. Noncontrast CT multiplanar reformation in the short-axis (*left*) and long-axis (*right*) views demonstrating focal area of low attenuation representing fat in the basal inferior segment (*arrows*).

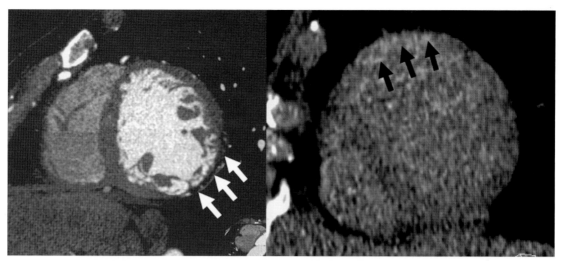

Fig. 4. Contrast-enhanced CCTA multiplanar reformation in the short-axis views demonstrating low attenuation of infarction region (*white arrows*) on early-phase, first-pass perfusion imaging (*left*) in a patient with inferolateral myocardial infarction, and high attenuation of the infarction region (*black arrows*) on late-phase imaging obtained approximately 10 minutes after contrast administration (*right*) in a different patient with an anterior myocardial infarction.

myocardial infarction and 100% of cases of chronic myocardial infarction. Thus early perfusion defects and delayed enhancement can be seen with myocardial infarction.[29]

Complications of myocardial infarction such as LV aneurysm can also be detected on CCTA. In the Coronary Artery Surgery Study, the rate of LV aneurysm in patient with acute myocardial infarction was 7.6%.[30] There are 2 types of aneurysms, true and false. The wall of true aneurysms is made up of infarcted myocardium (**Fig. 5**) whereas false aneurysms, which represent a contained rupture, are walled off by an external structure such as the pericardium. On CCTA, true aneurysms are often apical in location and commonly have a wide neck; in contrast, false aneurysms are often posterior diaphragmatic in location and commonly have a narrow neck (**Fig. 5**). Although pseudoaneurysms may require urgent surgical resection because of the likelihood of rupture, true aneurysms can often be managed medically. This difference makes an accurate diagnosis imperative.

Myocardial Ischemia

Complete assessment of myocardial states in coronary artery disease includes evaluation of

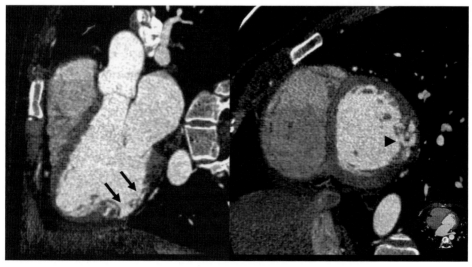

Fig. 5. Contrast-enhanced CCTA multiplanar reformation images demonstrating wide neck true aneurysm (*left, arrows*) and narrow neck pseudoaneurysm (*right, arrowhead*).

myocardial ischemia in addition to myocardial infarction. CCTA examination in conjunction with vasodilator stress challenge offers an important advantage in the ability to simultaneously visualize coronary anatomy and myocardial perfusion including ischemia. Vasodilator agents can help identify the myocardium supplied by coronary artery with critical flow-limiting stenosis because

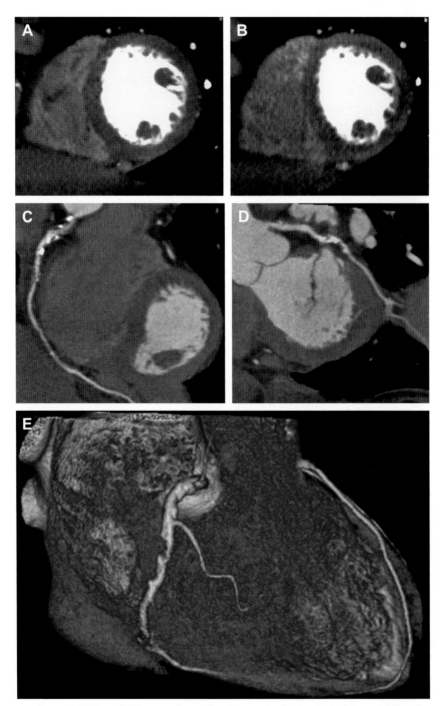

Fig. 6. Contrast-enhanced CCTA multiplanar reformation images in short axis during rest (*A*) and stress (*B*) perfusion with corresponding curved and volume-rendered reformations demonstrating coronary anatomy (*C–E*). (*Adapted from* George RT, Arbab-Zadeh A, Miller JM, et al. Adenosine stress 64- and 256-row detector CT angiography and perfusion imaging: a pilot study evaluating the transmural extent of perfusion abnormalities to predict atherosclerosis causing myocardial ischemia. Circ Cardiovasc Imaging 2009;2:179; with permission.)

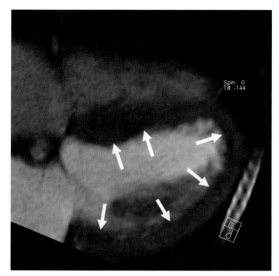

Fig. 7. Contrast-enhanced CCTA multiplanar reformation images in horizontal long-axis view demonstrating global increased LV wall thickness with diffuse subendocardial hypoattenuation (*arrows*) on early-phase imaging in a patient with cardiac amyloidosis.

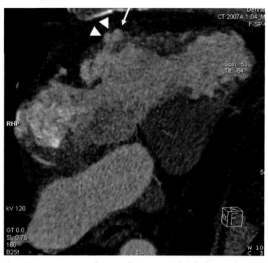

Fig. 9. Contrast-enhanced CCTA multiplanar reformation image demonstrating focal right ventricular aneurysm (*arrowheads*) with low-attenuation areas of the myocardium (*arrow*) suggestive of fibrofatty replacement of the myocardium characteristic for arrhythmogenic right ventricular cardiomyopathy/dysplasia.

the myocardium at risk will perfuse normally at baseline but will demonstrate hypoperfusion after vasodilator challenge (**Fig. 6**). In addition, the high spatial resolution and volumetric coverage provided by CCTA allows for improved detection of small areas of ischemia when compared with SPECT, PET, and CMR techniques.

Stress-perfusion CT using vasodilator agents has been shown to provide similar information as stress SPECT for the detection of ischemic myocardium,[31,32] with reported sensitivities of 79% to 96% and specificities of 73% to 92%.[33,34] Depending on the study protocol, additional information on coronary anatomy, rest perfusion, and late-phase enhancement may also

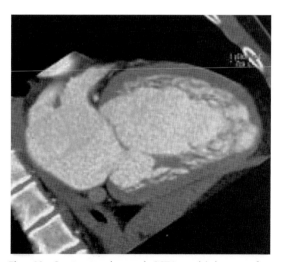

Fig. 10. Contrast-enhanced CCTA multiplanar reformation image in long-axis view demonstrating numerous deep trabeculations along the mid and apical LV myocardium consistent with noncompaction of the left ventricle. (*Reprinted from* Koh YY, Seo YU, Woo JJ, et al. Familial isolated noncompaction of the ventricular myocardium in asymptomatic phase. Yonsei Med J 2004;45:932; with permission.)

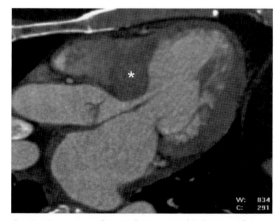

Fig. 8. Contrast-enhanced CCTA multiplanar reformation image in long axis demonstrating abnormal increased end-diastolic wall thickness of the basal septum (*asterisk*) in a pattern consistent with asymmetric septal hypertrophic cardiomyopathy.

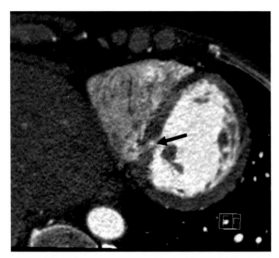

Fig. 11. Contrast-enhanced CCTA multiplanar reformation image in short-axis view demonstrating muscular ventricular septal defect (*arrow*).

be obtained in a single examination (**Fig. 6**). However, the potential benefits of a comprehensive CCTA protocol must be weighed against the inherent limitations including higher radiation-dose exposure, larger volume of iodinated contrast administration, and potential artifacts such as motion and beam hardening.

There have been a couple of small observational studies that noted the ability of rest CCTA to detect myocardial ischemia conventionally depicted by myocardial perfusion scintigraphy, with sensitivity 90% to 100% and specificity of 67% to 83%.[35,36] These studies suggest potential mechanisms for this effect including diminished capacitance of ischemic capillary microvessels in the subendocardium during systole,[35] intrinsic vasodilatory effect

of iodinated contrast material, differences in the myocardial distribution kinetics of the different contrast agents, and the wider dynamic range for different rates of myocardial perfusion when compared with SPECT.[36] However, resting perfusion CT abnormalities seem to underestimate the extent of ischemia depicted by stress/rest SPECT imaging,[35] and better agreement is likely to occur with the use of dedicated stress CT perfusion protocols.

Other Myocardial Abnormalities

Although myocardial ischemia and infarction related to coronary artery disease probably accounts for most myocardial abnormalities noted in patients with heart disease, a small subset of patients may present with other "nonischemic" myocardial diseases. A recent study demonstrated that approximately 1% of patients undergoing CCTA for evaluation of obstructive coronary artery disease were noted with unsuspected but clinically relevant cardiovascular abnormalities unrelated to coronary atherosclerosis, with 20% of these patients diagnosed with an underlying myocardial abnormality.[37]

As already mentioned, the ability of CCTA to evaluate the coronary arteries in addition to the myocardium is particularly useful for ruling out "ischemic" myocardial disease related to coronary artery lesions. In particular, myocardial fibrosis related to coronary artery disease often demonstrates a subendocardial or transmural pattern of fibrosis in the territory supplied by the diseased coronary artery. Consequently, based on prior CMR studies, nonischemic myocardial disease demonstrates no significant fibrosis, or a different

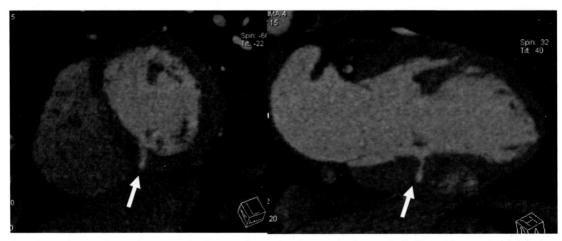

Fig. 12. Contrast-enhanced CCTA multiplanar reformation images in short-axis (*left*) and long-axis (*right*) views demonstrating single deep intramyocardial recess (*arrows*) at the mid inferior/inferoseptal junction consistent with left ventricular diverticulum.

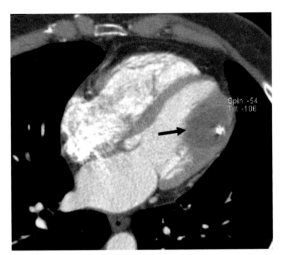

Fig. 13. Contrast-enhanced CCTA multiplanar reformation image in the horizontal long-axis view demonstrating well-circumscribed area of low attenuation within the mid to apical lateral wall of the left ventricle with focus of calcification within the lesion. These findings are suggestive of a benign tumor, as opposed to focal hypertrophy, and cardiac fibroma was found intraoperatively in this patient.

pattern of fibrosis, with midwall and/or subepicardial involvement, when compared with ischemic myocardial disease.[38,39] CCTA findings of nonobstructive coronary artery disease in combination with myocardial wall motion abnormalities and fibrosis in a nonischemic pattern is highly suggestive of a nonischemic cardiomyopathy. There have been scattered case reports of the use of CCTA for evaluating nonischemic myocardial abnormalities such as cardiac sarcoidosis,[40] cardiac amyloidosis (**Fig. 7**),[41,42] hypertrophic

cardiomyopathy (**Fig. 8**),[43,44] arrhythmogenic right ventricular dysplasia/cardiomyopathy (**Fig. 9**),[45,46] and LV noncompaction (**Fig. 10**).[47]

With the high spatial resolution of CCTA combined with its increased use for evaluation of coronary artery disease, incidental myocardial lesions such as ventricular septal defect (**Fig. 11**),[48] congenital ventricular diverticuli (**Fig. 12**),[49] and intramyocardial tumors (**Fig. 13**)[50] have been increasingly recognized. CCTA can also be used for primary myocardial evaluation of structure and function in congenital heart disease or cardiac masses, particularly when echocardiography or CMR is limited or unavailable (eg, pacemaker).[51,52]

FUTURE DIRECTIONS

In clinical practice, as discussed herein, ischemic or infarcted myocardium is diagnosed on qualitative evaluation. On early first-pass perfusion imaging, ischemic myocardium appears hypoattenuated because of decreased delivery of blood (which is mixed with iodinated contrast agent). Animal models and research studies have shown that by performing high temporal resolution first-pass perfusion imaging, ischemic myocardium demonstrates lower and more attenuated time-activity attenuation curves than normal myocardium.[14] Iodinated contrast is used in CT because of its ability to attenuate x-rays, and this attenuation is directly proportional to iodine content. However, there is inter- and intra-scanner variability in attenuation values, and hence conversion of CT attenuation values to iodine concentration (mg/mL) usually requires optimization with a phantom validation study. As a result, these quantitative techniques have not gained widespread use in clinical practice. Another

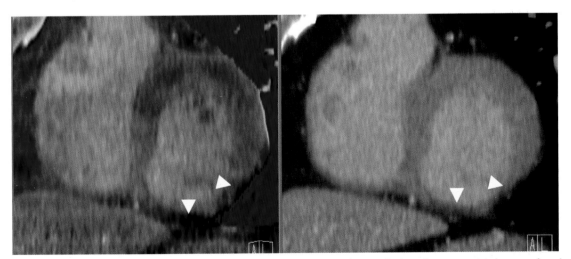

Fig. 14. Contrast-enhanced CCTA multiplanar reformation images in short-axis view demonstrating hypoperfused myocardial infarct (*arrowheads*) involving the inferior and inferolateral walls on early-phase dual-energy image (*left*) with corresponding single-energy (140 kV) image (*right*).

problem with quantitative CT perfusion imaging is the need for repeated acquisitions, which result in an increase in radiation dose to the patients.

Dual-energy techniques in which information from different x-ray spectra are generated by different kilovolt settings of the x-ray tubes is a technique that can enhance tissue differentiation by taking advantage of the different absorption characteristics shown by tissues when exposed to different x-ray spectra. Dual-energy techniques have been used to improve the conspicuity of myocardial perfusion abnormalities (**Fig. 14**).[53] The resultant low- and high-energy CT data can be postprocessed as image-based analyses, using a so-called 3-material decomposition algorithm (for these analyses, the 3 materials are fat, soft tissue, and iodine) to determine contribution of iodine to the contrast-enhanced CT image.[54] This contribution can be evaluated qualitatively and quantitatively in mg/mL. The role of dual-energy imaging in the assessment of myocardial ischemia and infarction is still under investigation, but seems promising.[36]

Finally, studies demonstrating the prognostic value of cardiac CT in the evaluation of myocardial abnormalities in ischemic and nonischemic disease are needed to further justify and validate its use, particularly given the additional radiation dose often accompanied by the methods used to obtain the additional information on myocardial structure, perfusion, and function beyond the assessment of the coronary arteries.

SUMMARY

In this article the authors review the role of cardiac CT in the evaluation of myocardial structure, perfusion, and function. When evaluated in conjunction with coronary anatomy, myocardial structure, perfusion, and function can provide additional information on the functional significance of coronary artery plaques. A single cardiac CT examination has the ability to not only discriminate between hemodynamically significant and insignificant stenoses but also identify which patients are likely to benefit most from revascularization versus optimized medical treatment. In addition, the use of cardiac CT in the evaluation of nonischemic myocardial disease is an area of active research with continued expansion of cardiac CT applications. Thus, cardiac CT will continue to play an increasingly important role in the diagnosis and management of patients with ischemic and nonischemic myocardial disease.

REFERENCES

1. Meijboom WB, Meijs MF, Schuijf JD, et al. Diagnostic accuracy of 64-slice computed tomography versus invasive coronary angiography a prospective, multicenter, multivendor study. J Am Coll Cardiol 2008;52: 2135–44.

2. Budoff MJ, Dowe D, Jollis JG, et al. Diagnostic performance of 64-multidetector row coronary computed tomographic angiography for evaluation of coronary artery stenosis in individuals without known coronary artery disease: results from the prospective multicenter ACCURACY (Assessment by Coronary Computed Tomographic Angiography of Individuals Undergoing Invasive Coronary Angiography) trial. J Am Coll Cardiol 2008;52:1724–32.

3. Hachamovitch R, Berman DS, Shaw LJ, et al. Incremental prognostic value of myocardial perfusion single photon emission computed tomography for the prediction of cardiac death: differential stratification for risk of cardiac death and myocardial infarction. Circulation 1998;97:535–43.

4. Hachamovitch R, Hayes SW, Friedman JD, et al. Comparison of the short-term survival benefit associated with revascularization compared with medical therapy in patients with no prior coronary artery disease undergoing stress myocardial perfusion single photon emission computed tomography. Circulation 2003;107:2900–7.

5. Bigi R, Bax JJ, van Domburg RT, et al. Simultaneous echocardiography and myocardial perfusion single photon emission computed tomography associated with dobutamine stress to predict long-term cardiac mortality in normotensive and hypertensive patients. J Hypertens 2005;23:1409–15.

6. Jahnke C, Nagel E, Gebker R, et al. Prognostic value of cardiac magnetic resonance stress tests: adenosine stress perfusion and dobutamine stress wall motion imaging. Circulation 2007;115:1769–76.

7. Steel K, Broderick R, Gandla V, et al. Complementary prognostic values of stress myocardial perfusion and late gadolinium enhancement imaging by cardiac magnetic resonance in patients with known or suspected coronary artery disease. Circulation 2009;120:1390–400.

8. Kim RJ, Fieno DS, Parrish TB, et al. Relationship of MRI delayed contrast enhancement to irreversible injury, infarct age, and contractile function. Circulation 1999;100:1992–2002.

9. Kim RJ, Wu E, Rafael A, et al. The use of contrast-enhanced magnetic resonance imaging to identify reversible myocardial dysfunction. N Engl J Med 2000;343:1445–53.

10. Gerber BL, Garot J, Bluemke DA, et al. Accuracy of contrast-enhanced magnetic resonance imaging in predicting improvement of regional myocardial function in patients after acute myocardial infarction. Circulation 2002;106:1083–9.

11. Beek AM, Kuhl HP, Bondarenko O, et al. Delayed contrast-enhanced magnetic resonance imaging for the prediction of regional functional improvement

after acute myocardial infarction. J Am Coll Cardiol 2003;42:895–901.

12. Gerber BL, Belge B, Legros GJ, et al. Characterization of acute and chronic myocardial infarcts by multidetector computed tomography: comparison with contrast-enhanced magnetic resonance. Circulation 2006;113:823–33.

13. Nieman K, Shapiro MD, Ferencik M, et al. Reperfused myocardial infarction: contrast-enhanced 64-section CT in comparison to MR imaging. Radiology 2008;247:49–56.

14. George RT, Jerosch-Herold M, Silva C, et al. Quantification of myocardial perfusion using dynamic 64-detector computed tomography. Invest Radiol 2007;42:815–22.

15. Hoffmann U, Millea R, Enzweiler C, et al. Acute myocardial infarction: contrast-enhanced multidetector row CT in a porcine model. Radiology 2004;231:697–701.

16. Mahnken AH, Koos R, Katoh M, et al. Assessment of myocardial viability in reperfused acute myocardial infarction using 16-slice computed tomography in comparison to magnetic resonance imaging. J Am Coll Cardiol 2005;45:2042–7.

17. Buecker A, Katoh M, Krombach GA, et al. A feasibility study of contrast enhancement of acute myocardial infarction in multislice computed tomography: comparison with magnetic resonance imaging and gross morphology in pigs. Invest Radiol 2005;40:700–4.

18. Lee IH, Choe YH, Lee KH, et al. Comparison of multidetector CT with F-18-FDG-PET and SPECT in the assessment of myocardial viability in patients with myocardial infarction: a preliminary study. Eur J Radiol 2009;72(3):401–5.

19. van der Vleuten PA, Willems TP, Gotte MJ, et al. Quantification of global left ventricular function: comparison of multidetector computed tomography and magnetic resonance imaging. A meta-analysis and review of the current literature. Acta Radiol 2006;47:1049–57.

20. Mahnken AH, Koos R, Katoh M, et al. Sixteen-slice spiral CT versus MR imaging for the assessment of left ventricular function in acute myocardial infarction. Eur Radiol 2005;15:714–20.

21. Juergens KU, Seifarth H, Maintz D, et al. MDCT determination of volume and function of the left ventricle: are short-axis image reformations necessary? AJR Am J Roentgenol 2006;186:S371–8.

22. Wu YW, Tadamura E, Yamamuro M, et al. Estimation of global and regional cardiac function using 64-slice computed tomography: a comparison study with echocardiography, gated-SPECT and cardiovascular magnetic resonance. Int J Cardiol 2008; 128:69–76.

23. Higgins CB, Sovak M, Schmidt W, et al. Uptake of contrast materials by experimental acute myocardial infarctions: a preliminary report. Invest Radiol 1978; 13:337–9.

24. Huber DJ, Lapray JF, Hessel SJ. In vivo evaluation of experimental myocardial infarcts by ungated computed tomography. AJR Am J Roentgenol 1981;136:469–73.

25. Gray WR, Buja LM, Hagler HK, et al. Computed tomography for localization and sizing of experimental acute myocardial infarcts. Circulation 1978; 58:497–504.

26. Ahn SS, Kim YJ, Hur J, et al. CT detection of subendocardial fat in myocardial infarction. AJR Am J Roentgenol 2009;192:532–7.

27. Sarwar A, Shapiro MD, Nasir K, et al. Evaluating global and regional left ventricular function in patients with reperfused acute myocardial infarction by 64-slice multidetector CT: a comparison to magnetic resonance imaging. J Cardiovasc Comput Tomogr 2009;3:170–7.

28. Gosalia A, Haramati LB, Sheth MP, et al. CT detection of acute myocardial infarction. AJR Am J Roentgenol 2004;182:1563–6.

29. Ko SM, Kim YW, Han SW, et al. Early and delayed myocardial enhancement in myocardial infarction using two-phase contrast-enhanced multidetector-row CT. Korean J Radiol 2007;8:94–102.

30. Faxon DP, Ryan TJ, Davis KB, et al. Prognostic significance of angiographically documented left ventricular aneurysm from the Coronary Artery Surgery Study (CASS). Am J Cardiol 1982;50:157–64.

31. Kurata A, Mochizuki T, Koyama Y, et al. Myocardial perfusion imaging using adenosine triphosphate stress multi-slice spiral computed tomography: alternative to stress myocardial perfusion scintigraphy. Circ J 2005;69:550–7.

32. Okada DR, Ghoshhajra BB, Blankstein R, et al. Direct comparison of rest and adenosine stress myocardial perfusion CT with rest and stress SPECT. J Nucl Cardiol 2009;17(1):27–37.

33. Blankstein R, Shturman LD, Rogers IS, et al. Adenosine-induced stress myocardial perfusion imaging using dual-source cardiac computed tomography. J Am Coll Cardiol 2009;54:1072–84.

34. George RT, Arbab-Zadeh A, Miller JM, et al. Adenosine stress 64- and 256-row detector computed tomography angiography and perfusion imaging: a pilot study evaluating the transmural extent of perfusion abnormalities to predict atherosclerosis causing myocardial ischemia. Circ Cardiovasc Imaging 2009;2:174–82.

35. Nagao M, Matsuoka H, Kawakami H, et al. Detection of myocardial ischemia using 64-slice MDCT. Circ J 2009;73:905–11.

36. Ruzsics B, Schwarz F, Schoepf UJ, et al. Comparison of dual-energy computed tomography of the heart with single photon emission computed tomography for assessment of coronary artery stenosis and of

the myocardial blood supply. Am J Cardiol 2009;104: 318–26.

37. Knickelbine T, Lesser JR, Haas TS, et al. Identification of unexpected nonatherosclerotic cardiovascular disease with coronary CT angiography. JACC Cardiovasc Imaging 2009;2:1085–92.

38. McCrohon JA, Moon JC, Prasad SK, et al. Differentiation of heart failure related to dilated cardiomyopathy and coronary artery disease using gadolinium-enhanced cardiovascular magnetic resonance. Circulation 2003;108:54–9.

39. Soriano CJ, Ridocci F, Estornell J, et al. Noninvasive diagnosis of coronary artery disease in patients with heart failure and systolic dysfunction of uncertain etiology, using late gadolinium-enhanced cardiovascular magnetic resonance. J Am Coll Cardiol 2005; 45:743–8.

40. Muth G, Daniel WG, Achenbach S. Late enhancement on cardiac computed tomography in a patient with cardiac sarcoidosis. J Cardiovasc Comput Tomogr 2008;2:272–3.

41. Marwan M, Pflederer T, Ropers D, et al. Cardiac amyloidosis imaged by dual-source computed tomography. J Cardiovasc Comput Tomogr 2008;2: 403–5.

42. Mikami Y, Funabashi N, Kijima T, et al. Focal fibrosis in the left ventricle of subjects with cardiac amyloidosis evaluated by multislice computed tomography. Int J Cardiol 2007;122:72–5.

43. Okayama S, Uemura S, Soeda T, et al. Role of cardiac computed tomography in planning and evaluating percutaneous transluminal septal myocardial ablation for hypertrophic obstructive cardiomyopathy. J Cardiovasc Comput Tomogr 2009;4(1):62–5.

44. Ghersin E, Lessick J, Litmanovich D, et al. Comprehensive multidetector CT assessment of apical hypertrophic cardiomyopathy. Br J Radiol 2006;79: e200–4.

45. Soh EK, Villines TC, Feuerstein IM. Sixty-four-multi-slice computed tomography in a patient with arrhythmogenic right ventricular dysplasia. J Cardiovasc Comput Tomogr 2008;2:191–2.

46. Wu YW, Tadamura E, Kanao S, et al. Structural and functional assessment of arrhythmogenic right ventricular dysplasia/cardiomyopathy by multi-slice computed tomography: comparison with cardiovascular magnetic resonance. Int J Cardiol 2007;115: e118–21.

47. Koh YY, Seo YU, Woo JJ, et al. Familial isolated noncompaction of the ventricular myocardium in asymptomatic phase. Yonsei Med J 2004;45:931–5.

48. Kantarci M, Duran C, Bozkurt M, et al. Cardiac multidetector computed tomography (MDCT) of spontaneously closed ventricular septal defect. Radiol Med 2009;114:370–5.

49. Srichai MB, Hecht EM, Kim DC, et al. Ventricular diverticula on cardiac CT: more common than previously thought. AJR Am J Roentgenol 2007;189:204–8.

50. van Beek EJ, Stolpen AH, Khanna G, et al. CT and MRI of pericardial and cardiac neoplastic disease. Cancer Imaging 2007;7:19–26.

51. Ho VB. ACR appropriateness criteria on suspected congenital heart disease in adults. J Am Coll Radiol 2008;5:97–104.

52. Hendel RC, Patel MR, Kramer CM, et al. ACCF/ACR/SCCT/SCMR/ASNC/NASCI/SCAI/SIR 2006 appropriateness criteria for cardiac computed tomography and cardiac magnetic resonance imaging: a report of the American College of Cardiology Foundation Quality Strategic Directions Committee Appropriateness Criteria Working Group, American College of Radiology, Society of Cardiovascular Computed Tomography, Society for Cardiovascular Magnetic Resonance, American Society of Nuclear Cardiology, North American Society for Cardiac Imaging, Society for Cardiovascular Angiography and Interventions, and Society of Interventional Radiology. J Am Coll Cardiol 2006;48:1475–97.

53. Petersilka M, Bruder H, Krauss B, et al. Technical principles of dual source CT. Eur J Radiol 2008;68: 362–8.

54. Johnson TR, Krauss B, Sedlmair M, et al. Material differentiation by dual energy CT: initial experience. Eur Radiol 2007;17:1510–7.

Computed Tomography Evaluation of Cardiac Valves: A Review

Dominik Ketelsen, MD[a], Elliot K. Fishman, MD[b],
Claus D. Claussen, MD[a], Jens Vogel-Claussen, MD[a,b,*]

KEYWORDS

- Computed tomography • Cardiac valves
- Heart disease • Angiography

Cardiac valve disease causes significant mortality and morbidity in the United States.[1,2] An estimated 20,891 patients died as a result of valvular heart disease in 2007, with aortic and mitral valve disease accounting for 13,137 and 2605 deaths, respectively.[3] Less common are disorders of the pulmonic and tricuspid valve. In 2006, the cost of valve replacement procedures was $141,120 per patient, with an in-hospital death rate of 5.0% in the United States.[3]

To assess the morphology and function of cardiac valves, various noninvasive imaging technologies are available. Usually, echocardiography is the standard technique for the noninvasive evaluation of the cardiac valves, because of its widespread accessibility and cost-effectiveness. Echocardiography typically provides all the information required for treatment planning.[4,5] However, its limitations are high interobserver variability, and low reliability in the measurement of the pulmonary valve and right-heart function, especially in patients with a restricted field of view (eg, in patients with emphysema, obese habitus, or with thoracic deformities). For evaluation of the cardiac valves in these patients, transesophageal echocardiography is a possibility, but there are several contraindications to this invasive technique (eg, recent esophageal surgery, unevaluated

gastrointestinal bleeding).[6] As an alternative imaging modality, cardiac magnetic resonance (MR) has evolved as a useful tool for the evaluation of valve anatomy and function, and for quantification of ventricular volumes with high temporal and spatial resolution without ionizing radiation.[1,7–9] However, the constrained availability, long imaging times, and several contraindications of MR imaging (eg, pacemaker, implantable defibrillators, claustrophobia) limit the widespread use of cardiac MR.[2]

Computed tomography (CT) coronary angiography has already been proven to be a valuable tool for the noninvasive assessment of coronary arteries, with a high negative predictive value.[10–12] Recent technical improvements and advances in temporal resolution allow a detailed anatomic and functional evaluation of the cardiac valves with retrospective electrocardiograph (ECG)-gated CT angiography, without relevant motion artifacts.[13–15] Currently, CT is not the first-line modality for assessment of the cardiac valves, but CT may be useful, particularly for patients in whom other more commonly used methods, such as echocardiography and MR imaging, fail to provide all the necessary information.

This article reviews the technical aspects and the latest advances in cardiac CT for the evaluation of

[a] Department of Diagnostic and Interventional Radiology, University Hospital Tuebingen, Eberhard-Karls-University Tuebingen, Hoppe-Seyler-Strasse 3, 72076 Tuebingen, Germany
[b] Russel H. Morgan Department of Radiology and Radiological Science, The Johns Hopkins Hospital, MRI, Room 143 (Nelson Basement), 600 North Wolfe Street, Baltimore, MD 21287, USA
* Corresponding author.
E-mail address: jclauss1@jhmi.edu

Radiol Clin N Am 48 (2010) 783–797
doi:10.1016/j.rcl.2010.04.007

the cardiac valves, and illustrates the CT findings of normal, pathologic, and postoperative cardiac valves.

TECHNICAL CONSIDERATIONS

The introduction of multidetector computed tomography (MDCT) permits high-resolution imaging with a short data acquisition time. The increased gantry rotation time, together with improved ECG-gated image reconstruction algorithms, allow the acquisition of high temporal resolution three-dimensional (3D) MDCT data sets.[12] With current single-source, 64-slice CT systems, the temporal resolution is approximately 90 to 180 milliseconds, whereas the introduced 64-slice and 128-slice dual-source scanner systems allow a temporal resolution of 83 milliseconds and 75 milliseconds, respectively.[2,10,12]

Using 64-slice MDCT, image acquisition for the evaluation of the cardiac valves is based on a protocol for CT coronary angiography. The scanning parameters include a collimation of 0.6 mm, a gantry rotation time of 330 milliseconds, a pitch of 0.2, a tube voltage of 120 kV, and a tube current of up to 800 mAs. Images are usually reconstructed with a small field of view (12–16 cm) for better visualization of the cardiac detail as a result of magnification and interpolation of the initial 3D MDCT dataset. The scan direction is usually from the carina to the apex of the heart.[2,16]

Depending on the inherent temporal resolution of the CT system, oral or intravenous β-blockers may be necessary to reduce the heart rate and to minimize valve and cardiac motion artifacts.

The synchronization of data acquisition and contrast enhancement can be evaluated by 2 different techniques. The test-bolus technique uses a small bolus (20 mL) of contrast agent for analysis of the enhancement time curve in the ascending aorta, followed by a straight bolus (60–80 mL) for the image acquisition. Alternatively, there is the so-called bolus-tracking technique, with real-time monitoring of the arrival of the straight bolus in the ascending aorta.

To achieve the optimal contrast, even in the right heart, a modified split-bolus protocol should be used, with an injection of 60 to 80 mL of an undiluted iodinated contrast agent at a flow rate of 5 mL/s, followed by a slower bolus infusion of 30 mL (100% contrast medium) and a saline flush to assess the tricuspid and pulmonic valve.[2,17]

To obtain static and cine images retrospectively, ECG-gated cardiac CT is recommended. For evaluation of the coronary arteries, the data set should be reconstructed in the phase of the systolic or diastolic cardiac rest period. For cardiac valve evaluation, 20 data sets at 5% increments or 10 data sets at 10% increments of the cardiac cycle are usually reconstructed using a 1-mm slice thickness.[18,19] In general, the number of reconstructed cardiac phases should be similar to the temporal resolution of the CT system used.

In our experience, it has been most practical for cardiac valve evaluation to upload the entire four-dimensional (4D) data set (0%–100% reconstruction at 10% or 5% intervals) and use thin-slab maximum intensity projection (MIP) or volume rendering to create reformatted images in any plane desired.[20] With the reverse ramp technique, the contrast-enhanced blood appears black and the soft-tissue-density valve leaflets are highlighted.[21] Some physicians use endoluminal 3D tools to display the anatomy of the cardiac valves.[1,3]

With current MDCT technology, volumetric ventricular measurements can also be performed using dedicated software. With this method, right and left ventricular function parameters can be calculated with high accuracy, compared with cardiac cine MR imaging.[22] For accurate right ventricle (RV) function measurements, optimized contrast opacification of the RV is required for better depiction of the blood pool-RV wall border. From biventricular stroke volume measurements, the regurgitant volume can then be calculated, which is useful in grading the severity of isolated valvular insufficiency.[23]

RADIATION EXPOSURE

Especially in younger patients, the radiation dose is a cause of concern. Although the individual cancer risk is low, the increasing medical radiation exposure in the general population may be a public health concern in the future.[24,25] With current single-source and dual-source scanners, the effective whole-body dose for a cardiac CT examination ranges between 13 and 15 mSv for men and 18 and 21 mSv for women.[26–29] ECG-controlled tube current modulation has the potential to reduce radiation exposure up to 45% by lowering the tube current in the systolic phase.[20] However, ECG-controlled tube current modulation can be disadvantageous for valve assessment because motion of the cardiac valves may be difficult to evaluate during the phase of reduced tube current.[2]

CT EVALUATION OF VALVE DISEASE
Normal Morphology and Function

Two semilunar (pulmonic and aortic) valves separate the ventricle from a great vessel, and 2 atrioventricular valves (mitral and tricuspid) regulate the blood flow in the 4 heart chambers. Controlled by pressure differences generated within the heart, the opening and closing functions of the valves control a unidirectional blood flow.[2]

Pathologic Conditions and Dysfunction

Degenerative and inherited cardiac valve diseases are the main causes of valvular disease in the Western world, whereas postrheumatic heart disease is the primary cause worldwide.[2,3,16,30] Heart valves can malfunction in several ways, including regurgitation, stenosis, or atresia. A valve stenosis is characterized by a constricted opening that inhibits the ability of the heart to pump blood into the body. Regurgitation indicates an incomplete closing function, causing the blood to flow backward rather than forward through the valve. Valvular stenosis can be due to calcifications, valve thickening, or congenital malformations. In valvular insufficiency (regurgitation), incomplete coaptation of valve cusps leads to retrograde blood flow.

AORTIC VALVE

The aortic valve, with 3 thin cusps (left, right, posterior), is located between the left ventricle and the aorta (**Fig. 1**). Occasionally, rather than being a tricuspid valve, the aortic valve can have 1, 2, or even 4 or 5 cusps.[31,32] Above the right and left cusp (coronary cusps), the right and left coronary arteries arise from the right and left coronary sinuses, respectively.[21,30,33] The morphology of the aortic valve can be assessed using multiplanar reformation (MPR) and multiphasic cine movie loops at the midsystolic (open valve) and the middiastolic phase (closed valve).[34] The causes of aortic valve pathology are listed in **Box 1**.

Aortic Stenosis

Aortic stenosis (AS) is defined as an obstruction of the left ventricular outflow tract at the level of the aortic valve. The stenosis can be subvalvular, supravalvular, or valvular. The valvular stenosis is the most frequent type, and can be classified as congenital or acquired.

Age-related degenerative calcified AS is the common cause of AS in adults and is associated with severe atherosclerosis of the aorta and the coronary arteries (**Fig. 2**). In a recent study, aortic valve calcification was independently associated with an increased severity of coronary artery calcification after controlling for demographic factors and cardiovascular risk factors.[35]

The most common congenital variant is bicuspid valves, occurring in 1% to 2% of people, with possible stenotic disease and commissural fusion, and 2 separate cusps of unequal size at birth

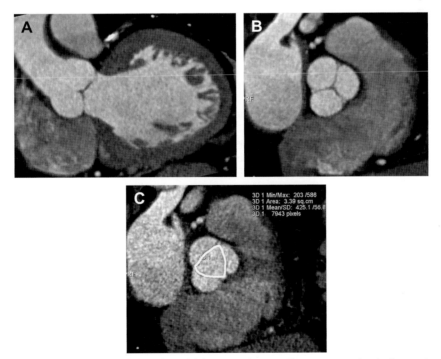

Fig. 1. Normal aortic valve. Coronal (*A*) and axial (*B*) CT MIP images show a normal valvular anatomy with thin cusps in end diastole (*B*) and end systole (*C*). Axial end-systolic image (*C*) displays a planimetric measurement of the aortic valve area of 3.4 cm^2.

Box 1
Causes of aortic valve disease

Aortic stenosis

Younger patients (<60 years):

- Congenital (bicuspid aortic valve)

Older patients (>60 years)

- Degenerative

Other:

Rheumatic heart disease

Aortic regurgitation

Acute disease:

- Infectious endocarditis
- Type A aortic dissection
- Thoracic trauma

Chronic disease:

- Degenerative
- Congenital (bicuspid aortic valve)
- Ascending aortic aneurysm
- Marfan syndrome
- Ehlers-Danlos syndrome
- Syphilis

(**Fig. 3**).[21,33] In general, degenerative AS in patients with a bicuspid aortic valve occurs at a younger age (<60 years), compared with AS stenosis in patients with a tricuspid aortic valve (>60 years). A bicuspid aortic valve is strongly associated with congenital abnormalities of the aorta (ie, coarctation, aortic root dilatation, patent ductus arteriosus). Particularly in these patients, routine evaluation of the thoracic aorta is mandatory, which is almost always included in the routine cardiac CT examination.

The pathophysiology of adult AS is characterized by a gradual decrease in valve area (normal values, 2.5–4.0 cm^2), in which initially nonhemodynamically relevant valve calcification progresses to a hemodynamically relevant obstruction of the left ventricular outflow (<1 cm^2). The physiologic response is compensatory left ventricular hypertrophy and dilatation of the aortic root.[33]

Cardiac CT findings in AS may include thickening and calcification of the aortic valve cusps. The cardiac CT 3D dataset can also be reconstructed in the aortic valve plane in systole for planimetric measurements of the aortic valve area to classify the severity of AS (see **Fig. 1**C). Even in patients with severe calcifications, planimetric measurements are not restricted as a result of artifacts, and correlate significantly with transesophageal echocardiography findings and mean transvalvular

pressure gradients.[36–39] The main advantage of ECG-gated CT angiography compared with echocardiography is the more accurate measurement of the valve orifice area, which, in CT, is not limited by hemodynamic factors, such as low cardiac output. CT gives a reproducible quantification of valve calcification that correlates with the severity of AS.[1,40] In addition, compensatory left ventricular hypertrophy and dilatation of the ascending aorta can be visualized.[2]

Aortic Regurgitation

Aortic insufficiency (AI) is characterized by blood reflux into the left ventricle during diastole, caused by a failure of the aortic valve to close properly due to a malcoaptation of the valve cusps.

The regurgitation can result from intrinsic valve disease, pathologic changes of the aortic root, or both. AI can be categorized by severity (mild to severe) and chronicity (acute vs chronic).

Intrinsic, chronic AI is commonly a result of atherosclerotic degeneration of a normal tricuspid aortic valve, or is due to a congenital bicuspid or multicusp valve.[32] Aortic valve closure can also be affected by an increased diameter of the ascending aorta, including a Stanford A aortic dissection, ascending aortic aneurysm, and Marfan and Ehlers-Danlos syndrome (**Fig. 4**, see also Movie 1 in online version of article at www.radiologic.theclinics.com). Acute AI is often the result of bacterial endocarditis (**Fig. 5**), Stanford A aortic dissection, or thoracic trauma. The most common cause of AI in older patients is idiopathic degeneration of the normal aortic valve, whereas aortic root dilatation secondary to Marfan syndrome is the most common cause in younger patients.[41]

In time, the left ventricular volume overload increases. This increase leads to a progressive dilatation of the left ventricle, as well as dilatation of the aortic root, with a high end-diastolic left ventricular volume. The left ventricular ejection fraction begins to deteriorate and symptoms occur.

Using cardiac CT, moderate to severe AI can be assessed qualitatively and quantitatively with a sensitivity and specificity higher than 95%, compared with transesophageal echocardiography. The anatomic regurgitant area of AI can be graded with transesophageal echocardiography, with a sensitivity and specificity of 85% and 97% up to 98% and 93% for mild and severe AI, respectively.[42] During mid- to end diastole, planimetric measurements can be performed to evaluate the central valvular leakage area, which correlates with the severity of AI diagnosed with echocardiography.[43,44] In addition, the underlying

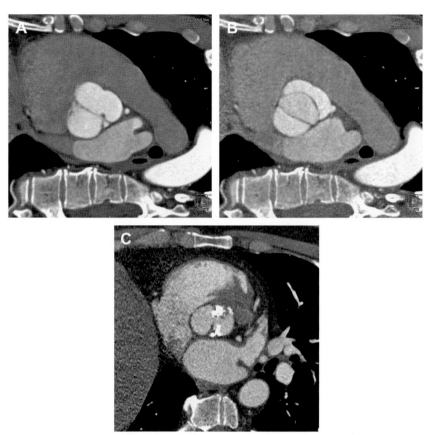

Fig. 2. Bicuspid aortic valve. Axial CT MIP (*A, B*) and volume rendering technique (VRT) images show a noncalcified (*A, B*) as well as a calcified bicuspid aortic valve in systole (*B*) and diastole (*A, C*).

disease can often be visualized by CT as shortened and thickened aortic cusps in intrinsic valve disease or a dilatation of the aortic root causing a malcoaptation of the valve cusps.

MITRAL VALVE

The bicuspid mitral valve, with 2 thin cusps (1 anterior and 1 crescentic posterior leaflet), is located between the left atrium and the left ventricle, with a normal area of the valve from 4.0 to 6.0 cm² (**Fig. 6**). The mitral valve complex involves the mitral leaflets, chordae tendinae, papillary muscles, and the mitral valve annulus.[21] The mitral valve can be evaluated using MPR and volume rendering technique (VRT) images in any desired plane. We routinely reconstruct 2-chamber and 4-chamber long-axis and short-axis planes using the 4D volume data set covering the whole cardiac cycle.[2,45,46] The causes of mitral valve pathology are listed in **Box 2**.

Mitral Stenosis

Mitral stenosis (MS) is defined as an obstruction of the left ventricular inflow tract, which prevents proper filling of the left ventricle during diastole.

The predominant cause of MS is rheumatic fever, especially in developing countries.[47] It has been shown that molecular mimicry between the *Streptococcus pyogenes* antigen and human proteins leads to humoral and cell-mediated autoimmune reactions, causing regurgitant fraction (RF)/rheumatic heart disease (RHD). Heart tissues, namely the valves, left atrial appendage (LAA), and myocardium, reveal variable amounts of infiltration by lymphocytes. Significant endocarditis and valvulitis is observed in these cases.[48] Apart from rheumatic fever, MS can be caused by congenital anomalies, mitral calcifications, left atrial tumors (eg, myxomas, **Fig. 7**), carcinoid syndrome, and an obstructive atrial thrombus.

MS ultimately leads to right-sided heart failure, with dilatation of the left atrium and RV and

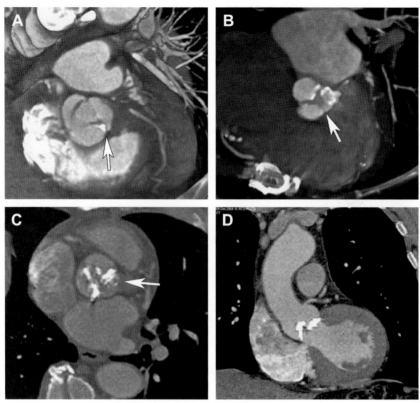

Fig. 3. Age-related degenerative aortic stenosis. Axial (*A–C*) and coronal (*D*) VRT (*A, B*) and MIP (*C, D*) CT images show minimal (*arrow* in *A*), moderate (*arrow* in *B*), and severe (*arrow* in *C, D*) aortic valve calcifications with a significant stenosis causing a compensatory left ventricular hypertrophy (*D*). (*From* Vogel-Claussen J, Pannu H, Spevak PJ, et al. Cardiac valve assessment with MR imaging and 64-section multidetector row CT. Radiographics 2006;26(6):1769–84; with permission.)

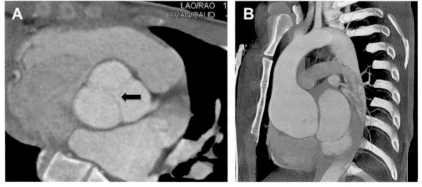

Fig. 4. Patient with Marfan syndrome. (*A*) Axial MIP image shows a malcoaptation (*arrow*) of the aortic cusps causing an aortic regurgitation (see also Movie 1). Note the severe dilatation of the aortic root in the coronal VRT image (*B*).

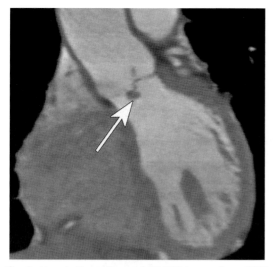

Fig. 5. Vegetations. Coronal CT MIP image from ECG-gated CT angiography shows a vegetation (*arrow*) of the aortic valve due to a bacterial endocarditis. (*From* Vogel-Claussen J, Pannu H, Spevak PJ, et al. Cardiac valve assessment with MR imaging and 64-section multidetector row CT. Radiographics 2006;26(6):1769–84; with permission.)

| Box 2 |
| **Causes of mitral valve disease** |

Mitral stenosis
Rheumatic heart disease (predominant)
Congenital anomalies
Degenerative
Carcinoid syndrome
Connective tissue disorder
Left atrial tumor (eg, myxoma)
Obstructive atrial thrombus

Mitral regurgitation
Rheumatic heart disease (predominant)
Infectious endocarditis
Degenerative
Mitral valve prolapse
Dilatative cardiomyopathy
Ischemic heart disease
Chronic left-heart failure
Postvalvuloplasty
Marfan syndrome
Ehlers-Danlos syndrome

a secondary tricuspidal and pulmonary insufficiency (PI).[21,49] A possible complication of MS is atrial fibrillation, which may decrease the quality of ECG-gated CT angiography.

CT findings include a stenotic mitral valve with thickened and calcified leaflets, left atrial dilatation, pulmonary edema, and right ventricular hypertrophy. On CT angiography during early diastole (about 75% R-R), the mitral valve area can be

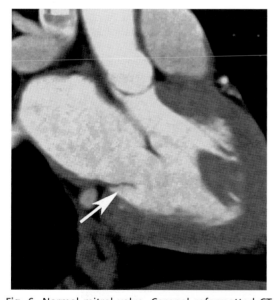

Fig. 6. Normal mitral valve. Coronal reformatted CT MIP image shows normal mitral valve leaflets (*arrow*) during diastole. (*From* Vogel-Claussen J, Pannu H, Spevak PJ, et al. Cardiac valve assessment with MR imaging and 64-section multidetector row CT. Radiographics 2006;26(6):1769–84; with permission.)

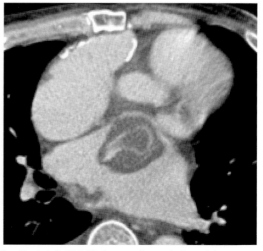

Fig. 7. Axial CT MIP image shows left atrial myxoma causing MS with dilatation of the left atrium.

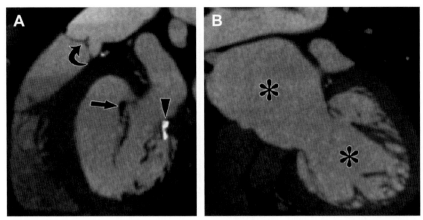

Fig. 8. Mitral regurgitation (*A, B*). Sagittal CT MIP image (*A*) shows calcification (*arrowhead*) and thickening (*straight arrow*) of mitral valve leaflets. Curved arrow displays a closed pulmonic valve during diastole. Coronal CT MIP image (*B*) shows left atrial and ventricular dilatation (∗) caused by mitral regurgitation. (*From* Chen JJ, Manning MA, Frazier AA, et al. CT angiography of the cardiac valves: normal, diseased, and postoperative appearances. Radiographics 2009;29(5):1393–412; with permission.)

measured with good reproducibility and correlation with transesophageal echocardiography.[50]

Mitral Regurgitation

Mitral insufficiency (MI) is defined as retrograde blood flow from the left ventricle to the left atrium during systole due to dysfunction of the mitral valve complex (ie, annular dilatation, leaflet retraction, calcifications, anomalies of the chordae tendinae, and dysfunction of the papillary muscles).

MI can be the result of primary leaflet dysfunction (ie, degenerative leaflet calcification), or can occur secondary to ischemic dyskinesia, papillary muscle rupture, or annular dilatation (**Fig. 8**). As in AI, mitral regurgitation can be classified as acute or chronic.

The most common cause of MI is mitral valve prolapse caused by myxomatous valve degeneration. This congenital defect, with abnormal fibroelastic connective tissue, causes an elongation and thickening of the mitral valve complex.[2] Another cause of MI is postrheumatic degeneration with a diffuse fibrosis and thickening of the mitral valve leaflets, but without calcifications or commissural fusion.[51–53] Malcoaptation of the mitral valve

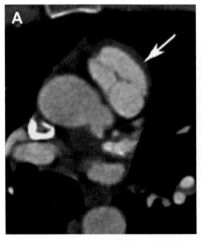
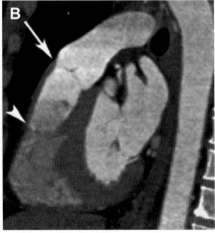

Fig. 9. Normal pulmonic valve. Axial (*A*) and sagittal (*B*) CT MIP images show a normal pulmonic valve (*arrow*) located anterior, superior, and to the left of the aortic valve. Because of the administration of a saline chaser to coronary CT angiography patients, there is reduced contrast in the RV (*B*) causing a difficult evaluation of the tricuspid valve (*arrowhead*). (*From* Vogel-Claussen J, Pannu H, Spevak PJ, et al. Cardiac valve assessment with MR imaging and 64-section multidetector row CT. Radiographics 2006;26(6):1769–84; with permission.)

can also be affected by endocarditis, dilated cardiomyopathy, ischemic heart disease, or Marfan syndrome.[54]

Acute MI is mainly caused by endocarditis or papillary muscle rupture. Papillary muscle rupture may occur in the clinical setting of acute myocardial infarction. Chronic mitral regurgitation is often due to mitral valve prolapse, dilated cardiomyopathy, or can be the result of the systolic anterior motion of the mitral valve that is often seen in patients with hypertrophic cardiomyopathy with significant left ventricular outflow tract obstruction.[55]

Pathophysiologically, the left atrium and the left ventricle dilate because of the regurgitant blood volume. Pulmonary edema may also be observed in severe cases.[2,21]

Similar to AS and MS, the size of the mitral orifice area, as measured by planimetric cardiac MDCT, correlates well with echocardiographic findings.[37] In addition, ECG-gated cardiac MDCT allows an exact evaluation of morphology, thickening, and calcifications of the mitral valve complex. Other findings, such as left-heart dilatation and pulmonary edema, can also be visualized.[2] In cases with isolated mitral regurgitation, cardiac CT is useful for grading the severity of mitral regurgitation, because its RF measurements, derived from right and left ventricular stroke volumes, correlate well with the results of two-dimensional transthoracic echocardiography. According to Lembcke and colleagues,[23] the severity of mitral regurgitation can be classified according to 4 grades: grade I (mild) RF of less than 20%; grade II (moderate) RF of 20% to less than 30%; grade III (moderately severe) RF of 30% to less than 44%; and grade IV (severe) RF of 44% or higher.

Box 3
Causes of pulmonic valve disease

Pulmonary stenosis

Congenital (nearly exclusive)

Associated disorders:

- Ventricle septal defect
- Fallot tetralogy
- Double outlet RV

Other:

RHD

Carcinoid syndrome

Pulmonary regurgitation

Secondary to pulmonary artery hypertension

Other:

- Infectious endocarditis
- Marfan syndrome
- Postvalvuloplasty
- Late complication of Fallot surgery
- Carcinoid syndrome
- Iatrogen

PULMONIC VALVE

The semilunar pulmonic valve, with 3 cusps (anterior, right, and left), is located between the RV and the pulmonary artery, with a normal valve area of about 2 cm² (**Fig. 9**). Because of lower right-heart pressures, the pulmonic and tricuspid valves are more delicate and cannot be easily seen on CT without adequate contrast opacification in the right ventricular outflow tract and main pulmonary artery. In general, if the cusps of the right-heart valves are easily visible, they are likely to be thickenend.[1,2,21] The causes of pulmonic valve pathology are listed in **Box 3**.

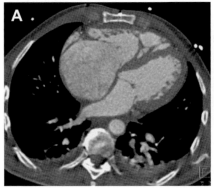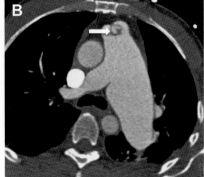

Fig. 10. PS. Axial CT MIP image (*A*) shows a dilated and mildly hypertrophied RV caused by PS. Axial CT MIP image (*B*) shows poststenotic dilatation of the main, as well as the left, pulmonary artery, with sparing of the right pulmonary artery. Also note the thickened pulmonary valve leaflets (*arrow in B*).

Box 4
Causes of tricuspid valve disease

Tricuspid stenosis
RHD (predominant)
Congenital anomalies
Right atrial tumors
Ebstein anomaly
Tricuspid regurgitation
RV failure
RHD
Infectious endocarditis
Congenital anomalies
Carcinoid syndrome
Ebstein anomaly

Pulmonary Stenosis

Pulmonary stenosis (PS) is defined as an obstruction of the right ventricular outflow tract at the level of the pulmonic valve. Like AS, the stenosis can be subvalvular, supravalvular, or valvular, with valvular stenosis being the most common (90%) and supravalvular being associated with congenital abnormalities, such as patent ductus arteriosus or tetralogy of Fallot.[21,33]

The cause of PS is congenital heart disease in 95% of cases. Acquired PS is a rare disease that may be caused by rheumatic fever or metastatic carcinoid syndrome.[2,21,33,56]

Moderate to severe PS causes compensatory right ventricular hypertrophy as a result of increased right ventricular pressure load, which can be assessed with cardiac MDCT. In addition, CT findings may include pulmonary valve thickening, as well as a systolic interventricular septal shift to the left due to increased right ventricular systolic pressure. Because of the 90° angle origin of the right pulmonary artery, primarily the main and left pulmonary artery show dilatation in patients with PS, because the poststenotic turbulent flow is directed toward the left main pulmonary artery (**Fig. 10**).[2]

Pulmonary Regurgitation

PI is defined as an incomplete closure of the pulmonic valve, which causes a blood leak backward into the RV. In progressive disease, PI leads to right-sided heart failure.

The most common cause of PI is dilatation of the valve ring, with resulting malcoaptation (ie, secondary to pulmonary hypertension or Marfan syndrome). In rare cases, PI can develop primarily due to RHD or infectious endocarditis.[2,21]

CT findings include a malcoaptation of the pulmonic valve cusps at end diastole, a right ventricular dilatation, and hypertrophy.

TRICUSPID VALVE

The tricuspid valve, with 3 cusps (septal anterior, superior, and inferior), is located between the right atrium and the RV. Similar to the mitral valve, the tricuspid valve complex involves the tricuspid leaflets, the chordae tendinae, the papillary muscles, and the tricuspid valve annulus. Because of low right-heart pressure, the tricuspid valve is thinner than the mitral valve.[2] Evaluation by ECG-gated CT angiography is more difficult and usually requires an intracardiac contrast opacification timing that optimizes right-heart structures, such

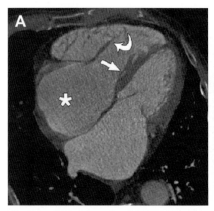
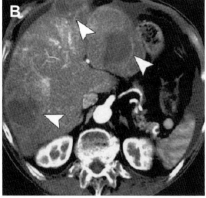

Fig. 11. Tricuspidal insufficiency caused by carcinoid syndrome secondary to liver metastasis from ileal primary tumor (*A, B*). Axial CT MIP image (*A*) displays thickening of the tricuspid leaflets (*straight arrow*) and chordae tendinae (*curved arrow*). Also note the dilated right atrium (*). Axial abdominal CT (*B*) shows multiple hypervascular carcinoid liver metastases (*arrowheads*). (*From* Ryan R, Abbara S, Colen RR, et al. Cardiac valve disease: spectrum of findings on cardiac 64-MDCT. AJR Am J Roentgenol 2008;190(5):W294–303; with permission.)

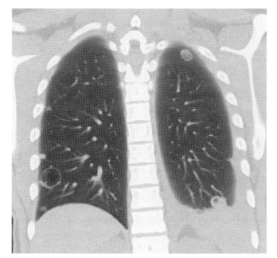

Fig. 12. Septic emboli. Coronal MPR CT image shows septic emboli as an additional diagnostic finding in a patient presenting with vegetation of the aortic valve (see **Fig. 5**) as a result of infectious endocarditis.

as an ECG-gated CT pulmonary angiogram protocol.[21] The causes of tricuspid valve pathology are listed in **Box 4**.

Tricuspid Stenosis

In most cases, tricuspid stenosis (TS) is due to RHD, which is stenotic and regurgitant. Rare causes include congenital disorders or infectious endocarditis.

CT findings include a narrowed valve annulus with a shortened and fused tricuspid valve complex, and signs of right-heart failure with enlargement of the superior and inferior vena cava, as well as dilatated hepatic veins.[2,21]

Tricuspid Regurgitation

The most common cause of tricuspid regurgitation is secondary to any cause of right ventricular failure, with a stretching of the leaflets and a resulting malcoaption of the tricuspid valve complex (**Fig. 11**). Another cause involving the right-heart structures are carcinoid tumors, with cardiac involvement of 50% to 60%, usually between 18 and 24 months after diagnosis. Right-heart valvular dysfunction is the most common abnormality in cardiac carcinoid disease, with the tricuspid valve affected in 97% of cases. Endocardial plaques of fibrous tissue are present on both sides of the tricuspid valve leaflets, resulting in marked thickening and retraction. Approximately 90% of patients with tricuspid valve involvement have moderate to severe regurgitation, whereas tricuspid valve stenosis is less common. The relative lack of involvement of the left heart is believed to be due to inactivation, by monoamine oxidase secreted by the pulmonary endothelium, of vasoactive substances released by carcinoid tumors. The left side of the heart is affected in less than 10% of patients, usually in cases of bronchogenic carcinoid tumors.[56]

Echocardiographic and CT findings show a valve thickening without calcification, reduced mobility, and a retraction of the tricuspid and pulmonary valve.[56]

VALVULAR TUMORS AND VEGETATIONS

In the United States, the incidence of community-acquired infectious valve endocarditis in adults is about 1.7 to 6.2 cases per 100,000 persons per

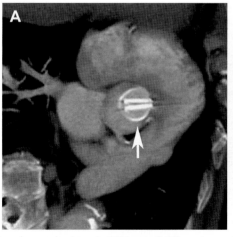
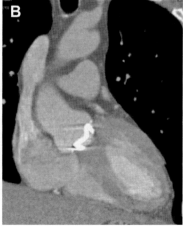

Fig. 13. Aortic valve replacement. ECG-gated CT angiography axial (A) and coronal (B) CT VRT images show a mechanical bileaflet valve (*arrow*) during diastole (B) and systole (A). (*From* Vogel-Claussen J, Pannu H, Spevak PJ, et al. Cardiac valve assessment with MR imaging and 64-section multidetector row CT. Radiographics 2006;26(6):1769–84; with permission.)

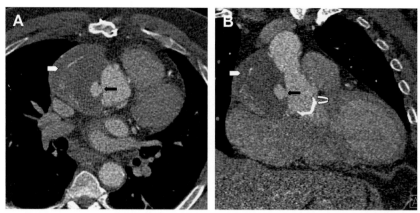

Fig. 14. Complication of aortic valve replacement. Axial (*A*) and coronal (*B*) MIP images show an aortic root pseudoaneurysm (*arrow*) with a hematoma (*arrowhead*) of the aortic root caused by postoperative perforation as a complication of aortic valve and root repair (*curved arrow*).

year, up to 150 to 2000 per 100,000 persons per year in high-risk populations.[57] Larger valve vegetations in endocarditis patients can be depicted routinely on ECG-gated CT angiography, with a good correlation with echocardiography (see **Fig. 5**). In addition, CT has the capacity to identify several complications, such as perivalvular abscess and extracardiac septic emboli (**Fig. 12**).[2]

The entity of cardiac masses ranges from non-neoplastic lesions to high-grade malignancies.[58] However, primary valvular tumors are rare and include papillary fibroelastoma, which mostly occurs on the aortic valve cusps. Other possible valve tumors are myxoma (see **Fig. 7**) and hamartoma.[2,58] ECG-gated CT angiography can help to detect these small tumors.

RADIATION-INDUCED VALVE DISEASE

Another rare cause, reported in a few case reports, is radiation-induced valve disease, including all cardiac valves with stenosis or regurgitation.[59–62] The underlying mechanism of postradiation cardiac disease is not clear, but seems to progress slowly. After significant mediastinal radiation (ie, for lymphoma treatment), individual case reports describe a marked fibrosis of the mediastinum, a hypertrophy of pericardium, and a valve thickening and retraction in irradiated patients with no history of rheumatic disease, which may lead to severe heart failure and death.[62]

VALVE SURGERY

Valve replacement procedures are usually performed for the aortic and mitral valves. CT is promising for the assessment of mechanical valves. Although fluoroscopy is used as the gold standard to assess the function of artificial valves,

ECG-gated CT angiography with multiphase data sets can be used to determine the leaflet motion and opening angle (**Fig. 13**, see also Movie 2 in the online version of this article at www.radiologic.theclinics.com).[2,63,64] CT can measure the size and function of mechanical valves with high interobserver agreement. The opening angle with CT strongly correlates with cinefluoroscopy.[16] Despite streak artifacts from surgical clips, CT angiography can assess prosthetic complications, such as thrombus, hemorrhage, valve dehiscence, or paravalvular abscess (**Fig. 14**).[2]

SUMMARY

Technical advances in ECG-gated multidetector row cardiac CT imaging allow an excellent visualization of normal and pathologic cardiac valve morphology and function, including the number of valve cusps, the thickness of the leaflets, and calcifications. It is not the current gold standard, but cardiac CT can be a helpful clinical tool for evaluation of the cardiac valves.

APPENDIX: SUPPLEMENTARY DATA

Supplementary data associated with this article can be found in the online version, at doi:10.1016/j.rcl.2010.04.007.

REFERENCES

1. Vogel-Claussen J, Pannu H, Spevak PJ, et al. Cardiac valve assessment with MR imaging and 64-section multi-detector row CT. Radiographics 2006;26(6):1769–84.
2. Chen JJ, Manning MA, Frazier AA, et al. CT angiography of the cardiac valves: normal, diseased, and

postoperative appearances. Radiographics 2009; 29(5):1393–412.

3. Lloyd-Jones D, Adams R, Carnethon M, et al. Heart disease and stroke statistics–2009 update: a report from the American Heart Association Statistics Committee and Stroke Statistics Subcommittee. Circulation 2009;119(3):480–6.

4. Bolger AF, Eigler NL, Maurer G. Quantifying valvular regurgitation. Limitations and inherent assumptions of Doppler techniques. Circulation 1988;78(5 Pt 1): 1316–8.

5. Simpson IA, Sahn DJ. Quantification of valvular regurgitation by Doppler echocardiography. Circulation 1991;84(3 Suppl):I188–92.

6. Ryan R, Abbara S, Colen RR, et al. Cardiac valve disease: spectrum of findings on cardiac 64-MDCT. AJR Am J Roentgenol 2008;190(5): W294–303.

7. Didier D, Ratib O, Lerch R, et al. Detection and quantification of valvular heart disease with dynamic cardiac MR imaging. Radiographics 2000;20(5): 1279–99 [discussion: 1299–301].

8. Didier D. Assessment of valve disease: qualitative and quantitative. Magn Reson Imaging Clin N Am 2003;11(1):115–34, vii.

9. Grothues F, Smith GC, Moon JC, et al. Comparison of interstudy reproducibility of cardiovascular magnetic resonance with two-dimensional echocardiography in normal subjects and in patients with heart failure or left ventricular hypertrophy. Am J Cardiol 2002;90(1):29–34.

10. Brodoefel H, Burgstahler C, Tsiflikas I, et al. Dual-source CT: effect of heart rate, heart rate variability, and calcification on image quality and diagnostic accuracy. Radiology 2008;247(2):346–55.

11. Heuschmid M, Burgstahler C, Reimann A, et al. Usefulness of noninvasive cardiac imaging using dual-source computed tomography in an unselected population with high prevalence of coronary artery disease. Am J Cardiol 2007;100(4): 587–92.

12. Schroeder S, Achenbach S, Bengel F, et al. Cardiac computed tomography: indications, applications, limitations, and training requirements: report of a Writing Group deployed by the Working Group Nuclear Cardiology and Cardiac CT of the European Society of Cardiology and the European Council of Nuclear Cardiology. Eur Heart J 2008; 29(4):531–56.

13. Ohnesorge B, Flohr T, Becker C, et al. Cardiac imaging by means of electrocardiographically gated multisection spiral CT: initial experience. Radiology 2000;217(2):564–71.

14. Weinreb JC, Larson PA, Woodard PK, et al. American College of Radiology clinical statement on noninvasive cardiac imaging. Radiology 2005; 235(3):723–7.

15. Willmann JK, Weishaupt D, Lachat M, et al. Electrocardiographically gated multi-detector row CT for assessment of valvular morphology and calcification in aortic stenosis. Radiology 2002;225(1): 120–8.

16. LaBounty TM, Agarwal PP, Chughtai A, et al. Evaluation of mechanical heart valve size and function with ECG-gated 64-MDCT. AJR Am J Roentgenol 2009;193(5):W389–96.

17. Kerl JM, Ravenel JG, Nguyen SA, et al. Right heart: split-bolus injection of diluted contrast medium for visualization at coronary CT angiography. Radiology 2008;247(2):356–64.

18. Alkadhi H, Bettex D, Wildermuth S, et al. Dynamic cine imaging of the mitral valve with 16-MDCT: a feasibility study. AJR Am J Roentgenol 2005; 185(3):636–46.

19. Baumert B, Plass A, Bettex D, et al. Dynamic cine mode imaging of the normal aortic valve using 16-channel multidetector row computed tomography. Invest Radiol 2005;40(10):637–47.

20. Hermann F, Martinoff S, Meyer T, et al. Reduction of radiation dose estimates in cardiac 64-slice CT angiography in patients after coronary artery bypass graft surgery. Invest Radiol 2008;43(4):253–60.

21. Manghat NE, Rachapalli V, Van Lingen R, et al. Imaging the heart valves using ECG-gated 64-detector row cardiac CT. Br J Radiol 2008;81(964): 275–90.

22. Raman SV, Shah M, McCarthy B, et al. Multi-detector row cardiac computed tomography accurately quantifies right and left ventricular size and function compared with cardiac magnetic resonance. Am Heart J 2006;151(3):736–44.

23. Lembcke A, Borges AC, Dushe S, et al. Assessment of mitral valve regurgitation at electron-beam CT: comparison with doppler echocardiography. Radiology 2005;236(1):47–55.

24. Brenner DJ, Hall EJ. Computed tomography–an increasing source of radiation exposure. N Engl J Med 2007;357(22):2277–84.

25. Einstein AJ, Henzlova MJ, Rajagopalan S. Estimating risk of cancer associated with radiation exposure from 64-slice computed tomography coronary angiography. JAMA 2007;298(3):317–23.

26. Ketelsen D, Thomas C, Werner M, et al. Dual-source computed tomography: estimation of radiation exposure of ECG-gated and ECG-triggered coronary angiography. Eur J Radiol 2010;73(2): 274–9.

27. Hunold P, Vogt FM, Schmermund A, et al. Radiation exposure during cardiac CT: effective doses at multi-detector row CT and electron-beam CT. Radiology 2003;226(1):145–52.

28. Kalra MK, Maher MM, Toth TL, et al. Strategies for CT radiation dose optimization. Radiology 2004; 230(3):619–28.

29. McCollough CH, Primak AN, Saba O, et al. Dose performance of a 64-channel dual-source CT scanner. Radiology 2007;243(3):775–84.

30. Wiant A, Nyberg E, Gilkeson RC. CT evaluation of congenital heart disease in adults. AJR Am J Roentgenol 2009;193(2):388–96.

31. Jacobs JE, Srichai M, Kim D, et al. Quadricuspid aortic valve: imaging findings on multidetector helical CT with echocardiographic correlation. J Comput Assist Tomogr 2006;30(4):569–71.

32. Meng Y, Zhang L, Zhang Z, et al. Cardiovascular magnetic resonance of quinticuspid aortic valve with aortic regurgitation and dilated ascending aorta. J Cardiovasc Magn Reson 2009;11(1):28.

33. Brickner ME, Hillis LD, Lange RA. Congenital heart disease in adults. First of two parts. N Engl J Med 2000;342(4):256–63.

34. Chun EJ, Choi SI, Lim C, et al. Aortic stenosis: evaluation with multidetector CT angiography and MR imaging. Korean J Radiol 2008;9(5):439–48.

35. Nasir K, Katz R, Al-Mallah M, et al. Relationship of aortic valve calcification with coronary artery calcium severity: the Multi-Ethnic Study of Atherosclerosis (Mesa). J Cardiovasc Comput Tomogr 2010;4(1):41–6.

36. Pouleur AC, le Polain de Waroux JB, Pasquet A, et al. Aortic valve area assessment: multidetector CT compared with cine MR imaging and transthoracic and transesophageal echocardiography. Radiology 2007;244(3):745–54.

37. Alkadhi H, Wildermuth S, Plass A, et al. Aortic stenosis: comparative evaluation of 16-detector row CT and echocardiography. Radiology 2006; 240(1):47–55.

38. LaBounty TM, Sundaram B, Agarwal P, et al. Aortic valve area on 64-MDCT correlates with transesophageal echocardiography in aortic stenosis. AJR Am J Roentgenol 2008;191(6):1652–8.

39. Laissy JP, Messika-Zeitoun D, Serfaty JM, et al. Comprehensive evaluation of preoperative patients with aortic valve stenosis: usefulness of cardiac multidetector computed tomography. Heart 2007;93(9):1121–5.

40. Koos R, Mahnken AH, Sinha AM, et al. Aortic valve calcification as a marker for aortic stenosis severity: assessment on 16-MDCT. AJR Am J Roentgenol 2004;183(6):1813–8.

41. Glockner JF, Johnston DL, McGee KP. Evaluation of cardiac valvular disease with MR imaging: qualitative and quantitative techniques. Radiographics 2003;23(1):e9.

42. Ozkan M, Ozdemir N, Kaymaz C, et al. Measurement of aortic valve anatomic regurgitant area using transesophageal echocardiography: implications for the quantitation of aortic regurgitation. J Am Soc Echocardiogr 2002;15(10 Pt 2):1170–4.

43. Feuchtner GM, Dichtl W, Muller S, et al. 64-MDCT for diagnosis of aortic regurgitation in patients referred to CT coronary angiography. AJR Am J Roentgenol 2008;191(1):W1–7.

44. Feuchtner GM, Dichtl W, Schachner T, et al. Diagnostic performance of MDCT for detecting aortic valve regurgitation. AJR Am J Roentgenol 2006; 186(6):1676–81.

45. Asante-Korang A, O'Leary PW, Anderson RH. Anatomy and echocardiography of the normal and abnormal mitral valve. Cardiol Young 2006;16(Suppl 3):27–34.

46. Ranganathan N, Lam JH, Wigle ED, et al. Morphology of the human mitral valve. II. The valve leaflets. Circulation 1970;41(3):459–67.

47. Roberts WC, Perloff JK. Mitral valvular disease. A clinicopathologic survey of the conditions causing the mitral valve to function abnormally. Ann Intern Med 1972;77(6):939–75.

48. Chopra P, Gulwani H. Pathology and pathogenesis of rheumatic heart disease. Indian J Pathol Microbiol 2007;50(4):685–97.

49. Braunwald E, Moscovitz HL, Amram SS, et al. The hemodynamics of the left side of the heart as studied by simultaneous left atrial, left ventricular, and aortic pressures; particular reference to mitral stenosis. Circulation 1955;12(1):69–81.

50. Messika-Zeitoun D, Serfaty JM, Laissy JP, et al. Assessment of the mitral valve area in patients with mitral stenosis by multislice computed tomography. J Am Coll Cardiol 2006;48(2):411–3.

51. Waller BF, Howard J, Fess S. Pathology of mitral valve stenosis and pure mitral regurgitation–Part II. Clin Cardiol 1994;17(7):395–402.

52. Virmani R, Atkinson JB, Forman MB. The pathology of mitral valve prolapse. Herz 1988; 13(4):215–26.

53. Barber JE, Kasper FK, Ratliff NB, et al. Mechanical properties of myxomatous mitral valves. J Thorac Cardiovasc Surg 2001;122(5):955–62.

54. Devereux RB, Jones EC, Roman MJ, et al. Prevalence and correlates of mitral valve prolapse in a population-based sample of American Indians: the Strong Heart Study. Am J Med 2001;111(9): 679–85.

55. Luckie M, Khattar RS. Systolic anterior motion of the mitral valve–beyond hypertrophic cardiomyopathy. Heart 2008;94(11):1383–5.

56. Sandmann H, Pakkal M, Steeds R. Cardiovascular magnetic resonance imaging in the assessment of carcinoid heart disease. Clin Radiol 2009;64(8): 761–6.

57. Mylonakis E, Calderwood SB. Infective endocarditis in adults. N Engl J Med 2001;345(18):1318–30.

58. Burke A, Jeudy J Jr, Virmani R. Cardiac tumours: an update. Heart 2008;94(1):117–23.

59. Raviprasad GS, Salem BI, Gowda S, et al. Radiation-induced mitral and tricuspid regurgitation with severe ostial coronary artery disease: a case report

with successful surgical treatment. Cathet Cardio-vasc Diagn 1995;35(2):146–8.

60. Bose AS, Shetty V, Sadiq A, et al. Radiation induced cardiac valve disease in a man from Chernobyl. J Am Soc Echocardiogr 2009;22(8):973 e971–3.

61. Aqel RA, Lloyd SG, Gupta H, et al. Three-vessel coronary artery disease, aortic stenosis, and constrictive pericarditis 27 years after chest radiation therapy: a case report. Heart Surg Forum 2006;9(4):E728–30.

62. Tamura A, Takahara Y, Mogi K, et al. Radiation-induced valvular disease is the logical consequence of irradiation. Gen Thorac Cardiovasc Surg 2007; 55(2):53–6.

63. Abbara S, Soni AV, Cury RC. Evaluation of cardiac function and valves by multidetector row computed tomography. Semin Roentgenol 2008;43(2):145–53.

64. Gilkeson RC, Markowitz AH, Balgude A, et al. MDCT evaluation of aortic valvular disease. AJR Am J Roentgenol 2006;186(2):350–60.

Computed Tomography of Cardiac Pseudotumors and Neoplasms

Nandan S. Anavekar, MD, Crystal R. Bonnichsen, MD,
Thomas A. Foley, MD, Michael F. Morris, MD,
Matthew W. Martinez, MD, Eric E. Williamson, MD,
James F. Glockner, MD, Dylan V. Miller, MD,
Jerome F. Breen, MD, Philip A. Araoz, MD*

KEYWORDS

- Cardiac masses • Cardiac neoplasm
- Computed tomography • Pseudotumor

"The heart is an organ too noble to be attacked by a primary tumor" was the contention made by de Senac, a prominent pathologist, in 1783.[1] Cardiac masses are uncommon entities; the prevalence of primary cardiac tumors ranges from 0.001% to 0.3% based on autopsy series.[2,3] Cardiac masses may be described as nonneoplastic or neoplastic. Nonneoplastic lesions, or pseudotumors, are tumorlike structures that may resemble a true neoplasm and include entities such as intracavitary thrombi or prominent normal anatomic variants such as a prominent crista terminalis. Neoplastic masses can be divided into metastatic, primary benign, and primary malignant tumors. Of the neoplastic disease that afflicts the heart, the most common is metastatic disease from malignancies arising from other organs. Metastases to the heart occurs 20 to 40 times more commonly than any primary cardiac neoplasm.[4–6] Of the primary cardiac neoplasms, 75% are considered benign.[6] The rarity of cardiac masses and their variability in clinical presentation makes their diagnosis challenging, and this has important implications for the therapeutic strategies available.

Traditionally, echocardiography, cardiac magnetic resonance (MR) imaging, and multidetector CT are the established imaging modalities for the diagnosis and surveillance of cardiac tumors. With recent advances in multidetector CT technology, there is an increased interest in its use and applicability in imaging of cardiac masses. CT can be used to accurately image the heart and surrounding mediastinum, can depict calcification and fat, can provide high level of soft tissue contrast, and, under certain circumstances, may allow for tissue diagnosis.[7] In this article, various cardiac masses are described, including pseudotumors and true cardiac neoplasms, and the CT imaging findings that may be useful in distinguishing these rare entities are presented.

IMAGING MODALITIES

For the initial evaluation of cardiac masses, echocardiography is widely available and provides a simple noninvasive technique. This imaging modality is especially useful in detection of a cardiac mass and the presence of any hemodynamic consequences such as outflow tract obstruction or source of emboli. Cardiac MR imaging[8,9] and CT[10] provide noninvasive high-resolution images of the heart. In cardiac tumor imaging, MR imaging is usually the preferred

Division of Cardiovascular Diseases, Department of Radiology, Mayo Clinic College of Medicine, 200 first Street South West, Rochester MN 55905, USA
* Corresponding author.
E-mail address: araoz.philip@mayo.edu

Radiol Clin N Am 48 (2010) 799–816
doi:10.1016/j.rcl.2010.04.002

modality as it provides a reflection of the chemical microenvironment within a tumor and its interaction with adjacent normal structures. This feature is especially useful in identifying the nature of the mass being investigated.

CT imaging has an equally important role in cardiac tumor imaging, specifically with regard to delineating precise anatomic relationships with the surrounding normal anatomic structures, at the submillimeter level. It is an extremely fast modality that can reconstruct images in any desired plane, can allude to some tissue characteristics such as presence of fat and calcification, and allows for staging of the tumor at the same time. The more widespread availability of CT scanners implies that this modality can be used in situations where MR imaging is contraindicated or not available. Under many circumstances, features observed on CT imaging combined with the clinical history serve to help identify the nature of the cardiac mass.

Within the realms of the diagnostic algorithm, cardiac mass evaluation requires an understanding of the clinical question to be answered to formulate the most appropriate CT examination to provide the most useful clinical information. Generally, high-resolution images are needed, necessitating the use of multidetector scanners. Electrocardiographic gating is required because cardiac masses, by definition, are affected by the cardiac motion in a predictable manner throughout the cardiac cycle. Noncontrast imaging is useful to identify calcification, followed by contrast arterial phase and delayed imaging to assess for the presence or absence of contrast enhancement, which in turn is useful in elucidating the nature of the mass being evaluated.

In general, a multimodality imaging approach is advocated when investigating a cardiac tumor. The goals of the initial evaluation of a patient with a suspected cardiac tumor should always be kept at the forefront. These goals are to ascertain whether a tumor is present, the location of the lesion within the heart, the extent and relation of the lesion to other anatomic structures, and distinguish between a benign and malignant lesion. Imaging of cardiac masses plays a pivotal role in the clinical decision-making algorithms because it allows for appropriate planning of necessary interventions.

PSEUDOTUMORS
Intracavitary Thrombi

Intracavitary thrombi are the most common cardiac mass. Thrombi form in areas of low or stagnant blood flow. Patients usually have a predisposing factor for thrombus formation such as atrial fibrillation, leading to left atrial appendage thrombi (**Fig. 1**A and B), or previous myocardial infarctions with dilated left ventricular cavity and a low-flow state that serves as a perfect nidus for thrombus formation as in the case of left ventricular apical thrombi (**Fig. 2**A and B). In the setting of atrial fibrillation, thrombi typically abut the posterolateral wall of the left atrium or occupy the left atrial appendage.[11] On CT imaging with contrast, thrombi appear as a filling defect within the cardiac chamber, which remains with delayed postcontrast imaging.[12,13] The absence of delayed contrast enhancement has been advocated for definitively demonstrating that a mass is avascular, and likely a thrombus.[14] Thrombi appear as circumscribed, noninfiltrative, nonenhancing masses, and a clinical history such as the presence of an atrial arrhythmia or the presence of a previous myocardial infarction makes the diagnosis more certain.

Lipomatous Hypertrophy of the Interatrial Septum

Lipomatous hypertrophy of the interatrial septum is a nonencapsulated, circumscribed, tumorlike fatty mass located within the cardiac interatrial septum, and was first described by Prior[15] in

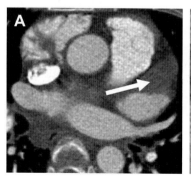 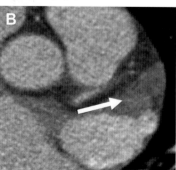

Fig. 1. ECG gated 64-detector dual-source CT scan with intravenous contrast (*A*) and delayed imaging (*B*) in a 51-year-old woman with a history of atrial fibrillation demonstrating a filling defect (*arrow*) in the left atrial appendage that likely represents thrombus.

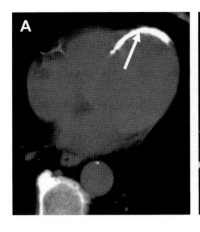
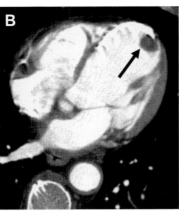

Fig. 2. Four-detector single-source CT (*A*) without and (*B*) with intravenous contrast in an 85-year-old man with a previous history of myocardial infarction. (*A*) Calcification in the region of the left ventricular apex (*arrow*). (*B*) With contrast, a filling (*arrow*) defect in the left ventricular apex is well visualized and is consistent with left ventricular apical thrombus in the setting of ischemic cardiomyopathy.

1964. Histologically it represents hyperplasia of adipose tissue, and is almost always benign with a usually silent clinical course. Lipomatous hypertrophy of the interatrial septum can contain brown fat, which is more metabolically active and for this reason can have increased uptake on fluorodeoxyglucose (FDG)-positron emission tomography (PET) imaging.[16] It is frequently associated with large deposits of fat elsewhere in the body and other parts of the heart. It has classically been described as having a bilobed appearance as a result of sparing of the fossa ovalis, with the area anterior to the fossa ovalis commonly involved, leading to the postulation that destruction of the anterior and middle internodal pathways may result in arrhythmias in these patients.[17,18] On CT imaging, lipomatous hypertrophy of the interatrial septum appears wedge shaped or shows diffuse septal thickening, and appears as a low-attenuation mass that is well circumscribed (**Fig. 3**). It varies in diameter from 1 to 8 cm and may be massive in size (**Fig. 4**). An important distinction must be made between lipomatous hypertrophy of the interatrial septum and liposarcomas, which are malignant and carry a poor prognosis. Liposarcomas are extremely rare and are more commonly metastatic to the heart rather than primary to the heart.[19] Liposarcomas tend to be infiltrative and usually do not occur in the region of the interatrial septum.

Prominent Crista Terminalis

The crista terminalis is a fibromuscular ridge formed by the junction of the sinus venosus and primitive right atrium. It is present on the interior of the atrium and appears as a vertical crest and represents a normal anatomic finding. When prominent it can be mistaken as an intracardiac mass (**Figs. 5** and **6**).

Pericardial Cyst

Pericardial cysts are benign mediastinal cysts and are almost always congenital in origin. They are thin-walled structures and lined with mesothelial cells that secrete a clear serous fluid. They rarely cause symptoms and are almost always diagnosed as an incidental finding (**Fig. 7**A and B) although there have been case reports of pericardial cysts causing hemodynamic compromise because of their atypical location[19] or because of hemorrhage into the cyst causing it to exert a mass effect.[20,21]

Pericardial cysts are most commonly located in the right cardiophrenic angle, where they

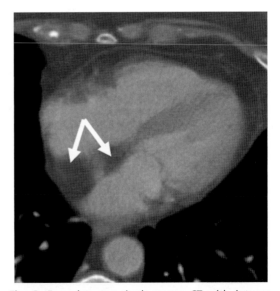

Fig. 3. Four-detector single-source CT with intravenous contrast in a 68-year-old woman presenting for evaluation of chest pain. Imaging demonstrated an incidental finding of lipomatous hypertrophy of the interatrial septum (*arrow*). Note the dumbbell shaped appearance centered around the fossa ovalis.

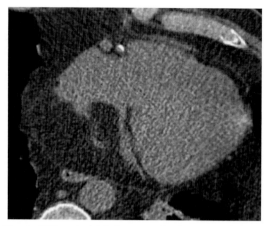

Fig. 4. ECG gated 64-detector single-source CT with intravenous contrast in a 65-year-old man performed to characterize an indeterminate mass seen on transthoracic echocardiography. Imaging was revealing for massive lipomatous hypertrophy of the interatrial septum with extension of fat intrapericardially along the posterior aspect of the right atrium and adjacent to the coronary sinus, resulting in mild deformity of the right atrium. Note the location of the mass in the region of the interatrial septum, the absence of contrast enhancement, and the fat attenuation, all findings consistent with lipomatous hypertrophy of the interatrial septum.

appear as a round fluid density.[22] They average 2 to 4 cm in diameter but can be much larger in size. Rarely, pericardial cysts become calcified or rupture.[23] Their well-defined circumference, fluid

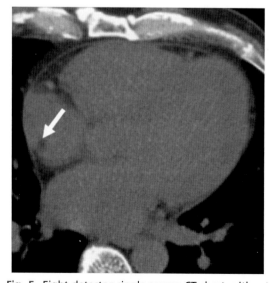

Fig. 5. Eight-detector single-source CT chest without intravenous contrast in a 48-year-old man being evaluated for dyspnea, which incidentally demonstrated the presence of a prominent crista terminalis seen as a focal area of low attenuation (*arrow*).

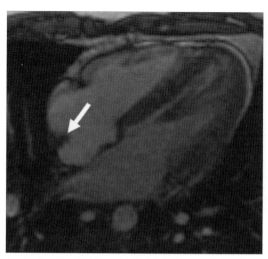

Fig. 6. Cardiac MR imaging with intravenous contrast performed to evaluate a right atrial mass seen on transthoracic echocardiogram in a 19-year-old woman demonstrating an early enhancing mass without delayed enhancement in the right atrium that represents a prominent crista terminalis (*arrow*).

attenuation, and pericardial location permit accurate identification on CT imaging, even when situated in atypical locations.[24] Occasionally encapsulated pericardial effusions and intrapericardial hematomas may exhibit similar imaging characteristics.[25]

Pericardial Hematoma

A hematoma is a collection of blood outside the confines of a blood vessel. A pericardial hematoma is such a collection of blood within the pericardium. The diagnosis of pericardial hematoma (**Fig. 8**) is usually made in concert with a clinical history that alludes to some form of pericardial trauma. Acutely, this can have the appearance of a pericardial effusion, but with chronicity, a rim of calcification may develop, which can aid in its definitive diagnosis. Localized pericardial and intramural hematomas have been described to compress various myocardial structures.[26,27] They are associated with trauma, cardiac surgery, mitral annular calcification, acute myocardial infarction, aortic valve disease, and aortic dissection.[26] Adhesions between the cardiac tissues and pericardium tend to contain hematomas and direct their spread along paths of least resistance. In the acute setting, pericardial or intramural hematomas can lead to hemodynamic compromise, because an expanding hematoma causing extrinsic compression of cardiac structures may impede the natural flow of blood.[28,29]

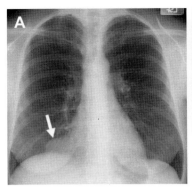

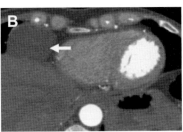

Fig. 7. Plain chest radiograph (*A*) of a 45-year-old woman who was being evaluated for chest pain, demonstrates a rounded opacity in the right cardiophrenic angle that is most likely a pericardial cyst (*arrow*). ECG gated 64-detector single-source CT imaging with intravenous contrast (*B*) confirms the diagnosis (*arrow*) by demonstrating a well-circumscribed fluid-filled structure in the right cardiophrenic angle that does not show contrast enhancement.

Endomyocardial Fibrosis

Endomyocardial fibrosis is a condition that can lead to a cardiomyopathy with restrictive features. It is associated with a pathophysiology that is not fully understood, but involves fibrotic changes in the endomyocardial surfaces with overlying thrombosis. It is a major cause of restrictive cardiomyopathy in North Africa and South America. The condition is associated with eosinophilia in about 50% of those afflicted, and is also known as Loeffler disease when encountered in North Africa. The recognition of endomyocardial fibrosis depends on a high level of clinical suspicion and characteristic imaging appearance.[30] Endomyocardial fibrosis shows masslike, nonneoplastic, apical lesions in the left ventricle (**Fig. 9**) resulting from a thrombotic fibrocalcific process.[31] These lesions are associated with restriction of left ventricular and right ventricular filling caused by obliteration of one or both cardiac apices. In addition to the unique appearance of the apices, the atria are strikingly enlarged and mitral and tricuspid regurgitation are often present. As the condition progresses, more and more of the left ventricular cavity is obliterated, leading to a progressively restrictive physiology. CT examination reveals the presence of endocardial,

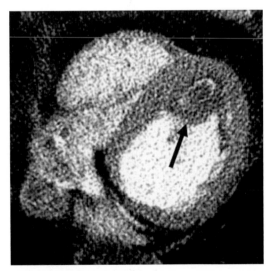

Fig. 8. ECG 64-detector dual-source CT without and with intravenous contrast in a 52-year-old man who was incidentally found to have a cardiac mass on transthoracic echocardiogram. CT demonstrates a heavily peripherally calcified pericardial hematoma (*arrow*) tracking along the right atrial ventricular groove with its epicenter at the level of the mid heart. The degree of calcification would suggest it has been present for years.

Fig. 9. ECG gated electron beam CT without and with contrast in a 72-year-old man who initially presented with progressive dyspnea. CT imaging demonstrates findings suggestive of endomyocardial fibrosis, specifically fibrocalcific changes involving the left ventricular apex and presence of nonenhancing filling defect (*arrow*) consistent with apical thrombus.

partially calcific soft tissue in strips of 2- to 10-mm thick involving the right and left ventricles with impingement on the ventricular cavity that can lead to cavity obliteration when severe.[32] Dynamic cine CT findings reveal the restrictive physiology associated with the disorder.

NEOPLASTIC HEART DISEASE
Secondary Tumors of the Heart

All types of malignant disease can involve the heart and no single type of malignant tumor has a tendency to metastasize preferentially to the heart with the possible exception of malignant melanoma, which can involve the myocardium in more than 50% of cases.[33] Cardiac metastases are more frequently carcinomas than sarcomas,[4] are usually associated with a widely disseminated tumor of origin, and their prevalence in patients with malignant tumors varies widely (1.5%–25%).[34,35]

Metastatic tumors reach the heart via 3 routes: lymphatic spread (**Fig. 10**), hematogeneous spread (**Figs. 11** and **12**), or direct invasion (**Fig. 13**). The epicardium is the site most often affected by metastases, and spread in this instance is mainly via a retrograde route through the mediastinal lymphatics leading to implantation in the epicardial surface of the heart.[36,37] Hematogeneous metastases in the heart and pericardium are normally accompanied by evidence of hematogeneous metastases in other organs. Melanomas and sarcomas usually spread hematogeneously to the myocardium and epicardium through the coronary arteries, or less commonly

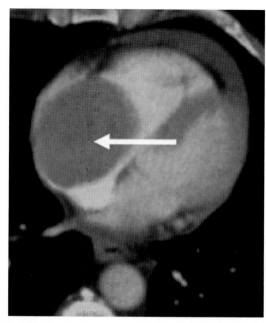

Fig. 11. Single-detector single-source CT chest with contrast in an 84-year-old man with known metastatic melanoma. CT demonstrates a right atrial mass (*arrow*).

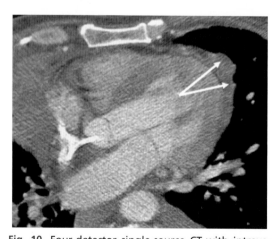

Fig. 10. Four-detector single-source CT with intravenous contrast performed to assess for pulmonary embolism in a 44-year-old man presenting with dyspnea and known history of rectal cancer. CT imaging demonstrates pericardial nodular metastases (*arrows*) as a result of lymphangitic spread of rectal cancer.

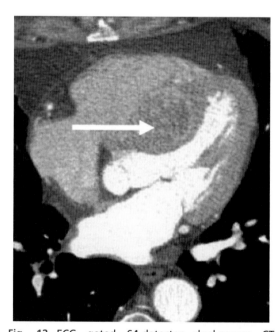

Fig. 12. ECG gated 64-detector dual-source CT without and with intravenous contrast in a 63-year-old man with metastatic renal cell carcinoma. CT imaging demonstrates renal cell carcinoma involving the interventricular septum (*arrow*) which enhances after contrast.

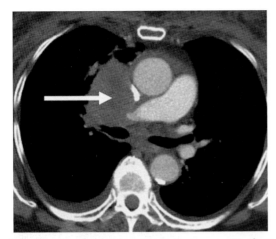

Fig. 13. Sixty-four–detector single-source CT chest with and without intravenous contrast in a 77-year-old man with known lung carcinoma. CT imaging demonstrates the lung mass (*arrow*) invading the superior vena cava resulting in superior vena cava syndrome.

by the implantation of cancer cells through the vena cava.[36,38] Direct extension can occur with thymic, bronchial, breast, and esophageal malignancies as a result of proximity of the primary lesions to the heart. Transvenous tumor spread relies on an extension of the tumor thrombus into the right atrium through the superior (see **Fig. 13**) and inferior vena cava (**Fig. 14**A, B, and C), or an extension into the left atrium via the pulmonary veins.[38]

Primary Benign Tumors of the Heart

Myxomas

Myxomas originate from a multipotent mesenchyme that is capable of neural and endothelial differentiation.[39] Histologically these tumors are composed of scattered cells within a mucopolysaccharide stroma.[39] Intracardiac myxomas are the most common benign tumors of the heart, constituting up to 50% of all such tumors.[38,40] More than 90% of these tumors have an atrial location and most are found in the left atrium (**Fig. 15**).[41] Children have a higher incidence of ventricular myxomas (**Fig. 16**).[42]

These tumors usually originate from the region of the fossa ovalis, in the left atrium, but can have a variable origin (**Fig. 17**). Atypical locations include the right atrium or the right or left ventricles. They are attached to the endocardium by either a narrow or broad base, usually pedunculated, polypoid, and variably friable, typically with smooth rounded surfaces. Grossly these tumors average 5 to 6 cm in size and are soft, gelatinous,

mucoid gray-white masses with areas of hemorrhage or thrombosis. Myxomas can occur at any age but are most commonly seen in the fourth to seventh decades with a female preponderance.[43] In familial series, multiple myxomas are seen with equal distribution on both sides of the heart and associated with a male preponderance.[44]

The cardiovascular manifestations depend on the location of the tumor within the heart and its effects on blood flow through the cardiac chambers; most commonly symptoms of mitral valve obstruction are observed.[45] In addition to the cardiovascular manifestations, patients with myxomas frequently have constitutional symptoms, and although the cause of these symptoms is unclear, it is thought to be related to the production and release of various cytokines from the tumor.[46]

The Carney complex is an inherited autosomal dominant disorder characterized by multiple tumors including atrial and extracardiac myxomas, schwannomas, and various endocrine tumors.[47,48] The cardiac myxomas tend to occur at an earlier age compared with sporadic tumors and have a tendency to recur. In additional, patients have a variety of pigmented lentigines and blue nevi on the face neck and trunk.[47,48]

Contrast-enhanced CT demonstrates the presence of a well-defined spherical or ovoid intracavitary mass with lobulated contours.[38] The tumor attenuation is lower than the unopacified blood pool, and contrast helps delineate the mass as a low-attenuation lesion surrounded by enhancing intracardiac blood.[38] Heterogeneity is a common imaging feature with areas of hemorrhage, necrosis, cyst formation, fibrosis, or calcification.[6,49] However, the most helpful feature is the narrow base of attachment (stalk) which is not seen with other neoplasms. A well-circumscribed neoplasm with a stalk, particularly in the atria can be confidently diagnosed as a myxoma.

Rhabdomyomas

Rhabdomyomas are lesions of striated muscle and are generally considered hamartomas, meaning tumorlike growth made up of normal mature cells in abnormal number or distribution. Rhabdoymyomas are the most frequently occurring primary cardiac tumor in infants and children.[40,50] There is a male preponderance and when detected it can be treated conservatively because of its tendency to regress spontaneously.[50] Surgical resection is required if symptoms can be ascribed to the presence of the tumor.[51] These symptoms are usually caused by obstruction of blood flow within a cardiac chamber. When they occur they are usually multiple and arise from the ventricular

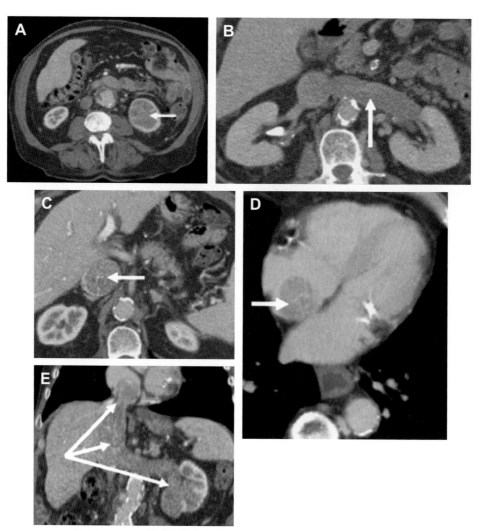

Fig. 14. Four-detector single-source CT chest and abdomen with intravenous contrast in an 84-year-old man. CT imaging demonstrates renal cell carcinoma (*A*) with transvenous spread into the inferior vena cava and extending into the right atrium (*B–D*). When reformatted in a pseudocoronal plane (*E*) the snakelike appearance of the renal mass extending into the right atrium can be well appreciated.

myocardium either projecting into the cavity or moving freely as a pedunculated mass. Rhabdoymyomas are associated with tuberous sclerosis in 80% to 90% of cases.[50,51] These tumors appear as hypodense areas within the myocardium on contrast CT imaging.[25]

Lipomas

Primary cardiac lipomas are benign neoplasms composed of mature adipose tissue and are histologically similar to extracardiac soft tissue lipomas, which are composed of benign fatty cells.[6,25,40] About half of these tumors occur in the subendocardial region with the remainder evenly distributed between the myocardial and subepicardial regions.[52] They can occur as solitary findings

(**Fig. 18**) or as multiple tumors (**Fig. 19**A and B), the latter being associated with tuberous sclerosis.[53] They may also occur on heart valves.[54] Generally, primary cardiac lipomas are rare entities that may be reported incidentally during autopsy and occur over a wide age range.[6] A distinction should be made between a lipoma that represents a true neoplasm and lipomatous hypertrophy of the interatrial septum, which is not a true neoplasm. Suspected pericardial lipomas should be distinguished from diaphragmatic hernias, which are more common.[55]

Lipomas may be massive and can occur throughout the heart including the pericardium.[6] Intramyocardial lipomas are usually small and well encapsulated, although lipomas elsewhere

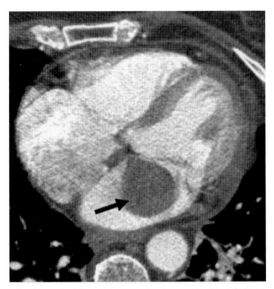

Fig. 15. Sixty-four–detector dual-source CT with intravenous contrast to assess for pulmonary thromboembolism in a 76-year-old woman presenting with pleuritic chest pain. CT imaging demonstrates a low-attenuation left atrial mass (*arrow*) with a pedunculated origin at the interatrial septum consistent with left atrial myxoma.

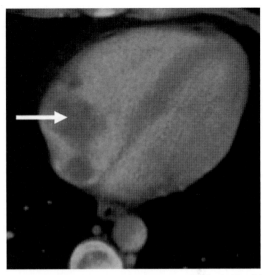

Fig. 17. Single-detector single-source helical CT with contrast in a 53-year-old man demonstrating a pedunculated multilobulated mass (*arrow*) that is nonenhancing and arising from the right atrial free wall and found to be right atrial myxoma.

may be massive. Lipoma-induced arrhythmias including atrial fibrillation, conduction abnormalities, and ventricular tachycardias are an unusual complication of primary cardiac lipomas.[7,56,57]

CT imaging can help identify fat with a high degree of specificity.[6] Lipomas that arise from the interatrial septum may be mistaken for

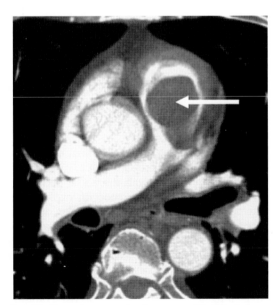

Fig. 16. Four-detector single-source CT with intravenous contrast to assess for pulmonary thromboembolism in a 69-year-old man presenting with dyspnea and with a right ventricular mass found on transthoracic echocardiogram. CT demonstrates a nonenhancing pedunculated mass (*arrow*) with an attachment in the right ventricle extending into the right ventricular outflow tract and found to be a myxoma after surgical resection.

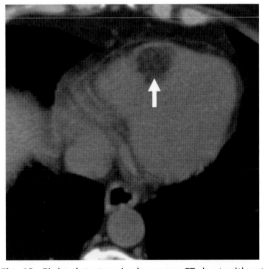

Fig. 18. Eight-detector single-source CT chest without intravenous contrast in a 60-year-old woman performed for surveillance of a pulmonary nodule incidentally demonstrated a solitary low-attenuation lesion in the right ventricle (*arrow*) that likely represents a lipoma.

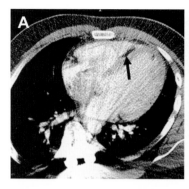
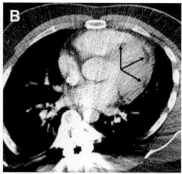

Fig. 19. ECG gated electron beam CT chest with and without intravenous contrast performed in a 31-year-old man with a history of ventricular arrhythmias. CT demonstrates multiple cardiac lipomas. (*A*) A large low-attenuation mass can be seen in the right ventricle near the apex (*arrow*). (*B*) Multiple low-attenuation masses (*arrows*) can be seen, intracavitary and intramyocardial.

a myxoma on echocardiography. However, at CT they are easily distinguished from myxomas because the lipoma is composed entirely of fat and their broad base of attachment and lack of mobility may be a useful distinguishing feature.[58] At CT, cardiac lipomas appear as homogeneous low-attenuation masses either in a cardiac chamber or in the pericardial space.

Fibromas

Histologically fibromas are composed of fibroblasts interspersed among large amounts of collagen.[6] They tend to be ventricular and intramural in location and can be calcified.[59] Primary cardiac fibromas (**Fig. 20**) are rare with a tendency to occur in infants and children.[40,60] The presence of a cardiac fibroma is associated with developmental disorders including cleft palate, cleft lip, and hydrocephalus.[61] Gorlin syndrome, the nevoid basal cell carcinoma syndrome (NBCCS), is a rare inherited multisystem disorder most commonly associated with multiple nevoid basal cell cancers and medulloblastomas.[62] Affected patients have

multiple developmental anomalies of which cardiac fibromas may also represent a common feature.[63]

Clinical presentation includes heart failure, arrhythmias, and chest pain. Sudden death may occur in up to 33% of patients and the contended mechanism is involvement of the conduction system by the tumor with the production of fatal arrythmias or as a result of left ventricular outflow tract obstruction.[60] By autopsy series, cardiac fibromas are the second most common primary benign cardiac tumor after rhabdomyoma, in children.

At gross examination the tumor appears as a firm, white, fibrous mass that arises within the myocardial wall; they are usually large with a mean diameter of 5 cm but may reach sizes that can totally obliterate the ventricular cavity. At CT, fibromas manifest as a homogeneous mass with soft tissue attenuation that may be either sharply marginated or infiltrative with areas of calcification.

Papillary fibroelastomas

Papillary fibroelastomas are the most commonly diagnosed tumor of the heart valves.[64] They arise from the heart valves, with the aortic and mitral valves the most common sites of involvement. Histologically they represent a collection of avascular fronds of dense connective tissue lined by endothelium. Their exact cause remains unclear, however, it is contended that they represent either a hamartoma or a response to previous endocardial damage.[65] After myxomas, papillary fibroelastomas (**Fig. 21**) are the second most common primary benign tumor of the heart, representing 10% of all primary cardiac tumors.[66]

They typically arise in patients more than 50 years of age with equal male to female distribution. When they affect the aortic valve, associated clinical features include angina, paroxysmal atrial fibrillation, myocardial infarction, or sudden death.[67] Occlusion of the right coronary artery

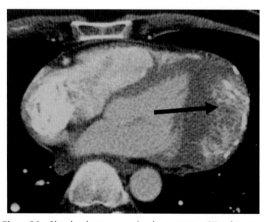

Fig. 20. Single-detector single-source CT demonstrating a large homogeneous mass (*arrow*) with soft tissue attenuation that was found to be a fibroma.

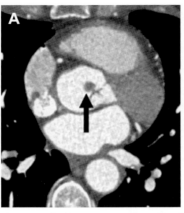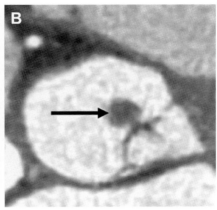

Fig. 21. ECG 64-detector dual-source gated cardiac CT coronary angiogram with intravenous contrast performed in a 53-year-old woman before noncardiac surgery demonstrating an incidentally found papillary fibroelastoma (*arrow*) in relation to other cardiac structures (*A*) and a magnified image (*B*) demonstrates the papillary fibroelastoma (*arrow*) arising from the right coronary cusp.

ostium has been reported.[68] Papillary fibroelastomas can embolize with consequent systemic effects.[67] Right-sided papillary fibroelastomas are usually asymptomatic.[69,70] Fibroelastomas are most easily detected using echocardiography; they appear as small mobile masses attached to valves by a short pedicle. Although they can be seen on CT imaging, this is not the primary mode of diagnosis because of their usual small size, high mobility, and attachment to the valves. At our institution, papillary fibroelastomas are being seen more frequently on CT than in the past, although CT is not the primary modality used to evaluate these lesions (see **Fig. 21**). This can be explained by the increasing trend toward using coronary CT angiography to evaluate the coronary arteries preoperatively in patients with known papillary fibroelastomas, as there is a desire to avoid disrupting the tumor with catheter angiography.

Paragangliomas

A paraganglionoma is a tumor that arises from paraganglia, which represent clusters of neuroendocrine cells widely distributed throughout the body, including the adrenal medulla, carotid, vagal and paraaortic bodies, and groups of cells associated with sympathetic ganglia. Patients range in age from the early teens to the mid-60s, but typically are young adults in their fourth and fifth decades of life.[71] They may occur over the base of the heart in the major region of the vagus nerve distribution, adjacent to or involving the left atrium[72] or from visceral paraganglia in the left atrium, most frequently in the posterior wall of the left atrium or the left atrial roof.[72] However, they may also arise from the interatrial septum.[72]

Biochemically these tumors are commonly positive for chromogranin, neuron-specific enolase, and methionine enkephalin.[73] Clinically patients may present with hypertension and dilated cardiomyopathy with complimentary biochemical evidence of catecholamine over production.[71]

These tumors are described as benign cardiac tumors, however, there have been reports of metastatic spread of cardiac paragangliomas, which may represent evolution of a benign neoplasm to one with metastatic potential and thus malignant nature. Because these tumors are highly vascular and tend to involve the coronary arteries, surgical resection is often difficult.[71,74] At gross examination, the tumors are soft, fleshy, usually tan or brown in color, and range from 3 to 8 cm in diameter.[75] The tumors may be encapsulated or infiltrative, necrosis is common, but calcification rarely occurs.[75] These tumors may be detected on nuclear octreotide scans, which then may lead to further evaluation with CT imaging. At CT, these tumors are well-circumscribed heterogeneous masses having a broad base of attachment, with low attenuation (**Fig. 22**A and B). Extracardiac extension and ill-defined infiltrative borders may also be seen.[75–77]

Primary Malignant Tumors of the Heart

Angiosarcoma

As mentioned earlier, primary malignant cardiac tumors are extremely rare, representing 25% of all primary cardiac tumors.[6] The most common primary malignant cardiac tumor is angiosarcoma.[78–80] Angiosarcomas (**Figs. 23** and **24**) are tumors of endothelial cell origin and comprise endothelial cells that line ill-defined anastomotic vascular spaces. These tumors show a slight

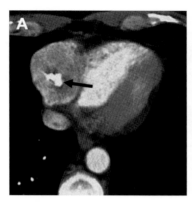
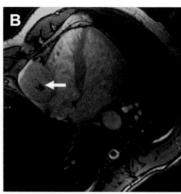

Fig. 22. ECG gated 64-detector dual-source CT with intravenous contrast (*A*) and MR imaging (*B*) in a 60-year-old male demonstrating a well-circumscribed heterogeneous mass with a broad base of attachment and areas of central calcification (*arrow*) representing a paraganglioma located at the base of the heart related to the anterior and posterior aspect of the right ventricle.

male preponderance occurring usually in the middle ages, however, with a wide age range.[81]

These tumors usually arise from the right atrium or pericardium, but may also arise from the pulmonary artery.[82] Up to 25% of these tumors are partly intracavitary and can cause valvular obstruction, right-sided heart failure, and pericardial tamponade with hemorrhagic fluid.

Two main morphologic types have been described in angiosarcoma.[80] The first is a well-defined mass protruding into a cardiac chamber; the second is a diffusely infiltrative mass extending along the pericardium. The incidence of metastatic

disease varies from 66% to 89% and can involve the lungs, liver, cerebellum, skin, and bone.[79,80] Prognosis is poor with treatment aimed at palliation rather than cure, which may reflect delay in diagnosis.

On CT imaging, a low-attenuation intracavitary mass, which may be irregular or nodular and usually arising from the right atrial free wall with areas of necrosis, may be seen.[83,84] Tumor infiltration of the myocardium, compression of the cardiac chambers, direct extension into the pericardium with features of pericardial thickening or effusions, and involvement of the great vessels

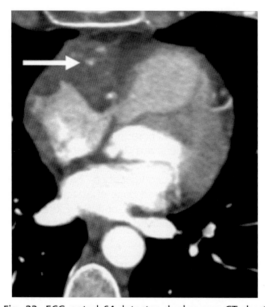

Fig. 23. ECG gated 64-detector dual-source CT chest with intravenous contrast in a 44-year-old woman with chest pain and known cardiac mass detected on transthoracic echocardiogram. CT demonstrates a right atrial angiosarcoma (*arrow*) which is heterogeneous in nature with areas of internal calcification, located along the margin of the atrioventricular groove with invasion of the overlying pericardium.

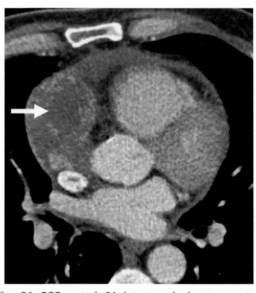

Fig. 24. ECG gated 64-detector dual-source gated cardiac CT with intravenous contrast, performed to evaluate a cardiac mass detected on transthoracic echocardiogram in a 67-year-old man. CT imaging demonstrates a malignant-appearing heterogeneous mass that enhances with contrast, causing complete obstruction of the right atrial cavity (*arrow*) and features suggestive of right atrial angiosarcoma.

are other features discernible on CT imaging. Contrast shows a heterogeneous enhancement pattern.[85]

Undifferentiated sarcoma

Undifferentiated sarcomas are malignant neoplasms without specific histologic features and with diverse clinical manifestations.[6] There is a large age variation ranging from neonates to the elderly.[86] Outcome, which is generally poor, is not different in patients with undifferentiated sarcomas versus those with differentiated sarcomas.[66] On CT, (**Fig. 25**) these tumors appear as large, irregular, low-attenuation intracavitary lesions.[87] Tumor infiltration of the myocardium may appear as thickening and irregularity. The tumor may also manifest as a hemorrhagic mass replacing the pericardium, similar to angiosarcoma. Several reports have demonstrated a tendency to involve the valves.[88,89]

Rhabdomyosarcoma

Rhabdomyosarcoma (see **Fig. 25**) is a malignant tumor of striated muscle. Rhabdomyosarcomas represent 4% to 7% of cardiac sarcomas,[66] but are the most common cardiac malignancy in infants and children.[6] There is a slight male predilection, but because there is no predilection for any cardiac chamber, clinical signs and symptoms vary. Rhabdomyosarcomas may arise anywhere in the myocardium and are more likely than other sarcomas to involve or arise from cardiac valves.[90] They are often multiple and may invade the pericardium.[90]

In contrast to angiosarcomas, rhabdomyosarcomas tend to always involve the myocardium, and when they involve the pericardium, the appearance is that of nodular masses rather than sheetlike thickening of the pericardium.[90] The gross specimens may be gelatinous and friable,[91] firm and fleshy,[92] or cystlike.[93] CT imaging may demonstrate a smooth or irregular low-attenuation mass in a cardiac chamber. CT is also useful in identifying extracardiac extension of the tumor.[94,95]

Osteosarcoma

Osteosarcomas (**Fig. 26**) of the heart are a heterogeneous group of tumors that contain malignant bone-producing cells. They may be predominantly osteoblastic or may have chondroblastic or fibroblastic differentiation. Cardiac osteosarcomas represent 3% to 9% of all cardiac sarcomas.[6] Osteosarcomas that are metastatic to the heart tend to occur in the right atrium.[96] By contrast, primary cardiac osteosarcomas tend to occur in the left atrium and their obstructive nature results

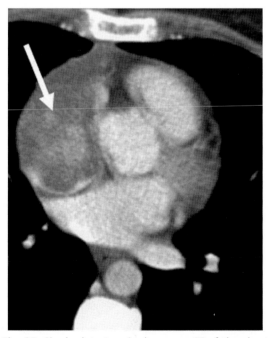

Fig. 25. Single-detector single-source CT of the chest with intravenous contrast performed in a 42-year-old woman. CT imaging demonstrates an irregular mass starting at the confluence of the superior vena cava and right atrium extending to completely involve the right atrium (*arrow*). At pathology this mass was found to be a rhabdomyosarcoma.

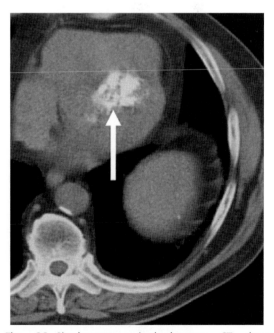

Fig. 26. Single-source single-detector CT chest without and with intravenous contrast in a 70-year-old man with suspected pulmonary malignancy demonstrates a heavily calcified left ventricular mass that was found to be a cardiac osteosarcoma (*arrow*).

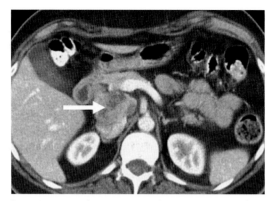

Fig. 27. Four-detector single-source CT chest, abdomen, and pelvis with contrast using a multidetector scanner performed for staging purposes in a 62-year-old woman. CT imaging shows the primary tumor to be a leiomyosarcoma (*arrow*) of the inferior vena cava.

in signs and symptoms of congestive heart failure.[96] As with other cardiac sarcomas, the overall prognosis is poor. Grossly, these tumors are highly calcified and may be described as stone hard.[97]

CT imaging demonstrates dense calcifications within a low-attenuation mass.[98] Because these tumors are most commonly observed in the left atrium, they may be confused with atrial myxomas, especially in the early stages, when calcifications may be absent. Distinguishing features on imaging that are more suggestive of an osteogenic sarcoma include a broad base, an aggressive growth pattern such as extension into the pulmonary veins, invasion of the atrial septum, or infiltrative growth along the epicardium.[6] It has been contended that primary cardiac osteosarcoma should be in the differential diagnosis of all atypical left atrial myxomas.[96]

Leiomyosarcoma

Leiomyosarcomas (**Fig. 27**) are malignant tumors with smooth muscle differentiation. They may arise from smooth muscle bundles lining the subendocardium, but many cardiac leiomyosarcomas may arise from the smooth muscle of the pulmonary veins and arteries, and then spread into the heart.[6]

Cardiac leiomyosarcomas constitute 8% to 9% of all cardiac sarcomas, they have a predilection for the left atrium, and manifest commonly with congestive heart failure signs and symptoms. On gross examination, leiomyosarcomas appear as gelatinous sessile masses. On CT, they usually appear as lobulated, irregular, low-attenuation masses in the left atrium, most commonly arising from the posterior wall, a feature that distinguishes them from left atrial myxomas. Additional imaging findings include a tendency to invade the pulmonary veins and mitral valve, the former with the appearance of a low-attenuation filling defect.[99]

Cardiac lymphoma

A primary cardiac lymphoma is defined as that which is mostly confined to the heart or pericardium. This definition helps distinguish primary cardiac lymphoma from the more common cardiac spread of non-Hodgkin lymphoma.[100] Almost all primary cardiac lymphomas are aggressive B-cell lymphomas.[101–103] These tumors have variable presentation including arrhythmias,[104,105] superior vena caval obstruction,[106] and cardiac tamponade.[103] These tumors are seen more frequently in those who are immunocompromised.[107]

As opposed to other primary cardiac malignancies, primary cardiac lymphomas have a favorable response to chemotherapy.[101] The tumor has a tendency to arise from the right side of the heart

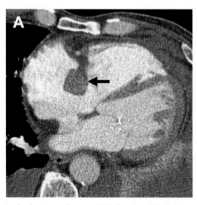
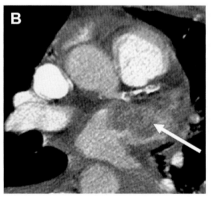

Fig. 28. ECG gated electron beam CT chest with intravenous contrast performed to assess for pulmonary thromboembolism in an 80-year-old patient. CT imaging reveals 2 intracardiac masses: (*A*) a mass attached to the tricuspid valve (*arrow*); (*B*) a polypoid appearing mass in the left atrial appendage (*arrow*). Surgical pathology revealed primary cardiac lymphoma.

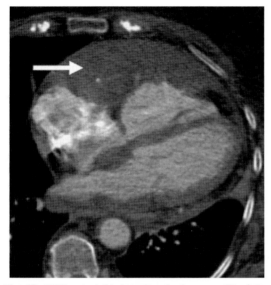

Fig. 29. ECG gated 64-detector dual-source CT of the chest with intravenous contrast performed for surveillance purposes in a 73-year-old woman with known cardiac lymphoma. The mass extends from the AV atrioventricular (AV) groove and is contained by the pericardium (*arrow*).

with the right atrium being reported as the most common site (**Fig. 28**A).[101,102] Pericardial effusions are frequently seen, are often large in nature, and may be the only finding on imaging that points to the diagnosis.[101] Primary cardiac lymphomas are less likely than sarcomas to have necrosis, involve the valve, or extend into the cardiac chambers. Findings on CT are nonspecific.[6] Variable morphologic types have been described, with either circumscribed polypoid masses (see **Fig. 28**B), or ill-defined infiltrative lesions (**Fig. 29**) reported.

SUMMARY

Important features of cardiac masses can be clearly delineated on cardiac CT imaging. This modality is useful in identifying the presence of a mass, its relationship with cardiac and extracardiac structures, and in demonstrating features that distinguish one type of mass from another. A multimodality approach to the evaluation of cardiac tumors is advocated, with the use of echocardiography, CT imaging and MR imaging as appropriately indicated.

REFERENCES

1. Primary cardiac tumours. Scott Med J 1975;20(3): 103–4.
2. McAllister HA Jr. Primary tumors of the heart and pericardium. Pathol Annu 1979;14(Pt 2):325–55.
3. Sutsch G, Jenni R, von Segesser L, et al. [Heart tumors: incidence, distribution, diagnosis. Exemplified by 20,305 echocardiographies]. Schweiz Med Wochenschr 1991;121(17):621–9 [in German].
4. Deloach JF, Haynes JW. Secondary tumors of heart and pericardium; review of the subject and report of one hundred thirty-seven cases. AMA Arch Intern Med 1953;91(2):224–49.
5. Prichard RW. Tumors of the heart; review of the subject and report of 150 cases. AMA Arch Pathol 1951;51(1):98–128.
6. Araoz PA, Eklund HE, Welch TJ, et al. CT and MR imaging of primary cardiac malignancies. Radiographics 1999;19(6):1421–34.
7. Conces DJ Jr, Vix VA, Tarver RD. Diagnosis of a myocardial lipoma by using CT. AJR Am J Roentgenol 1989;153(4):725–6.
8. Gulati G, Sharma S, Kothari SS, et al. Comparison of echo and MRI in the imaging evaluation of intracardiac masses. Cardiovasc Intervent Radiol 2004; 27(5):459–69.
9. Kaminaga T, Takeshita T, Kimura I. Role of magnetic resonance imaging for evaluation of tumors in the cardiac region. Eur Radiol 2003; 13(Suppl 6):L1–10.
10. Bleiweis MS, Georgiou D, Brundage BH. Detection of intracardiac masses by ultrafast computed tomography. Am J Card Imaging 1994;8(1):63–8.
11. Freedberg RS, et al. The contribution of magnetic resonance imaging to the evaluation of intracardiac tumors diagnosed by echocardiography. Circulation 1988;77(1):96–103.
12. Martinez MW, Williamson EE, Lin G, et al. Multidetector computed tomography with delay imaging for detection of left atrial thrombus. J Cardiovasc Comput Tomogr 2009;3(5):354–5.
13. Martinez MW, Lin G, Williamson EE, et al. Dual source computed tomography with delayed imaging for left atrial appendage thrombus compared with transoesophageal echocardiography. Heart 2009;95(6):460.
14. Krauser DG, Cham MD, Tortolani AJ, et al. Clinical utility of delayed-contrast computed tomography for tissue characterization of cardiac thrombus. J Cardiovasc Comput Tomogr 2007;1(2):114–8.
15. Prior JT. Lipomatous hypertrophy of cardiac interatrial septum. A lesion resembling hibernoma, lipoblastomatosis and infiltrating lipoma. Arch Pathol 1964;78:11–5.
16. Kuester LB, Fischman AJ, Fan CM, et al. Lipomatous hypertrophy of the interatrial septum: prevalence and features on fusion 18F fluorodeoxyglucose positron emission tomography/CT. Chest 2005;128(6):3888–93.
17. Hutter AM Jr, Page DL. Atrial arrhythmias and lipomatous hypertrophy of the cardiac interatrial septum. Am Heart J 1971;82(1):16–21.

18. Basu S, et al. Lipomatous hypertrophy of the intra-atrial septum. Cardiovasc Surg 1994;2(2):229–31.

19. Cunningham KS, Veinot JP, Feindel CM, et al. Fatty lesions of the atria and interatrial septum. Hum Pathol 2006;37(10):1245–51.

20. Ng AF, Olak J. Pericardial cyst causing right ventricular outflow tract obstruction. Ann Thorac Surg 1997;63(4):1147–8.

21. Borges AC, Gellert K, Dietel M, et al. Acute right-sided heart failure due to hemorrhage into a peri-cardial cyst. Ann Thorac Surg 1997;63(3):845–7.

22. Feigin DS, Fenoglio JJ, McAllister HA, et al. Peri-cardial cysts. A radiologic-pathologic correlation and review. Radiology 1977;125(1):15–20.

23. King JF, Crosby I, Pugh D, et al. Rupture of pericar-dial cyst. Chest 1971;60(6):611–2.

24. Schvartzman PR, White RD. Imaging of cardiac and paracardiac masses. J Thorac Imaging 2000; 15(4):265–73.

25. Restrepo CS, Largoza A, Lemos DF, et al. CT and MR imaging findings of benign cardiac tumors. Curr Probl Diagn Radiol 2005;34(1):12–21.

26. Gologorsky E, Gologorsky A, Galbut DL, et al. Left atrial compression by a pericardial hematoma pre-senting as an obstructing intracavitary mass: a diffi-cult differential diagnosis. Anesth Analg 2002; 95(3):567–9 [table of contents].

27. Kochar GS, Jacobs LE, Kotler MN. Right atrial compression in postoperative cardiac patients: detection by transesophageal echocardiography. J Am Coll Cardiol 1990;16(2):511–6.

28. Pepi M, Doria E, Fiorentini C. Cardiac tamponade produced by a loculated pericardial hematoma simulating a right atrial mass. Int J Cardiol 1990; 29(3):383–6.

29. Tardif JC, Taylor K, Pandian NG, et al. Right ventricular outflow tract and pulmonary artery obstruction by postoperative mediastinal hema-toma: delineation by multiplane transesophageal echocardiography. J Am Soc Echocardiogr 1994; 7(4):400–4.

30. Acquatella H, Schiller NB. Echocardiographic recognition of Chagas' disease and endomyocar-dial fibrosis. J Am Soc Echocardiogr 1988;1(1): 60–8.

31. Acquatella H, Schiller NB, Puigbo JJ, et al. Value of two-dimensional echocardiography in endomyo-cardial disease with and without eosinophilia. A clinical and pathologic study. Circulation 1983; 67(6):1219–26.

32. Mousseaux E, Hernigou A, Azencot M, et al. Endo-myocardial fibrosis: electron-beam CT features. Radiology 1996;198(3):755–60.

33. Mousseaux E, Meunier P, Azancott S, et al. Cardiac metastatic melanoma investigated by magnetic resonance imaging. Magn Reson Imaging 1998; 16(1):91–5.

34. Abraham KP, Reddy V, Gattuso P. Neoplasms metastatic to the heart: review of 3314 consecu-tive autopsies. Am J Cardiovasc Pathol 1990; 3(3):195–8.

35. Kutalek SP, Panidis IP, Kotler MN, et al. Meta-static tumors of the heart detected by two-dimen-sional echocardiography. Am Heart J 1985; 109(2):343–9.

36. Klatt EC, Heitz DR. Cardiac metastases. Cancer 1990;65(6):1456–9.

37. Lam KY, Dickens P, Chan AC. Tumors of the heart. A 20-year experience with a review of 12,485 consecutive autopsies. Arch Pathol Lab Med 1993;117(10):1027–31.

38. Kim EY, Choe YH, Sung K, et al. Multidetector CT and MR imaging of cardiac tumors. Korean J Ra-diol 2009;10(2):164–75.

39. Pucci A, Gagliardotto P, Zanini C, et al. Histopath-ologic and clinical characterization of cardiac myxoma: review of 53 cases from a single institu-tion. Am Heart J 2000;140(1):134–8.

40. Burke A, Virmani R. Tumors of the heart and great vessels. Atlas of tumor pathology: 3rd series. Fascicle 16. Washing, DC: American Registry of Pathology; 1996. p. 1–98.

41. Keeling IM, Oberwalder P, Anelli-Monti M, et al. Cardiac myxomas: 24 years of experience in 49 patients. Eur J Cardiothorac Surg 2002;22(6): 971–7.

42. Morgan DL, Palazola J, Reed W, et al. Left heart myxomas. Am J Cardiol 1977;40(4):611–4.

43. Peters MN, Hall RJ, Cooley DA, et al. The clinical syndrome of atrial myxoma. JAMA 1974;230(5): 695–701.

44. Powers JC, Falkoff M, Heinle RA, et al. Familial cardiac myxoma: emphasis on unusual clinical manifestations. J Thorac Cardiovasc Surg 1979; 77(5):782–8.

45. Pinede L, Duhaut P, Loire R. Clinical presentation of left atrial cardiac myxoma. A series of 112 consecutive cases. Medicine (Baltimore) 2001; 80(3):159–72.

46. Sakamoto H, Sakamaki T, Kanda T, et al. Vascular endothelial growth factor is an autocrine growth factor for cardiac myxoma cells. Circ J 2004; 68(5):488–93.

47. Vatterott PJ, Seward JB, Vidaillet HJ, et al. Syndrome cardiac myxoma: more than just a sporadic event. Am Heart J 1987;114(4 Pt 1): 886–9.

48. Vidaillet HJ Jr, Seward JB, Fyke FE 3rd, et al. "Syndrome myxoma": a subset of patients with cardiac myxoma associated with pigmented skin lesions and peripheral and endocrine neoplasms. Br Heart J 1987;57(3):247–55.

49. Tsuchiya F, Kohno A, Saitoh R, et al. CT findings of atrial myxoma. Radiology 1984;151(1):139–43.

50. Beghetti M, Gow RM, Haney I, et al. Pediatric primary benign cardiac tumors: a 15-year review. Am Heart J 1997;134(6):1107–14.

51. Bosi G, Lintermans JP, Pellegrino PA, et al. The natural history of cardiac rhabdomyoma with and without tuberous sclerosis. Acta Paediatr 1996; 85(8):928–31.

52. Hananouchi GI, Goff WB 2nd. Cardiac lipoma: six-year follow-up with MRI characteristics, and a review of the literature. Magn Reson Imaging 1990;8(6):825–8.

53. Winterkorn EB, Dodd JD, Inglessis I, et al. Tuberous sclerosis complex and myocardial fat-containing lesions: a report of four cases. Clin Genet 2007;71(4):371–3.

54. Benvenuti LA, Mansur AJ, Lopes DO, et al. Primary lipomatous tumors of the cardiac valves. South Med J 1996;89(10):1018–20.

55. Colagrande L, De Paulis R, Seddio F, et al. Anterior diaphragmatic hernia misinterpreted by X-ray, echocardiography, computed tomography scanning and magnetic resonance imaging. J Cardiovasc Surg (Torino) 2000;41(4):643–5.

56. Grande AM, Minzioni G, Pederzolli C, et al. Cardiac lipomas. Description of 3 cases. J Cardiovasc Surg (Torino) 1998;39(6):813–5.

57. Vanderheyden M, De Sutter J, Wellens F, et al. Left atrial lipoma: case report and review of the literature. Acta Cardiol 1998;53(1):31–2.

58. Mousseaux E, Idy-Peretti I, Bittoun J, et al. MR tissue characterization of a right atrial mass: diagnosis of a lipoma. J Comput Assist Tomogr 1992; 16(1):148–51.

59. Burke AP, Rosado-de-Christenson M, Templeton PA, et al. Cardiac fibroma: clinicopathologic correlates and surgical treatment. J Thorac Cardiovasc Surg 1994;108(5):862–70.

60. Reul GJ Jr, Howell JF, Rubio PA, et al. Successful partial excision of an intramural fibroma of the left ventricle. Am J Cardiol 1975;36(2):262–5.

61. de Leon GA, Zaeri N, Donner RM, et al. Cerebral rhinocele, hydrocephalus, and cleft lip and palate in infants with cardiac fibroma. J Neurol Sci 1990; 99(1):27–36.

62. Gorlin RJ, Goltz RW. Multiple nevoid basal-cell epithelioma, jaw cysts and bifid rib. A syndrome. N Engl J Med 1960;262:908–12.

63. Rahbari H, Mehregan AH. Basal cell epithelioma (carcinoma) in children and teenagers. Cancer 1982;49(2):350–3.

64. Edwards FH, Hale D, Cohen A, et al. Primary cardiac valve tumors. Ann Thorac Surg 1991; 52(5):1127–31.

65. Rubin MA, Snell JA, Tazelaar HD, et al. Cardiac papillary fibroelastoma: an immunohistochemical investigation and unusual clinical manifestations. Mod Pathol 1995;8(4):402–7.

66. Tazelaar HD, Locke TJ, McGregor CG. Pathology of surgically excised primary cardiac tumors. Mayo Clin Proc 1992;67(10):957–65.

67. Grinda JM, Couetil JP, Chauvaud S, et al. Cardiac valve papillary fibroelastoma: surgical excision for revealed or potential embolization. J Thorac Cardiovasc Surg 1999;117(1):106–10.

68. Prahlow JA, Barnard JJ. Sudden death due to obstruction of coronary artery ostium by aortic valve papillary fibroelastoma. Am J Forensic Med Pathol 1998;19(2):162–5.

69. Ganjoo AK, Johnson WD, Gordon RT, et al. Tricuspid papillary fibroelastoma causing syncopal episodes. J Thorac Cardiovasc Surg 1996;112(2): 551–3.

70. Scalia D, Basso C, Rizzoli G, et al. Should right-sided fibroelastomas be operated upon? J Heart Valve Dis 1997;6(6):647–50.

71. Jeevanandam V, Oz MC, Shapiro B, et al. Surgical management of cardiac pheochromocytoma. Resection versus transplantation. Ann Surg 1995; 221(4):415–9.

72. Orringer MB, Sisson JC, Glazer G, et al. Surgical treatment of cardiac pheochromocytomas. J Thorac Cardiovasc Surg 1985;89(5):753–7.

73. Johnson TL, Shapiro B, Beierwaltes WH, et al. Cardiac paragangliomas. A clinicopathologic and immunohistochemical study of four cases. Am J Surg Pathol 1985;9(11):827–34.

74. Rosamond TL, Hamburg MS, Vacek JL, et al. Intrapericardial pheochromocytoma. Am J Cardiol 1992;70(6):700–2.

75. Hamilton BH, Francis IR, Gross BH, et al. Intrapericardial paragangliomas (pheochromocytomas): imaging features. AJR Am J Roentgenol 1997; 168(1):109–13.

76. Gomi T, Ikeda T, Sakurai J, et al. Cardiac pheochromocytoma. A case report and review of the literature. Jpn Heart J 1994;35(1):117–24.

77. Lewis IH, Yousif D, Mullis SL, et al. Case 2–1994. Management of a cardiac pheochromocytoma in two patients. J Cardiothorac Vasc Anesth 1994; 8(2):223–30.

78. Makhoul N, Bode FR. Angiosarcoma of the heart: review of the literature and report of two cases that illustrate the broad spectrum of the disease. Can J Cardiol 1995;11(5):423–8.

79. Glancy DL, Morales JB Jr, Roberts WC. Angiosarcoma of the heart. Am J Cardiol 1968;21(3):413–9.

80. Janigan DT, Husain A, Robinson NA. Cardiac angiosarcomas. A review and a case report. Cancer 1986;57(4):852–9.

81. Rosenkranz ER, Murphy DJ Jr. Diagnosis and neonatal resection of right atrial angiosarcoma. Ann Thorac Surg 1994;57(4):1014–5.

82. Totaro M, Miraldi F, Ghiribelli C, et al. Cardiac angiosarcoma arising from pulmonary artery:

endovascular treatment. Ann Thorac Surg 2004; 78(4):1468–70.

83. Matheis G, Beyersdorf F. Primary cardiac angiosarcoma. A case report. Cardiology 1995;86(1):83–5.

84. Shin MS, Kirklin JK, Cain JB, et al. Primary angiosarcoma of the heart: CT characteristics. AJR Am J Roentgenol 1987;148(2):267–8.

85. Bruna J, Lockwood M. Primary heart angiosarcoma detected by computed tomography and magnetic resonance imaging. Eur Radiol 1998;8(1):66–8.

86. Lazarus KH, D'Orsogna DE, Bloom KR, et al. Primary pericardial sarcoma in a neonate. Am J Pediatr Hematol Oncol 1989;11(3):343–7.

87. Baumgartner RA, Das SK, Shea M, et al. The role of echocardiography and CT in the diagnosis of cardiac tumors. Int J Card Imaging 1988;3(1):57–60.

88. Itoh K, Matsumura T, Egawa Y, et al. Primary mitral valve sarcoma in infancy. Pediatr Cardiol 1998; 19(2):174–7.

89. Ludomirsky A, Vargo TA, Murphy DJ, et al. Intracardiac undifferentiated sarcoma in infancy. J Am Coll Cardiol 1985;6(6):1362–4.

90. Raaf HN, Raaf JH. Sarcomas related to the heart and vasculature. Semin Surg Oncol 1994;10(5):374–82.

91. Sholler GF, Hawker RE, Nunn GR, et al. Primary left ventricular rhabdomyosarcoma in a child: noninvasive assessment and successful resection of a rare tumor. J Thorac Cardiovasc Surg 1987;93(3):465–8.

92. Poole GV Jr, Breyer RH, Holliday RH, et al. Tumors of the heart: surgical considerations. J Cardiovasc Surg (Torino) 1984;25(1):5–11.

93. Becker RC, Hobbs RE, Ratliff NB. Cardiac rhabdomyosarcoma: case report with review of clinical and pathologic features. Cleve Clin Q 1984;51(1): 83–8.

94. Rheeder P, Simson IW, Mentis H, et al. Cardiac rhabdomyosarcoma in a renal transplant patient. Transplantation 1995;60(2):204–5.

95. Jack CM, Cleland J, Geddes JS. Left atrial rhabdomyosarcoma and the use of digital gated computed tomography in its diagnosis. Br Heart J 1986;55(3):305–7.

96. Burke AP, Virmani R. Osteosarcomas of the heart. Am J Surg Pathol 1991;15(3):289–95.

97. Schneiderman H, Fordham EW, Goren CC, et al. Primary cardiac osteosarcoma: multidisciplinary aspects applicable to extraskeletal osteosarcoma generally. CA Cancer J Clin 1984;34(2):110–7.

98. Chaloupka JC, Fishman EK, Siegelman SS. Use of CT in the evaluation of primary cardiac tumors. Cardiovasc Intervent Radiol 1986;9(3):132–5.

99. Takamizawa S, Sugimoto K, Tanaka H, et al. A case of primary leiomyosarcoma of the heart. Intern Med 1992;31(2):265–8.

100. Roberts WC, Glancy DL, DeVita VT Jr. Heart in malignant lymphoma (Hodgkin's disease, lymphosarcoma, reticulum cell sarcoma and mycosis fungoides). A study of 196 autopsy cases. Am J Cardiol 1968;22(1):85–107.

101. Ceresoli GL, Ferreri AJ, Bucci E, et al. Primary cardiac lymphoma in immunocompetent patients: diagnostic and therapeutic management. Cancer 1997;80(8):1497–506.

102. Nakchbandi IA, Day HJ. Primary cardiac lymphoma: initial symptoms suggestive of gastrointestinal disease. South Med J 1997;90(5):539–43.

103. Aboulafia DM, Bush R, Picozzi VJ. Cardiac tamponade due to primary pericardial lymphoma in a patient with AIDS. Chest 1994;106(4):1295–9.

104. Murphy PT, Sivakumaran M, Coleby P. Primary cardiac lymphoma: death from cardiac asystole after attaining second complete remission. Clin Lab Haematol 1998;20(1):57–9.

105. Nakayama Y, Uchimoto S, Tsumura K, et al. Primary cardiac lymphoma with infiltration of the atrioventricular node: remission with reversal of the atrioventricular block induced by chemotherapy. Cardiology 1997;88(6):613–6.

106. Versluis PJ, Lamers RJ, van Belle AF. Primary malignant lymphoma of the heart: CT and MRI features. Rofo 1995;162(6):533–4.

107. Levine AM. Lymphoma complicating immunodeficiency disorders. Ann Oncol 1994;5(Suppl 2): 29–35.

Computed Tomography of Adult Congenital Heart Disease

Douglas Hughes Jr, MD, Marilyn J. Siegel, MD*

KEYWORDS

• Computed tomography • Congenital heart disease • Adults

Congenital heart disease (CHD) is one of the most common inborn defects, occurring in approximately 0.8% of newborn infants.[1] Patients with CHD are living longer as a result of surgical interventional in early life and many of them will require lifelong care. It is estimated that there are approximately 800,000 adults with CHD in the United States and the number is increasing.[1,2] An understanding of the computed tomography (CT) findings of CHDs and their postoperative complications is important for the radiologist because patients with palliated or repaired CHD continue to be seen for long-term follow-up.[3]

IMAGING ALGORITHMS

The initial imaging algorithm for patients with suspected CHD includes a chest radiograph and subsequent transthoracic echocardiography (TTE).[4] TTE is readily available, portable, and noninvasive. It can provide detailed anatomic information and characterization of hemodynamic parameters through Doppler flow studies. However, the technique is operator-dependent and limited by acoustic window parameters (thoracic deformities, air-filled lung, sternal wires, and obesity) and inability to depict extracardiac vascular structures. Transesophageal echocardiography (TEE) offers higher spatial resolution than TTE, but it is a more invasive procedure and it still has limitations in examining the systemic and pulmonary vascular systems. Cardiac catheterization was previously the gold standard for cardiac evaluation, but its high cost and invasive nature have limited its widespread application although it still has a role in the diagnosis of complex heart diseases.[4]

Magnetic resonance imaging (MRI) provides noninvasive visualization of the morphologic changes in patients with CHD, overcoming the limitations of sonography. It offers excellent anatomic and functional information and is particularly valuable in the evaluation of valvular and myocardial function, but it is time-consuming and it is contraindicated in patients with pacemakers and in some with implantable cardioverter-defibrillators.[5–8]

There are several advantages of CT compared with MRI. CT is more available and less time-consuming than MRI.[9–12] The use of multidetector CT technology shortens examination times, increases spatial resolution, and enables superb reconstructions. CT allows a more complete evaluation of lung parenchyma than does MRI. CT, unlike MRI, is not hampered by postoperative metal artifacts. On the other hand, CT lacks the functional capabilities of MRI, but all patients with repaired CHD have complete echocardiographic evaluation, which often can provide the necessary functional data. CT also has the disadvantage of radiation exposure as well as the necessity for intravenous administration of contrast material. Nevertheless, CT is enjoying broader use because of its ease of use and

Washington University School of Medicine, Mallinckrodt Institute of Radiology, 510 South Kingshighway Boulevard, Saint Louis, MO 63110, USA
* Corresponding author.
E-mail address: siegelm@mir.wustl.edu

Radiol Clin N Am 48 (2010) 817–835
doi:10.1016/j.rcl.2010.04.005
0033-8389/10/$ – see front matter © 2010 Published by Elsevier Inc.

radiologic.theclinics.com

widespread availability. Thus, an understanding of the CT features of CHD is essential to ensure a correct diagnosis.

This article discusses and illustrates the technique of multidetector CT in the evaluation of adults with CHD and the pre- and postoperative CT appearances of common congenital heart malformations in adults.

CARDIAC CT TECHNIQUES IN ADULTS

Cardiac CT requires fast scan times and contrast enhancement. We perform our contrast-enhanced CT examinations of the heart using a pulmonary embolism protocol. A large-gauge venous catheter needs to be placed. Contrast-enhanced studies are performed with 150 mL of nonionic contrast agent (320 mgI/mL), which is administered with a power injector at a rate of 3 to 4 mL/s. To reduce artifacts from undiluted contrast material and to reduce the total amount of contrast material, a saline bolus chasing technique can be used.

We determine scan delay time with an automatic bolus tracking system using a region of interest and a threshold level of 100 to 120 HU for triggering the scan. The region of interest is usually placed in the ascending aorta. Noncontrast axial scans may be obtained in postoperative patients to identify dystrophic calcification and stents.

The contrast-enhanced CT examination is performed with thin collimation (<1 mm), fast table feed (pitch>1), tube voltage of 120 kV, tube current of approximately 200 mAs (or mAs appropriate for body size), and gantry rotation time <0.5 seconds. Scans are performed in a craniocaudal direction during a single breath-hold. Administration of a β-blocker is generally not needed for evaluation of patients with CHD, unless concurrent evaluation of the coronary arteries is needed.

Although electrocardiographic (ECG) gating can reduce motion artifacts, diagnostic quality scans can usually be obtained with nongated scanning. ECG gating is definitely needed if the coronary arteries, cardiac valves, and small vessels are areas of interest. Prospective gating is valuable for reducing radiation exposure, but requires a regular rhythm and a low heart rate.[13] Additional radiation reduction strategies including automated real-time anatomy-based dose regulation can be used to reduce radiation exposure.

The acquired image data are reformatted with a thickness of 2 mm (increment of 1- to 1.5 mm) and a medium (soft tissue) reconstruction kernel. Data sets are reconstructed at 1.0 mm (increment of 0.8 mm) for assessing the cardiac valves and coronary arteries. Review of axial images is important for accurate diagnosis. Multiplanar and three-dimensional (3D) reformatted images are useful to assess extracardiac vascular anomalies. Multiplanar images also can be helpful for visualizing atrioventricular septal defects.

VIEWING PLANES FOR CARDIAC CT ANGIOGRAPHY
Transverse, Coronal and Sagittal Views

CT images are routinely reviewed in the transverse plane, which provides information about the relationships of the great vessels and cardiac chambers and anatomy of the aortic and pulmonary valves and proximal parts of the coronary arteries. Supplemental coronal and sagittal multiplanar reformations have been shown to be valuable for evaluation and display of the ventricular outflow tracts and their valves, the connections of the superior and inferior vena cavae to the right atrium, the entrance of the pulmonary veins into the left atrium, and the diaphragmatic surface of the left ventricle.

Long and Short Axis Views

Long and short axis views may help in displaying intra- and extracardiac anatomy.

Vertical long axis plane (2-chamber view)

Because the heart lies obliquely in the thoracic cavity, the true vertical long axis of the heart is oriented approximately 45° to the midsagittal plane of the thoracic spine. Images parallel to this line produce the vertical long axis plane. This plane is prescribed from a transverse image. Images are acquired through the longest oblique diameter of the left ventricle (**Fig. 1**). The vertical long axis plane or 2-chamber view is used to evaluate the left and right heart structures and their respective outflow

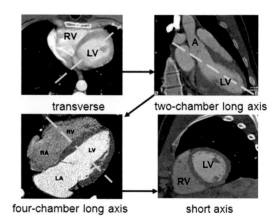

Fig. 1. Cardiac viewing planes. The axes (*dashed lines*) through which classic cardiac planes can be found. A, aorta; LA, left atrium; LV, left ventricle; RA, right atrium; RV, right ventricle.

tracts. It also reveals information about the anatomic relationship of structures superoinferior and anteroposterior to the heart.

Horizontal Long Axis Plane (4-Chamber View)

The horizontal long axis plane or 4-chamber view is prescribed from the vertical long axis (2-chamber) view. Images are acquired parallel to the long axis of the left ventricle (see **Fig. 1**). This plane displays the relationship of the 4-cardiac chambers to each other on a single image and is ideal for the assessment of atrial and septal defects and the tricuspid and mitral valves. This image plane can also be obtained by prescribing oblique transverse images from the short axis scout.

Short Axis Plane

The short axis plane is prescribed from the horizontal long axis (4-chamber) view. Images are prescribed perpendicular to the long axis of the left ventricle. This plane shows the true cross-sectional dimensions of the cardiac chambers and can also be used to evaluate wall thickness (see **Fig. 1**).

NORMAL ANATOMY

The diagnosis of cardiac anomalies requires identification and evaluation of 3 cardiac segments (atria, ventricles, and great arteries) and identification and evaluation of the atrioventricular and ventriculoarterial connections and any associated anomalies.

Atria

The right atrium is characterized by the right atrial appendage and the crista terminalis (**Fig. 2**). The right atrial appendage is a curved triangular structure that lies lateral and slightly anterior to the ascending aorta, with the superior vena cava slightly posterior. The crista terminalis divides the right atrium into a moderately trabeculated anterior portion and a smoother posterior portion. The systemic venous blood from the superior and inferior vena cavae and cardiac venous blood from the coronary sinus drain into the right atrium.

The left atrium is a quadrangular structure posterior to the ascending aorta, directly anterior to the vertebral body. The walls of the left atrium are smooth. The ligament of Marshall may be noted indenting the left atrium between the left atrial appendage and superior left pulmonary vein (see **Fig. 2**). The pulmonary veins drain into the left atrium.

Ventricles

The ventricular septum coursing from the right to the left anteriorly between the 2 ventricles is easily

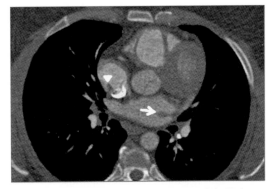

Fig. 2. Normal atrial anatomy. Transaxial CT image shows the crista terminalis (*arrowhead*), a ridge of fibromuscular tissue, along the posterior and lateral aspect of the right atrium. The ligament of Marshall (*arrow*) is seen in the left atrium. The ligament contains sympathetic nerve fibers, blood vessels, and myocardial fibers.

seen on CT (**Fig. 3**). In the right ventricle, a trabeculation known as the moderator band crosses from the ventricular septum to the free wall and carries the right branch of the atrioventricular bundle of the conducting system. The left ventricle has large papillary muscles that originate from the free wall. Typically, the right ventricle is more trabeculated than the left. In the presence of ventricular hypertrophy these trabeculations become more prominent and can mimic mass or

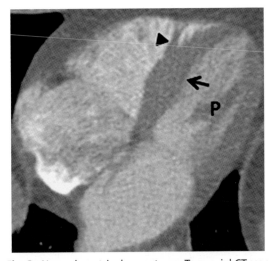

Fig. 3. Normal ventricular anatomy. Transaxial CT scan shows the interventricular septum (*arrow*), a prominent papillary muscle (P) in the left ventricle, and a thin moderator band (*arrowhead*) crossing from the interventricular septum to the right ventricle free wall. Both structures have an enhancement pattern similar to that of myocardium. These structures can mimic mass or thrombus, but the latter does not enhance.

thrombus. Normal morphologic structures enhance to the same degree as the myocardium, whereas thrombus does not enhance.

Cardiac Valves

The main pulmonary valve has 3 cusps: right, left, and anterior (**Fig. 4**). The aortic valve consists of the right, left, and noncoronary cusps, the last being in a posterior location. The tricuspid valve is slightly more apical in location than the mitral valve. The tricuspid valve consists of the septal, anterior, and posterior leaflets, whereas the mitral valve consists of the aortic and mural leaflets.

Great Arteries and Connections

The main pulmonary artery lies entirely within the pericardium. It divides into the right and left pulmonary arteries behind and to the left of the ascending aorta. The thoracic aorta can be divided into 5 segments: aortic root, ascending aorta, aortic arch, aortic isthmus, and descending thoracic aorta (**Fig. 5**).

In the normal relationship of the great arteries, the aorta lies to the right of, and posterior to the pulmonary artery. The term ventriculoarterial concordance refers to a morphologic right ventricle giving rise to a pulmonary valve and artery and a morphologic left ventricle giving rise to an aortic valve and aorta. In transposition of the great vessels, there is ventriculoarterial discordance. The term atrioventricular concordance refers to normal atrial and ventricular connections (ie, right

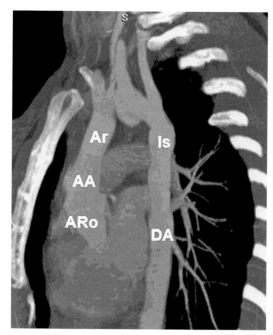

Fig. 5. Aortic anatomy. Thoracic aorta and branches, normal anatomy. Sagittal reformation shows the 5 aortic segments: aortic root (ARo), ascending aorta (AA), aortic arch (Ar), aortic isthmus (Is), and descending aorta (DA).

atrium to right ventricle and left atrium to left ventricle). Atrioventricular discordance refers to right atrial blood flowing to the left ventricle and left atrial blood flowing to the right ventricle.

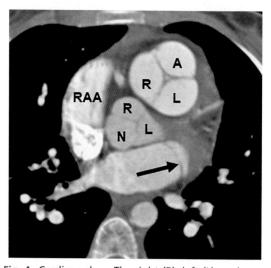

Fig. 4. Cardiac valves. The right (R), left (L), and non-coronary (N) cusps of the aortic valve and right (R), left (L), and anterior (A) cusps of the pulmonic valve are shown. Again note the triangular right atrial appendage (RAA). Arrow, mitral valve.

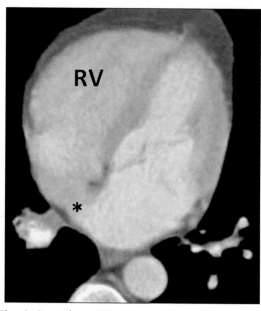

Fig. 6. Secundum ASD. Transaxial CT shows a large communication (*asterisk*) between the right and left atria, consistent with a secundum septal defect. Also note the mildly enlarged right ventricle (RV).

Great Veins

The superior vena cava, inferior vena cava, and coronary sinus join the right atrium. The 4 pulmonary veins (2 superior and 2 inferior) join the left atrium. The superior pulmonary veins drain the upper lobes, the middle lobe vein drains the right middle lobe vein commonly joins the superior right pulmonary vein.

CT OF CHD

CHD in the adult can be classified into shunt lesions, simple obstructive lesions, and complex CHD.[14–16]

Shunt Lesions

Atrial septal defect

Atrial septal defect (ASD) is the most common congenital heart defect in adults and accounts for about one-third of CHD detected in adults.[14,17–19] Left-to-right shunting at the interatrial level occurs at a level proportional to the size of the defect. Right-sided volume overload with resulting pulmonary hypertension can develop, especially in women and patients more than 40 years of age.

There are 4 major types of ASD, classified by their location in the interatrial septum: ostium secundum in the region of the fossa ovalis (midseptum) (**Fig. 6**); sinus venosus in the upper aspect of the atrial septum at the right atrial-superior vena caval junction or in the lower aspect of the atrial septum above the coronary sinus orifice (**Fig. 7**); ostium primum in the lower part of the atrial septum directly above the atrioventricular valves (**Fig. 8**); and unroofed coronary sinus defect in the posteroinferior atrial septum. Ostium secundum defects account for 75% of all ASDs, ostium primum defects make up 10% of lesions, and sinus venosus defects make up 10%.[18] Additional abnormalities may occur with these defects, including partial anomalous drainage of the

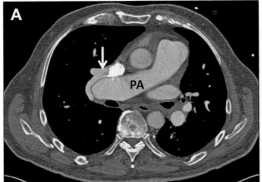
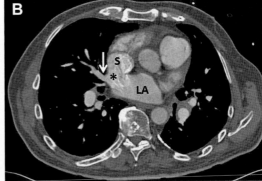
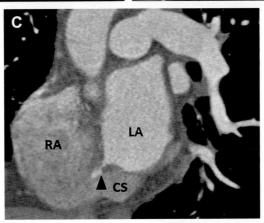

Fig. 7. Sinus venosum ASD. (*A*) Superior sinus venosus ASD. Transaxial CT image at the level of the superior vena cava shows an anomalous vein (*arrow*) from the right upper lobe draining into the lateral wall of the cava. Also notice the enlarged pulmonary artery (PA). (*B*) Transaxial CT slightly more caudal shows a communication (*asterisk*) between the right atrial-superior vena caval junction and left atrium (LA). The right middle lobe pulmonary vein straddles the defect (*arrow*). S, superior vena cava. (*C*) Inferior sinus venosus ASD. Sagittal oblique multiplanar reformatted CT image of another patient showing a small communication (*arrowhead*) between the left atrium (LA) and right atrium (RA), representing the inferior sinus venosus ASD just above the coronary sinus (CS).

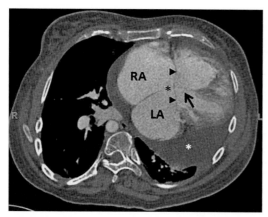

Fig. 8. Ostium primum defect. Transaxial CT scan through the level of the lower atrial septum shows communication (*black asterisk*) between the right atrium (RA) and left atrium (LA) just above a single valve (*black arrowheads*). Also note a VSD (*black arrow*). The combination of a primum ASD and inlet VSD is consistent with a complete atrioventricular septal (or canal) defect. A large pericardial effusion is also present (*white asterisk*).

pulmonary veins into the vena cava or right atrium (with sinus venosus defects), cleft mitral valve and endocardial cushion defect (with ostium primum defect), and persistent left superior vena cava (with unroofed coronary sinus defects). Primum defects with endocardial cushion (atrioventricular canal) defects are usually diagnosed in the neonatal period. The other lesions are not uncommon in adults.

Transcatheter closure with a septal occluder device is the preferred treatment of small to moderate secundum defects (**Fig. 9**).[20] Surgical

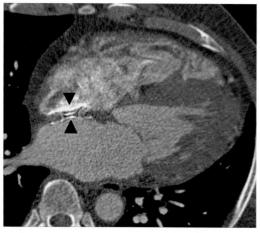

Fig. 9. Amplatzer septal occluder device. Transaxial CT shows the Amplatzer occluder (*arrowheads*) in the interatrial septum. The occluder has 2 flat discs.

closure is often necessary for other types of septal defects.

The secundum ASD should not be confused with a patent foramen ovale (PFO), in which incomplete fusion between the septum primum and septum secundum creates a flaplike opening at the foramen ovale (**Fig. 10**). There is no structural deficiency of septal tissue. The patent foramen is small and acts like a flaplike valve. It stays closed as long as left atrial pressure is greater than right atrial pressure, but it can reopen when right atrial pressure increases, such as with a Valsalva maneuver, coughing, or sneezing. In this case, blood may flow from the right to left atrium.

Ventricular septal defect

Ventricular septal defect (VSD) is the most common CHD in the pediatric population and the second most common defect in the adult population.[14,17,21] VSDs are classified into 4 types based on their location in the ventricular septum: perimembranous (70%–80% of defects) located in the membranous portion of the septum beneath the aortic valve (**Fig. 11**), muscular/trabecular (20%) in the muscular portion of the septum (**Fig. 12**), supracristal/outlet (5%) just below the pulmonic valve, and inlet (5%) below the junction of the mitral and tricuspid valves (causing the so-called atrioventricular canal defects).[17]

Functional effects depend on shunt volume and pressure gradient across the defect. Small- and moderate-size VSDs are generally restrictive, meaning that a pressure gradient between the left and right ventricles is maintained. Large defects are usually nonrestrictive with equalization of ventricular pressures.

Small VSDs may close spontaneously. VSDs that fail to close spontaneously may be closed with a percutaneous septal occluder device or a surgically placed patch graft.

Patent ductus arteriosus

Patent ductus arteriosus (PDA) in the fetus connects the proximal descending aorta with the proximal left pulmonary artery.[14,17] Normally this closes soon after birth. If the ductus does not spontaneously close, there is continuous flow from the aorta to the pulmonary arteries. Most adult patients with PDA are asymptomatic and the lesion is usually diagnosed by the discovery of a murmur.

At CT, the ductus is visualized as a tubular structure extending from the underside of the aortic arch just below the origin of the left subclavian artery to the left pulmonary artery (**Fig. 13**).[22] The communication between the pulmonary artery is

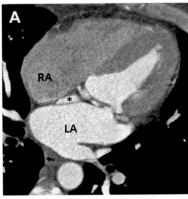
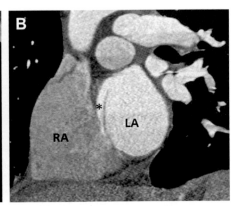

Fig. 10. PFO. (*A*) Transaxial CT image shows a small pocket of contrast (*asterisk*) interposed between the right atrium (RA) and left atrium (LA). (*B*) Oblique sagittal multiplanar reformatted CT image shows a small blush of contrast crossing from the left atrium to the right atrium across the PFO.

best seen on sagittal or oblique reformations. The ductus arteriosus may become aneurysmal and calcified, which may lead to rupture.[17]

Treatment is transcatheter device closure. Calcification may be noted in the ligamentum arteriosum after spontaneous ductal closure.

Other shunt lesions

Partial anomalous venous connection of 1 or more lobes produces a left-to-right shunt because the abnormal vein enters either the right heart or the systemic circulation.[23] This anomaly may occur in isolation or with other cardiovascular defects. Isolated anomalous drainage in an otherwise healthy individual is usually asymptomatic. The lesion is detected because of a murmur or associated pulmonary hypertension related to the left-to-right shunt.

There are 3 common patterns of anomalous drainage: anomalous right superior pulmonary venous drainage to the superior vena cava, anomalous left superior pulmonary venous return into the left brachiocephalic vein or innominate vein, and anomalous right lower lobe drainage into the inferior vena cava or portal vein. The CT diagnosis of anomalous return is based on recognition of the abnormal course of the intraparenchymal

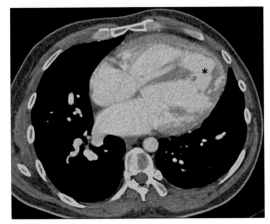

Fig. 11. Perimembranous VSD. Oblique axial multiplanar reformatted CT image shows a small communication (*arrow*) between the right (RV) and left (LV) ventricles at the level of the subaortic septum. Aneurysmal wind-sock deformity of the membranous septum (*arrowhead*) is also present. A, aorta; LA, left atrium.

Fig. 12. Muscular VSD. Transaxial CT shows a large communication (*asterisk*) in the muscular part of the interventricular septum at the apex of the heart.

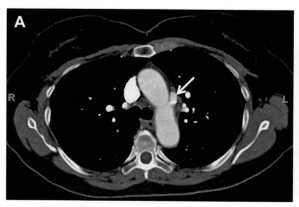
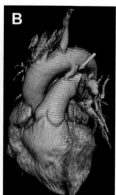

Fig. 13. PDA. (*A*) Transaxial CT image shows an enhancing tubular structure (*arrow*) extending inferolaterally from the undersurface of the aortic arch. (*B*) Sagittal 3D volume-rendered image shows the course of the PDA (*arrow*) and its relationship to the pulmonary artery and aortic arch.

pulmonary vein (**Fig. 14**). This situation is especially well seen on 3D reconstructions.[24] If the pulmonary-to-systemic shunt is severe enough, surgical repair involving reimplantation of the anomalous draining vein into the left atrium may be indicated.

Simple Obstructive Lesions

Aortic coarctation

Aortic coarctation refers to a constriction of the aortic arch in the region of the embryologic ductus arteriosus. The narrowing can be long-segment or focal, and may be located in the preductal or postductal region. Preductal coarctation, which usually presents in infancy with congestive heart failure, occurs proximal to the ductus arteriosus and is

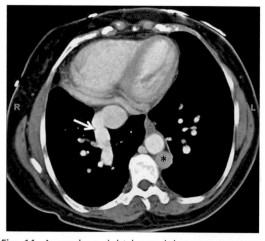

Fig. 14. Anomalous right lower lobe venous return. Transaxial CT scan shows an anomalous vessel (*arrow*) in the right lower lobe, a small right lung, and rightward mediastinal shift in this patient with scimitar syndrome. This patient also has hemiazygous continuation of the inferior vena cava (*asterisk*).

associated with hypoplasia of the aortic isthmus. There is a strong association with other congenital lesions, including PDA, VSD, and subaortic obstruction. In extreme cases, interruption of the aortic arch may occur.[25]

Postductal coarctation, which usually presents after the neonatal period, occurs distal to the insertion of the ductus arteriosus, and is likely the result of muscular ductal extension into the aorta. Most adults with aortic coarctation are asymptomatic and the diagnosis is made on routine physical examination, when systemic arterial hypertension is noted in the arms with diminished femoral arterial pulses.

At CT, the coarctation is visible as an indentation of the aorta, with prestenotic and poststenotic dilatation of the aorta (**Fig. 15**).[26,27] Between 50% and 85% of patients with coarctation have a bicuspid aortic valve.[15] Collateral vessels form to maintain blood flow to the lower body if the coarctation is hemodynamically significant. Collateral circulation is usually via the internal mammary arteries and the intercostal arteries. Increased collateral flow through intercostal vessels can cause notching of the posterior third to eighth ribs.

Treatment of coarctation includes endovascular stents and angioplasty. CT can be used to show residual stenosis and complications, such as restenosis, aneurysm formation, and dissection.[28]

Pseudocoarctation of the aorta is a condition in which the aorta is markedly dilated and distorted. Periductal kinking or buckling is present, but does not produce a pressure gradient. Therefore, there is no formation of collateral vessels (**Fig. 16**).

Aortic valvular stenosis

Aortic stenosis is the most common form of valvular stenosis. Stenotic aortic valves are usually bicuspid and less frequently dysplastic as a result of fusion of the 3-valve commissures, resulting in

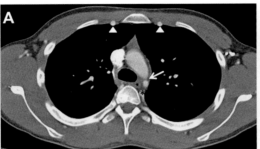
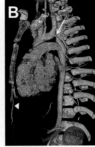

Fig. 15. Postductal aortic coarctation. (*A*) Transaxial CT image shows short segment narrowing of the proximal aortic arch (*arrow*). White arrowheads = dilated internal mammary arteries. Black asterisk = dilated intercostals artery. (*B*) Sagittal 3D image showing the focal coarctation (*arrow*) with aortic dilatation proximal and distal to the site of narrowing. White arrowhead, dilated internal mammary artery. Dilated posterior intercostal arteries are also noted.

leaflet rigidity and reduction of the aortic orifice. The incidence of bicuspid aortic valve is 1% to 2% in the general population.[12] Adults with bicuspid valves are often asymptomatic and the diagnosis is suspected on physical examination or it may be an incidental detection on imaging studies.

On CT, the valve has 2 cusps, which may be equal in size or more commonly 1 cusp is larger than other. The larger cusp often contains a ridge or raphe, which is the site of congenital fusion of the original commissures. Calcification may be seen at the site of fusion of the commissures. Associated findings include poststenotic vessel dilatation and left ventricular hypertrophy (**Fig. 17**).[29] Doming of the valve leaflets may be seen during ventricular systole.

Treatment of aortic valve stenosis includes percutaneous balloon valvuloplasty, surgical valvotomy, prosthetic valve replacement, and the Ross procedure. In the Ross procedure, the stenotic aortic valve is replaced with the native pulmonary valve, annulus, and outflow trunk (autograft transplantation), and the pulmonary valve and right ventricular outflow tract are replaced with a cadaveric homograft.

Pulmonary valvular stenosis

Pulmonary stenosis is valvular in about 90% of patients and in the remainder it is supravalvular or subvalvular.[17] Typically, the pulmonic valve is domed and characterized by a narrow central opening but preserved mobile leaflets.[30] About 10% of valves are dysplastic with thickened poorly

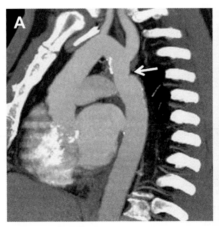
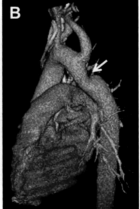

Fig. 16. Pseudocoarctation. (*A*) Sagittal reformatted thick slab maximum-intensity projection image shows a high and tortuous aortic arch with buckling of the proximal descending aorta (*arrow*) immediately distal to the origin of the left subclavian artery. There are no collateral intercostals vessels to suggest hemodynamically significant stenosis. (*B*) Sagittal 3D volume-rendered image also showing the pseudocoarctation (aortic buckling, *arrow*).

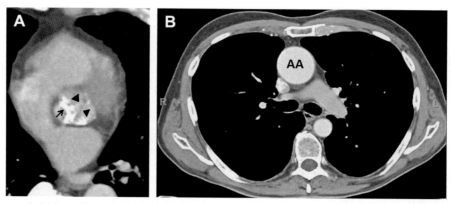

Fig. 17. Congenital bicuspid aortic valve. (*A*) Oblique axial multiplanar reformatted CT image shows a bicuspid aortic valve with 2 thickened cusps or leaflets (*arrowheads*) and a calcified ridge, also called a raphe (*arrow*), which is the site of fusion of the original commissures. (*B*) Transaxial CT of the chest near the level of the tracheal carina showing a dilated ascending aorta (AA).

mobile leaflets, unicuspid or bicuspid.[17,30] In classic valvular stenosis, CT shows poststenotic dilatation of the main and left pulmonary artery and right ventricular hypertrophy (**Fig. 18**).

Treatment of pulmonic valve stenosis includes percutaneous balloon valvuloplasty and more recently percutaneous valve replacement.

Complex Cyanotic Heart Disease

Most adult patients with complex cyanotic heart disease have undergone palliative shunt or definitive repair of their lesions in infancy or early childhood.[31–37] Patients come to clinical attention in later life because of postoperative complications. CT plays a role in delineating the underlying anatomy and characterizing the complications before therapy is instituted.[31–37] The CT findings of the morphologic abnormalities in the common complex CHDs are discussed in this section. Details of palliative and corrective surgical procedures are described later. With the exception of Ebstein anomaly, primary findings of CHDs in adults on CT are seen only if there has been palliative surgery.

Ebstein anomaly

Ebstein anomaly is a rare defect in which the septal and posterior leaflets of the tricuspid valve are inferiorly displaced into the right ventricle.[16,38,39] The anterior leaflet is normally located, but may be enlarged and/or possess abnormal attachments. This partitions the right heart into a right atrium, an atrialized portion of the right ventricle, and a functional right ventricle, which is small (**Fig. 19**). The tricuspid valve is usually regurgitant, but it may be stenotic. An interatrial communication (ASD or

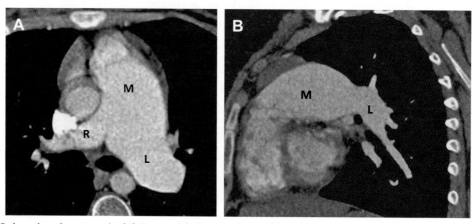

Fig 18. Pulmonic valve stenosis. (*A*) Transaxial CT scan shows dilated main (M) and left (L) pulmonary arteries. Note a normal caliber right pulmonary artery (R). (*B*) Sagittal multiplanar reformation shows dilated main (M) and left (L) pulmonary arteries.

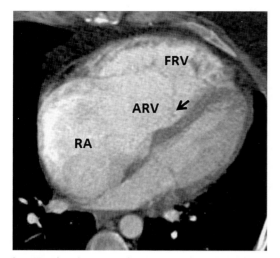

Fig. 19. Ebstein anomaly. Transaxial CT scan shows a dilated right atrium (RA), atrialized right ventricle (ARV), and small functional right ventricle (FRV). Note the apical displacement of the tricuspid valve septal leaflet (*arrow*).

PFO) is present in 80% to 94% of patients who come to operation.[38,39]

Patients with severe leaflet displacement present in the neonatal period with cyanosis caused by right-to-left shunting at the atrial level and/or right-sided heart failure. Arrhythmia is the dominant clinical presentation in adults. However, adults with mild tricuspid leaflet displacement can have normal valvular function and be symptom free, with the anomaly discovered incidentally on an imaging study.

Treatment of more severe Ebstein anomaly is reduction and plication of the right atrial free wall and tricuspid valve reconstruction or replacement. Patients with milder malformations may need no intervention.

Tetralogy of Fallot
Tetralogy of Fallot is the most common cyanotic cardiac condition, accounting for about 10% of all congenital heart defects.[12] The classic components include subpulmonic stenosis, VSD, overriding of the aorta, and right ventricular hypertrophy (**Fig. 20**). Associated anomalies include a right-sided aortic arch with mirror imaging branching (25% of cases), an ASD (10% of cases, referred to as pentalogy of Fallot), coronary artery anomalies (10% of cases), and stenosis of the peripheral pulmonary arteries.[16,38]

Most adult patients have undergone intervention in childhood. Palliative surgery for tetralogy of Fallot is usually a Blalock-Taussig shunt. Total surgical repair requires right ventriculotomy with right ventricular outflow tract reconstruction to

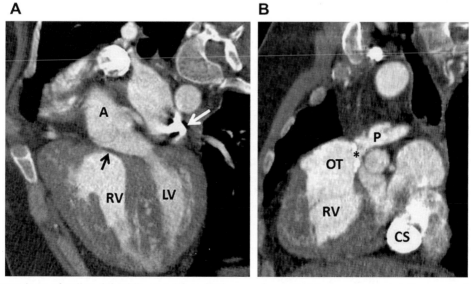

Fig. 20. Tetralogy of Fallot. (*A*) Oblique axial multiplanar reformatted image shows malalignment of the perimembranous septum, which has been repaired (*black arrow*), with an overriding aorta (A). The right ventricle (RV) myocardium is thickened. This patient has a persistent left superior vena cava (*white arrow*). LV, left ventricle. (*B*) Oblique sagittal multiplanar reformatted image in the same patient who has undergone patch graft repair of the right ventricle (RV) outflow tract (OT). Notice the hypoplastic calcified pulmonary valves (*asterisk*) and diminutive main pulmonary artery (P). Dense contrast is seen in the dilated coronary sinus (CS) related to the persistent left superior vena cava.

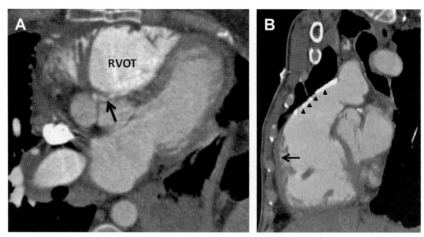

Fig. 21. Repaired tetralogy of Fallot. (*A*) Axial multiplanar reformatted image shows a high-density VSD patch (*arrow*) beneath the aortic valve. Notice the dilatation of the right ventricular outflow tract (RVOT) with bowing of the interventricular septum toward the left ventricle. (*B*) Sagittal multiplanar reformatted image of another patient showing a calcified, aneurysmally dilated right ventricular outflow tract (*arrowheads*). Notice the thickened right ventricle myocardium (*arrow*) and dilated right ventricle in this patient with pulmonic regurgitation following repair of the outflow tract.

relieve obstruction, as well as VSD patch closure (**Fig. 21**).[32,34,38,40] Complications of total repair include pulmonic valve regurgitation, right ventricular dilatation, aneurysmal dilatation (see **Fig. 21**) or stenosis of the right ventricular outflow tract, and leak in the VSD patch.[30,36]

Tricuspid atresia

Tricuspid atresia is a rare congenital heart defect involving failure of tricuspid valve formation with absence of direct communication between the right atrium and right ventricle.[41] In type I, the great arteries are normally related; in type II, the vessels are dextro (D)-transposed (20%); and in type III, the vessels are levo (L)-transposed (10%). CT findings include fat deposition in the right atrioventricular groove, small right ventricle, large right atrium, and supracristal VSD (**Fig. 22**).[42] Complications include right heart failure with nutmeg liver, mural thrombus, and dilatation of cardiac/systemic veins.

Surgical repair has included the Glenn shunt, bidirectional Glenn shunt, and Fontan shunt.[34,37]

Transposition of the great arteries

D-transposition of the great arteries Complete or D-transposition of the great arteries (D-TGA) is a cyanotic condition that accounts for 5% to 7% of cases of CHD.[12] This anomaly is characterized by ventriculoarterial discordance and atrioventricular concordance. The aorta arises from the morphologic right ventricle and is anterior and to the right of the pulmonary artery, which arise from the morphologic left ventricle (**Fig. 23**).[16,43]

The pulmonary and systemic circulations are independent circulations in parallel, rather than being in series.

Survival during the first few days of life depends on a PDA or associated defects such as an ASD or VSD which allow intracardiac mixing of blood. Early surgical intervention is necessary for long-term survival.

Currently, an arterial switch operation (Jatene procedure) is the surgical procedure of choice in neonates with D-TGA.[34,37,44] However, this is

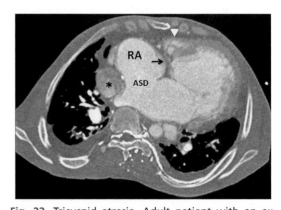

Fig. 22. Tricuspid atresia. Adult patient with an extracardiac total cavopulmonary shunt for tricuspid atresia who presents with increasing cyanosis. MDCT was performed to evaluate anatomy. Axial CT scan shows fat in the atrioventricular groove (*arrow*). The right atrium (RA) is enlarged and a large ASD is noted. The right ventricle is hypoplastic (*white arrowhead*). A VSD (not shown) in this patient allows the right ventricle to fill with contrast. Asterisk = extracardiac Fontan conduit.

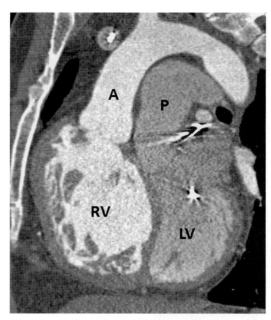

Fig. 23. D-transposition of the great vessels. Patient with acute chest pain who had a Mustard procedure in infancy. MDCT was performed to evaluate for pulmonary embolus. Oblique sagittal multiplanar reformatted image shows pulmonary trunk (P) arising from the smooth left ventricle (LV) and aorta (A) arising from the trabeculated right ventricle (RV), typical of D-transposition. Pacemaker lead is inserted in the left ventricle, causing metallic artifact.

a new operation and most adult patients with D-transposition of the great vessels have undergone the older atrial switch operation, either a Mustard and colleagues[45] or Senning procedure.

L-transposition of the great arteries Congenitally corrected or L-transposition of the great arteries (L-TGA) accounts for 0.5% of congenital heart lesions, and is characterized by atrioventricular and ventriculoarterial discordance (double discordance). The morphologic right ventricle is located to the left of the morphologic left ventricle and gives rise to the aorta, which is anterior and to the left of the main pulmonary artery (**Fig. 24**). As a result, blood flow through the pulmonary and systemic circuits occurs in normal series fashion. Associated defects are common, including VSD, pulmonary stenosis, tricuspid valve malformations, and atrioventricular conduction abnormalities. In the absence of associated anomalies, patients may be asymptomatic and the lesion is detected incidentally on echocardiography, CT, or MRI. Right heart failure is a late complication related to the high resistance systemic arterial circulation that this ventricle encounters.

Double-outlet ventricle
A double-outlet ventricle requires that more than 50% of both great arteries arise from either the morphologic right or left ventricle.[30] An artery is

considered to be connected to a ventricle when more than half of its semilunar valve is connected to that ventricle. Double-outlet right ventricle, in which the ascending aorta and the pulmonary trunk arise from the morphologic right ventricle, is more common than double-outlet left ventricle, in which both arteries originate from the morphologic left ventricle. A VSD is always present and pulmonic stenosis is frequently present.

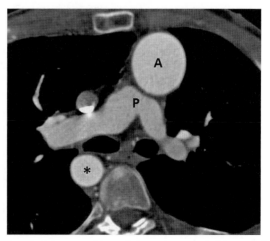

Fig. 24. L-transposition of the great vessels. Transaxial CT scan shows the aorta (A) lying to the left and anterior to the pulmonary artery (P). *, right sided descending aorta.

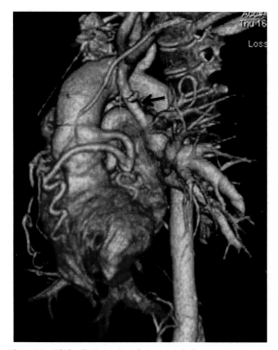

Fig. 25. Blalock-Taussig shunt. Adult woman with tetralogy of Fallot who had undergone palliative Blalock-Taussig shunt in infancy. Sagittal 3D volume-rendered image shows patent Blalock-Taussig shunt (*arrow*) extending from the left subclavian artery to the left pulmonary artery.

INTERVENTIONAL AND SURGICAL PROCEDURES
Palliative Shunts

The most common palliative shunts to increase pulmonary venous flow for the relief of cyanosis

are the Blalock-Taussig, Glenn, and Fontan shunts.[31,34,37,46] These shunts allow systemic venous blood to enter the pulmonary circulation directly, bypassing the right ventricle. Imaging plays a role in evaluating the patency of these shunts as well as their complications.

The Blalock-Taussig shunt is a communication between the proximal subclavian artery and pulmonary artery. This shunt has been used in the setting of tetralogy of Fallot. Originally, this shunt was performed on the side opposite the aortic arch. The distal subclavian artery was sacrificed, with restitution of flow in the ipsilateral upper limb being dependent on collateral vessel formation. Disadvantages of the classic shunt included distortion and kinking of the pulmonary artery and possible abnormal growth of the arm ipsilateral to the shunt (steal phenomenon).[31] In the more recent modified approach, a synthetic Gore-Tex graft is used to create a side-to-side shunt without subclavian artery takedown (**Fig. 25**). Advantages of the modified shunt include less distortion of the pulmonary arteries and better growth of the pulmonary tree, preserved blood flow to the ipsilateral arm, and technical ability to perform the shunt on either side of the aorta.[31,37] A not uncommon complication of the modified Blalock-Taussig shunt is thrombosis.[31]

The Glenn shunt is a conduit from the superior vena cava to the pulmonary artery. The shunt is used primarily in the setting of tricuspid atresia and pulmonary atresia with intact ventricular septum.[31,37] The original Glenn shunt was an anastomosis of the transected right pulmonary

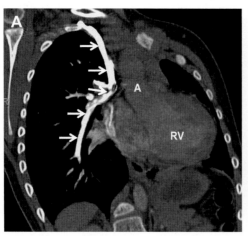
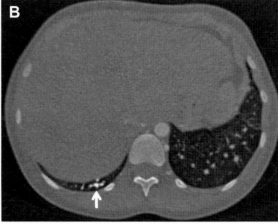

Fig. 26. Glenn shunt. (*A*) Adult patient with Glenn shunt for double-outlet right ventricle who presents with increasing cyanosis. Coronal oblique multiplanar reformatted image shows Glenn shunt (*white arrows*), which extends from superior vena cava to right pulmonary artery. Also note the aorta (A) arising from the right ventricle (RV). (*B*) Transaxial image of the lung bases shows a small pulmonary arteriovenous malformation (*arrow*) on the same side as the shunt.

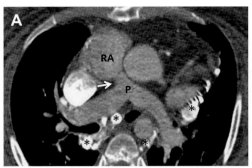

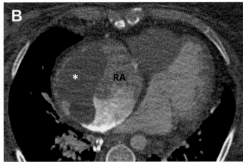

Fig. 27. Fontan shunt. (A) Adult with tricuspid and pulmonary atresia who had Fontan shunt placement. Transaxial images show the Fontan shunt (*arrow*) from right atrial appendage (RA) to pulmonary artery (PA). Multiple venovenous collateral vessels are seen around the bronchi, aorta, and pericardium (*black asterisks*). (B) Transaxial image in the same patient shows a complication of the Fontan shunt with thrombus formation (*white asterisk*) in the right atrium (RA).

artery to the superior vena cava, providing perfusion only to the right lung (**Fig. 26**). The modified procedure, termed the bidirectional Glenn shunt, involves an end-to-side anastomosis of the superior vena cava to the main pulmonary artery, which maintains continuity of both pulmonary arteries and provides bidirectional flow to the lungs. Complications of the Glenn shunt are pulmonary arteriovenous malformations and development of decompressing venous collaterals resulting in reduced oxygen saturation.[37]

The Fontan procedure was originally used for tricuspid atresia and connected the right atrium or right atrial appendage to the base of the pulmonary artery (**Fig. 27**). Complications include pulmonary hypertension, arrhythmias, right atrial enlargement and thrombus formation, right heart failure, venous collateral vessel formation, protein-losing enteropathy, and hepatomegaly.[31,37,47]

A more recent modification of the Fontan procedure is the bidirectional total cavopulmonary shunt.[31,37] The Fontan cavopulmonary pathway can now be used as a palliative procedure in any heart with single ventricle physiology, including tricuspid atresia and single ventricle physiology syndromes (hypoplastic left heart, hypoplastic right ventricle with pulmonary atresia, and double-inlet ventricle). This procedure consists of

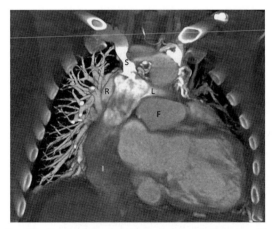

Fig. 28. Total cavopulmonary shunt. Adult man with tricuspid atresia who had undergone cavopulmonary repair and presents with dyspnea on exertion. Coronal 3D volume-rendered image shows opacified superior vena cava (S) and unopacified inferior vena cava (I), which are directly connected with the right (R) and left (L) pulmonary arteries. The patient had a prior Fontan shunt (F), which was taken down for the total shunt.

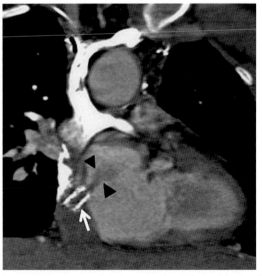

Fig. 29. Fenestrated Fontan shunt (lateral tunnel type). Oblique coronal reformatted CT image showing total cavopulmonary circulation and stented (*white arrow*) fenestrated lateral tunnel with a jet of unopacified blood flowing into the dilated right atrium (*black arrowheads*).

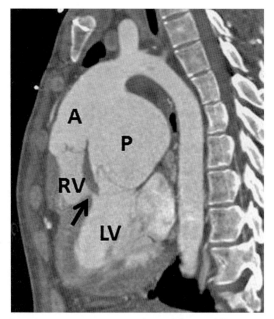

Fig. 30. Damus-Kaye-Stansel procedure. Oblique sagittal multiplanar reformatted image from a patient with tricuspid atresia and L-transposition of the great vessels. The pulmonary artery (P) arising from the left ventricle (LV) has been anastomosed with the aorta (A), which arises from the hypoplastic right ventricle (RV). The bulboventricular foramen (*arrow*) provides communication between the 2 ventricles.

a bidirectional Glenn shunt that is followed by an inferior vena cava to left pulmonary conduit that can be either intracardiac (lateral tunnel) or extracardiac (**Fig. 28**). The lateral tunnel method may be fenestrated to allow for decompression of

increased pulmonary arterial system pressures (**Fig. 29**). The major complication is conduit stenosis.

Aortopulmonary anastomoses include the Waterston-Cooley and Potts shunts. The Waterston-Cooley shunt connects the ascending aorta to the right pulmonary artery, whereas the Potts shunt connects the descending aorta to the left pulmonary artery. These procedures are no longer used because of the long-term sequelae of pulmonary hypertension, pulmonary artery distortion, and congestive heart failure secondary to excessive pulmonary flow.[31,34]

The Damus-Kaye-Stansel operation is a palliative procedure for patients with a dominant left ventricle giving rise to the pulmonary artery and rudimentary right ventricle giving rise to the aorta (such as double-inlet left ventricle and tricuspid atresia with TGA).[31] The proximal pulmonary artery is divided near its bifurcation and anastomosed to the side of the ascending aorta, thus bypassing any systemic outflow obstruction (**Fig. 30**).[31] Blood flow to the distal pulmonary arteries is reestablished by a Blalock-Taussig or cavopulmonary shunt. Complications include pulmonary valvular regurgitation and stenosis at the site of aorta-to-pulmonary artery anastomosis.[31]

Complex Corrective Surgeries

In the Ross procedure for isolated aortic valve disease, the aortic valve is replaced with the patient's own pulmonary valve, and the coronary arteries are reimplanted into the neoaortic root. A cadaveric pulmonary valve is then used to replace the patient's own pulmonary valve. Complications

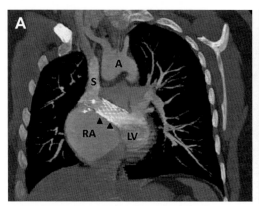
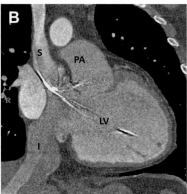

Fig. 31. Mustard procedure. (*A*) Multiplanar reformatted image shows opacified superior limb (S) (superior vena cava to left ventricle) of the systemic baffle with metallic stent (*arrowheads*) in place. RA, right atrium; LV, left ventricle; A, aorta. (*B*) Coronal multiplanar reformatted image in another patient shows opacified superior vena cava (S) with a pacemaker extending through to superior limb into the left ventricle. The pulmonary artery (PA) arises from the left ventricle (LV). Inferior limb (I) (inferior vena cava to left ventricle) of the systemic baffle is poorly opacified because contrast medium was injected via an antecubital approach. If visualization of the inferior limb is of clinical concern, delayed imaging or a second injection in a lower extremity is required.

include ascending neoaortic aneurysm and aortic valve regurgitation, caused by incompetence of the pulmonary valve homograft.

The Mustard and Senning procedures were originally used for the physiologic correction of D-transposition of the great arteries at the atrial level (atrial switch operation).[31,34,36] In this procedure, an atrial baffle redirects venous blood from the pulmonary veins to the right ventricle and aorta and systemic venous blood from the superior and inferior vena cava to the left ventricle (**Fig. 31**). The Mustard technique uses pericardial tissue, whereas the Senning approach uses infolding of the atrial walls. Although a physiologically corrected circulation is achieved, anatomic relations remain abnormal and the right ventricle remains exposed to systemic loading. Complications include baffle obstruction and leakage (usually the systemic limb), resulting in retrograde flow and pulmonary venous hypertension and edema; atrial and ventricular arrhythmias; and right ventricular (systemic) failure.[31,36] The atrial switch is no longer routinely used.

Currently, the Jatene arterial switch operation is the surgical treatment of choice for neonates with D-transposition of the great arteries.[34,36] In this procedure, the great vessels are transected above the semilunar valves and switched back to their normal positions, with the aorta connecting to the left ventricle and the pulmonary artery connecting to the right ventricle. The coronary arteries are separated from the right side and reattached to the new left-sided aorta. On imaging, the branches of the pulmonary artery are seen wrapping around the aorta in a Dutch hat configuration (**Fig. 32**). The

arterial switch prevents the development of right ventricular failure because it becomes the pulmonary ventricle and the left ventricle becomes the systemic ventricle. Complications include supravalvular pulmonary stenosis, dilatation of the neoaortic root with valve regurgitation, and coronary artery stenosis at the reimplantation site.[31,36]

REFERENCES

1. Gatzoulis MA, Webb GD. Adults with congenital heart diseases: a growing population. In: Gatzoulis MA, Webb GD, Daubeney PEF, editors. Diagnosis and management of adult congenital heart disease. Edinburgh (UK): Churchill Livingstone; 2003. p. 3–5.
2. Warnes CA, Liberthson R, Danielson GK, et al. Task force 1: the changing profile of congenital heart disease in adult life. J Am Coll Cardiol 2001;37:1170–5.
3. Deanfield J, Thaulow E, Warnes C, et al. Management of grown up congenital heart disease. Eur Heart J 2003;24:1035–84.
4. Kaemmerer H, Stern H, Fratz S, et al. Imaging in adults with congenital cardiac disease (ACCD). Thorac Cardiovasc Surg 2000;48:328–35.
5. Boxt LM. MR imaging and computed tomographic evaluation of congenital heart disease. J Magn Reson Imaging 2004;19:827–47.
6. de Roos A, Roest AAW. Evaluation of congenital heart disease by magnetic resonance imaging. Eur Radiol 2000;10:2–6.
7. Gutierrez FR, Siegel MJ, Fallah JH, et al. Magnetic resonance imaging of cyanotic and noncyanotic congenital heart disease. Magn Reson Imaging Clin N Am 2002;10:209–35.
8. Haramati LB, Glickstein FS, Issenberg HF, et al. MR imaging and CT of vascular anomalies and connections in patients with congenital heart disease. Radiographics 2002;22:337–49.
9. Gilkeson RC, Ciancibello L, Zahka K. Multidetector CT evaluation of congenital heart disease in pediatric and adult patients. AJR Am J Roentgenol 2003;180:973–80.
10. Goo HW, Park I-S, Ko JK, et al. CT of congenital heart disease: normal anatomy and typical pathologic conditions. Radiographics 2003;23:S147–65.
11. Leschka S, Oechslin E, Jusmann L, et al. Pre- and postoperative evaluation of congenital heart disease in children and adults with 64-section CT. Radiographics 2007;27:829–46.
12. Wiant A, Nyberg E, Gilkeson RC. CT evaluation of congenital heart disease in adults. AJR Am J Roentgenol 2009;193:388–96.
13. Earls JP, Berman EL, Urban BA. Prospectively gated transverse coronary CT angiography versus retrospectively gated helical technique: improved image

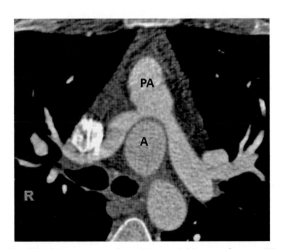

Fig. 32. Jatene procedure. Transaxial image from a CT scan after an arterial switch procedure shows characteristic draping of the pulmonary arteries (PA) over the aorta (A).

quality and reduced radiation dose. Radiology 2008; 246:742–53.

14. Sommer RJ, Hijazi ZM, Rhodes JF. Pathophysiology of congenital heart disease in the adult: part I: shunt lesions. Circulation 2008;117:1090–9.

15. Rhodes JF, Hijazi ZM, Sommer RJ. Pathophysiology of congenital heart disease in the adult, part II: simple obstructive lesions. Circulation 2008;117:1228–37.

16. Sommer RJ, Hijazi ZM, Rhodes JF. Pathophysiology of congenital heart disease in the adult: part III: complex congenital heart disease. Circulation 2008;117:1340–50.

17. Brickner ME, Hillis LD, Lange RA. Congenital heart disease in adults. First of two parts. N Engl J Med 2000;3342:256–63.

18. Jacobs JP, Quintessenza JA, Burke RP, et al. Congenital heart surgery nomenclature and database project: atrial septal defect. Ann Thorac Surg 2000;69:S18–24.

19. Rigby ML. Atrial septal defect. In: Gatzoulis MA, Webb GD, Daubeney PE, editors. Diagnosis and management of adult congenital heart disease. Edinburgh (UK): Churchill Livingstone; 2003. p. 163–70.

20. Ko SF, Liang CD, Yip HK, et al. Amplatzer septal occluder closure of atrial septal defect: evaluation of transthoracic echocardiography, cardiac CT, and transesophageal echocardiography. AJR Am J Roentgenol 2009;193:1522–9.

21. Jacobs JP, Quintessenza JA, Burke RP, et al. Congenital heart surgery nomenclature and database project: ventricular septal defect. Ann Thorac Surg 2000;69:S25–35.

22. Goitein O, Fuhrman CR, Lacomis JM. Incidental finding on MDCT of patent ductus arteriosus: use of CT and MRI to assess clinical importance. AJR Am J Roentgenol 2005;184:1924–31.

23. Zylak CJ, Eyler WR, Spizarny DL, et al. Developmental lung anomalies in the adult: radiologic-pathologic correlation. Radiographics 2002;22:S25–43.

24. Zwetsch B, Wicky S, Meuli R, et al. Three-dimensional image reconstruction of partial anomalous pulmonary venous return to the superior vena cava. Chest 1995;108:1743–5.

25. Kaemmerer H. Aortic coarctation and interrupted aortic arch. In: Gatzoulis MA, Webb GD, Daubeney PEF, editors. Adult congenital heart disease. Edinburgh (UK): Churchill Livingstone; 2003. p. 253–64.

26. Becker C, Soppa C, Fink U, et al. Spiral CT angiography and 3D reconstruction in patients with aortic coarctation. Eur Radiol 1997;7:1473–7.

27. Sebastia C, Quiroga S, Boye R, et al. Aortic stenosis spectrum of diseases depicted at multisection CT. Radiographics 2003;23:S79–91.

28. Shih MC, Tholpady A, Kramer CM, et al. Surgical and endovascular repair of aortic coarctation: normal findings and appearance of complications on CT angiography and MR angiography. AJR Am J Roentgenol 2006;187:W302–12.

29. Vogel-Claussen J, Pannu H, Spevak PJ, et al. Cardiac valve assessment with MR imaging and 64-section multi–detector row CT. Radiographics 2006;26:1769–84.

30. Bashore TM. Adult congenital heart disease: right ventricular outflow tract lesions. Circulation 2007; 115:1933–47.

31. Gaca A, Jaggers JJ, Dudley T, et al. Repair of congenital heart disease: a primer-Part 1. Radiology 2008;247:617–31.

32. Gaca A, Jaggers JJ, Dudley T, et al. Repair of congenital heart disease: a primer-Part 2. Radiology 2008;248:44–60.

33. Gatzoulis MA. Tetralogy of Fallot. In: Gatzoulis MA, Webb GD, Daubeney PEF, editors. Diagnosis and management of adult congenital heart disease. Edinburgh (UK): Churchill Livingstone; 2003. p. 315–26.

34. Rodriguez E, Soler R, Fernandez R, et al. Postoperative imaging in cyanotic congenital heart diseases: part 1, normal findings. AJR Am J Roentgenol 2007; 189:1353–60.

35. Siegel MJ, Bhalla S, Guitterez FR, et al. MDCT of post-operative anatomy and complications in adults with cyanotic heart disease. AJR Am J Roentgenol 2005;184:241–7.

36. Soler R, Rodriguez E, Alvarez M, et al. Postoperative imaging in cyanotic congenital heart diseases: part 2, complications. AJR Am J Roentgenol 2007;189:1361–9.

37. Spevak PJ, Johnson PT, Fishman EK. Surgically corrected congenital heart disease: utility of 64-MDCT. AJR Am J Roentgenol 2008;191:854–61.

38. Brickner ME, Hillis LD, Lange RA. Congenital heart disease in adults. Second of two parts. N Engl J Med 2000;342:334–42.

39. Dearani JA, Danielson GK. Congenital heart surgery nomenclature and database project: Ebstein's anomaly and tricuspid disease. Ann Thorac Surg 2000;69:S106–17.

40. Touati GD, Vouhe PR, Amodeo A, et al. Primary repair of tetralogy of Fallot in infancy. J Thorac Cardiovasc Surg 1990;99:396–402 [discussion: 402–3].

41. Thorne S. Atrioventricular valve atresia. In: Gatzoulis MA, Webb GD, Daubeney PEF, editors. Adult congenital heart disease. Edinburgh (UK): Churchill Livingstone; 2003. p. 405–11.

42. Mochizuki T, Ohtani T, Higashino H, et al. Tricuspid atresia with atrial septal defect, ventricular septal defect, and right ventricular hypoplasia demonstrated

by multidetector computed tomography. Circulation 2000;102:e164–5.

43. Warnes CA. Transposition of the great arteries. Circulation 2006;114:2699–709.

44. Gutgesell HP, Massaro TA, Kron IL. The arterial switch operation for transposition of the great arteries in a consortium of university hospitals. Am J Cardiol 1994;74:959–60.

45. Mustard WT, Keith JD, Trusler GA, et al. The surgical management of transposition of the great vessels. J Thorac Cardiovasc Surg 1964;48:953–8.

46. Mavroudis C, Backer CL, Deal BJ. Venous shunts and the Fontan circulation in adult congenital heart disease. In: Gatzoulis MA, Webb GD, Daubeney PEF, editors. Adult congenital heart disease. Edinburgh (UK): Churchill Livingstone; 2003. p. 79–83.

47. Feeedom RM, Li J, Yoo S-J. The complications following the Fontan operation. In: Gatzoulis MA, Wevbb GD, Daubeney PEF, editors. Adult congenital heart disease. Edinburgh (UK): Churchill Livingstone; 2003. p. 85–91.

Index

Note: Page numbers of article titles are in **boldface** type.

radiologic.theclinics.com